IMMUNOLOGICAL ASPECTS OF CANCER

DEVELOPMENTS IN ONCOLOGY

F.J. Cleton and J.W.I.M. Simons, eds. Genetic origins of Tumour Cells. 90-247-2272-1

J. Aisner and P. Chang, eds. Cancer Treatment Research. 90-247-2358-2

B.W. Ongerboer de Visser, D.A. Bosch and W.M.H. van Woerkom-Eykenboom, eds. Neuro-oncology: Clinical and Experimental Aspects. 90-247-2421-X

K. Hellman, P. Hilgard and S. Eccles, eds. Metastasis: Clinical and Experimental Aspects. 90-247-2424-4

H.F. Seigler, ed. Clinical Management of Melanoma. 90-247-2584-4

P. Correa and W. Haenszel, eds. Epidemiology of Cancer of the Digestive Tract. 90-247-2601-8

L.A. Liotta and I.R. Hart, eds. Tumour Invasion and Metastasis. 90-247-2611-5

J. Banoczy, ed. Oral Leukoplakia. 90-247-2655-7

C. Tijssen, M. Halprin and L. Endtz, eds. Familial Brain Tumours. 90-247-2691-3

F.M. Muggia, C.W. Young and S.K. Carter, eds. Anthracycline Antibiotics in Cancer. 90-247-2711-1

B.W. Hancock, ed. Assessment of Tumour Response. 90-247-2712-X

D.E. Peterson and S.T. Sonis, eds. Oral Complications of Cancer Chemotherapy. 0-89838-563-6

R. Mastrangelo, D.G. Poplack and R. Riccardi, eds. Central Nervous System Leukemia. Prevention and Treatment. 0-89838-570-9

A. Polliack, ed. Human Leukemias. Cytochemical and Ultrastructural Techniques in Diagnosis and Research. 0-89838-585-7

W. Davis, C. Maltoni and S. Tannenberger, eds. The Control of Tumour Growth and its Biological Bases. 0-89838-603-9

A.P.M. Heintz, C.Th. Griffiths and J.B. Trimbois, eds. Surgery in Gynecological Oncology. 0-89838-604-7

M.P. Hacker, E.B. Douple and I. Krakoff, eds. Platinum Coordination Complexes in Cancer Chemotherapy. 0-89838-619-5

M.J. van Zwieten. The Rat as Animal Model in Breast Cancer Research: A Histopathological Study of Radiation- and Hormone-Induced Rat Mammary Tumour. 0-89838-624-1

B. Lowenberg and A. Hagenbeek, eds. Minimal Residual Disease in Acute Leukemia. 0-89838-630-6

I. van der Waal and G.B. Snow, eds. Oral Oncology. 0-89838-631-4

IMMUNOLOGICAL ASPECTS OF CANCER

edited by B.W. HANCOCK
A. MILFORD WARD

MARTINUS NIJHOFF PUBLISHING
A MEMBER OF THE KLUWER ACADEMIC PUBLISHERS GROUP

Boston / Dordrecht / Lancaster

Distributors:

for North America

for all other countries

Kluwer Academic Publishers
190 Old Derby Street
Hingham, MA 02043

Kluwer Academic Publishers Group
Distribution Centre
P.O. Box 322
3300 AH Dordrecht
The Netherlands

Library of Congress Cataloging in Publication Data
Main entry under title:

Immunological aspects of cancer.

   (Developments in oncology)
   Includes index.
   1. Cancer—Immunological aspects. I. Hancock, Barry W. II. Ward, A. Milford (Anthony Milford)
III. Series.
   [DNLM: 1. Neoplasms—immunology. W1 DE998N / QZ 200 I337]
   RC268.3.I4626   1984   616.99′4079   84-8162

   ISBN-13: 978-1-4612-9607-2   e-ISBN-13: 978-1-4613-2557-4
   DOI: 10.1007/978-1-4613-2557-4

CONTENTS

CONTRIBUTING AUTHORS

S.A. Ali
Research Associate, Department of Virology
University of Sheffield Medical School
Beech Hill Road
Sheffield S10 2RX
UNITED KINGDOM

A.R. Bradwell
Director, Immunodiagnostic Research Laboratory
Department of Immunology
Medical School
Birmingham B15 2TH
UNITED KINGDOM

A. Clark
Senior Lecturer in Medical Microbiology
Sheffield University Medical School
Beech Hill Road
Sheffield S10 2RX
UNITED KINGDOM

M.A.H. French
Lecturer
University Department of Medicine
Northern General Hospital
Sheffield S5 7AU
UNITED KINGDOM

B.W. Hancock
Senior Lecturer in Medicine
University of Sheffield
Honorary Consultant Physician
Royal Hallamshire and Weston Park Hospitals
Sheffield S10 2JF
UNITED KINGDOM

R.F. Hinchliffe
Senior Chief Medical Laboratory Scientific Officer
Department of Haematology
The Children's Hospital
Sheffield S10 2TH
UNITED KINGDOM

J.S. Lilleyman
Consultant Haematologist
Department of Haematology
The Children's Hospital
Sheffield S10 2TH
UNITED KINGDOM

I.H. Manifold
Senior Registrar in Radiotherapy and Oncology
Weston Park Hospital
Sheffield S10 2SJ
UNITED KINGDOM

C.W. Potter
Professor, Department of Virology
University of Sheffield Medical School
Beech Hill Road
Sheffield S10 2RX
UNITED KINGDOM

T.J. Priestman
Consultant Radiotherapist and Oncologist
Queen Elizabeth Hospital
Edgbaston
Birmingham B15 2TH
UNITED KINGDOM

R.C. Rees
Senior Lecturer, Department of Virology
University of Sheffield Medical School
Beech Hill Road
Sheffield S10 2RX
UNITED KINGDOM

K. Sikora
Director and Honorary Consultant Radiotherapist and Oncologist
Ludwig Institute for Cancer Research
MRC Centre
Hills Road
Cambridge
UNITED KINGDOM

H. Smedley
Senior Registrar in Radiotherapy and Oncology
Addenbrooke's Hospital
Cambridge
UNITED KINGDOM

J.C.E. Underwood
Professor
Honorary Consultant Histopathologist
Department of Pathology
University of Sheffield Medical School
Beech Hill Road
Sheffield S10 2RX
UNITED KINGDOM

A. Milford Ward
Senior Lecturer in Immunology
Director of Supraregional Protein Reference Unit
Royal Hallamshire Hospital
Sheffield S10 2JF
UNITED KINGDOM

PREFACE

Many books have been written about cancer immunology. However, the subject is still in its infancy regarding full understanding of the complex mechanisms and interactions involved and their relevance to the clinical situation. Exciting developments are being seen in the fields of research, involving, for example, monoclonal antibodies and biological response modifiers. We, therefore, feel fully justified in introducing this new text, which is intended for clinical oncologists wishing to know more about the status of immunology in cancer and as a source of reference for workers, in all branches of oncology research, seeking up-to-date reviews. Contributors have, therefore, given both explanatory and more detailed accounts of developments in their particular fields of expertise.

IMMUNOLOGICAL ASPECTS OF CANCER

1. BASIC IMMUNOLOGY

A. MILFORD WARD

INTRODUCTION

The immune response represents the normal physiological process by which the body maintains homeostasis in the response to infection or to introduction of foreign material. The immune system that generates this response is complex in that it exerts its action by means of circulating cellular and humoral components capable of acting at sites far distant from their site of formation and by its interaction with a variety of biological effector systems.

CELLS OF THE IMMUNE SYSTEM

The major cell types of the immune system are the macrophages and the lymphocytes. Macrophages, as nonantigen-specific cells, are responsible for concentrating and presenting antigen to the lymphocyte in the generation of antigen-specific responses. They are also responsible for the production and secretion of biologically active components that modify or modulate lymphocyte responsiveness and initiate increased production of nonspecific factors such as the acute phase reactant proteins. Lymphocytes are the antigen-specific cells of the system acting via antigen-specific receptors on their cell surface. Lymphocytes responsible, in the main, for the cellular responses of delayed-type hypersensitivity are of thymic origin and termed *T-cells*, whilst those that mature into antibody-forming cells are bone-marrow derived and termed *B-cells*. These two major classes of lymphocyte differ in their surface membrane and functional characteristics.

B.W. Hancock and A.M. Ward (eds.), Immunological Aspects of Cancer. Copyright © 1985, Martinus Nijhoff Publishing, Boston/Dordrecht/Lancaster.

Functional subpopulations of lymphocytes

Lymphocytes, in common with macrophages, polymorphs, and erythrocytes, originate from the primordial haematopoetic cell. Lymphocyte precursors originate from the primitive haematopoetic foci in the fetal liver and bone marrow to populate the thymus and secondary lymphoid organs, where they proliferate and undergo the initial stages of maturation. During this stage of maturation, surface membrane characteristics are acquired that allow the identification of the various functional subpopulations of lymphocytes.

As cellular components of the thymus and peripheral lymphoid organs, the lymphocytes are not a static population but pursue a continual recirculating course from the lymphoid organs through the lymphatics to the vascular system and back via interstitial tissues or directly through the postcapillary venules to the lymphoid organs. This continual migration is an essential feature of the antigen-searching and -entrapment function system and explains why immune reactions assume a generalised character despite localised antigenic stimulation.

Different subpopulations of lymphocytes can be defined by their capacity to undergo transformation in response to mitogenic stimulation and by their surface membrane characteristics (table 1–1). The advent of monoclonal antibodies to cell surface antigens specific to the subpopulations and to different functional subsets has allowed this division to be further refined. Three major commercial sources of these antisera are now readily available; the interrelationship of the sera is shown on table 1–2.

T-lymphocytes

The lymphocyte precursor that populates the thymus acquires specific alloantigens and matures into a thymocyte. This maturation process continues in the medulla of the thymus to give rise to the T-lymphocyte, which is then ready to join the recirculating pool and populate the peripheral lymphoid system. The thymic environment does not seem to be essential for this maturation process, as uncommitted lymphocytes can be stimulated to T-cell maturation by exposure to thymic hormone in vitro.

The next stage of differentiation of the T-lymphocyte is dependent on antigen contact. Antigen contact or stimulation gives rise to the development of functionally and phenotypically distinct subsets: those that assist or cooperate in antibody production by B-lymphocytes—the T-helper or inducer cells—and those that modulate or control T-inducer cell function—the T-suppressor cells. A third subset of T-cells, the cytotoxic

Table 1–1. Surface membrane characteristics of T-cells and B-cells

	T-cells	B-cells
Sheep erythrocyte rosette forming cells	+	−
Mouse erythrocyte rosette forming cells	−	+
EAC rosette forming cells	−	+
Surface immunoglobulin	−	+
PHA transformation	+	−

Table 1-2. Monoclonal antibodies from commerical sources
used for the definition of functional subsets of lymphocytes

Pan T-cell	OKT3, OKT1, T101, Leu-1, Leu-4
T-helper/inducer cell	OKT4, T4, Leu-3
T-suppressor/cytotoxic cell	OKT8, OKT5, T8, Leu-2
E-rosette receptor	OKT11, Leu-5
Thymocyte	OKT6, Leu-6
NK/K-cell	Leu-7
Monocyte/macrophage	OKT1a1, OKM-1, LeuM1-3, HLA-DR
B-cell	OKT1a1, HLA-DR, Leu-10

T-cells, which can lyse target cells by direct contact, are also recognised. The cytolytic action of cytotoxic T-lymphocytes is the basis of the in vitro mixed lymphocyte culture (MLC) reaction, is antigen-specific in its initial phase, and does not require the presence of antibody or complement.

Helper-suppressor ratios

The relative proportion of T-helper inducer cells to T-suppressor cytotoxic cells in the peripheral circulation is fairly constant. With the advent of monoclonal antibodies for the definition of the T-cell subsets, this has become referred to as the T4:T8 ratio. In the normal state the T4:T8 ratio is in the order of 2.0:2.5. In infection the T4 numbers are reduced and the ratio reversed. T4-reactive cells are very low or absent in chronic or persistent viral infection and in acquired immunodeficiency syndromes. The T4:T8 ratio is also reversed in graft versus host disease and in transplant rejection, but this is a reflection of the absolute increase in T-suppressor cells rather than of a reduction in T-helper cells.

Natural killer cells

Antibody-dependent cell-mediated cytotoxicity (ADCC) is the function of further subsets of lymphocytes, killer cells (K-cells), and natural killer cells (NK-cells). The precise lineage of these cells, whether they are T-cell or B-cell related, is not clear, and the distinction between the two is not absolute. These cells act by virtue of Fc receptors on their surface membrane binding to antibody-coated target cells. NK-cells would appear to be of particular importance in nonspecific defense against viral infection and are believed to have an immune surveillance role in preventing the development of some tumours.

B-lymphocytes

The primordial B-lymphocyte undergoes its formative stages of differentiation within the bone marrow, from whence it emerges to populate the thymic independent areas of peripheral lymphoid tissue. These areas include the follicles and medulla of lymph nodes, follicles of the gut-associated lymphoid tissue, and the periphery of the white pulp of the spleen. The mature B-cell is an essentially sedentary cell of restricted longevity. It bears antigen receptors on its surface membrane in the form of IgD and monomeric IgM. On exposure to antigen it undergoes transformation in a blast-type cell and proceeds to undergo a number of maturation divisions to give rise to the final antibody-producing cell, the plasma cell.

For the majority of antigens this B-cell activation requires both antigen stimulation and the cooperation of the T-inducer cell. Antigens that are capable of activation of B-cells without this cellular interaction are termed *thymus-independent antigens*. The evoked immune response results in the formation of IgM antibody but allows no switch to IgG antibody production and no generation of immunologic memory. The cooperation of the T-inducer cell with B-cell maturation allows the amplification of the IgM antibody response and also the cellular switch to synthesis of IgG, IgA, and IgE class antibody. Some activated B-cells do not mature to form plasma cells but revert to the morphological form of small lymphocytes. These B-memory cells differ from unstimulated B-cells in that they are no longer sedentary but join the recirculating pool and have a much increased longevity. These B-cells are responsible for the rapid increase in antibody synthesis of the secondary immune response.

EFFECT OF IMMUNOSUPPRESSIVE AGENTS ON THE IMMUNE SYSTEM

Immunosuppression by anticancer drugs or agents may be profound. The extent and selectivity of the suppression depends on various factors:

1.   Pharmacological characteristics of the drug.
2.   Cellular characteristics of the immune response.
3.   Temporal relationship between antigenic stimulation and drug administration.

The immunosuppressive effect on the anticancer drugs is the result of selective effects on specific cells and factors altering the regulation of this complex cellular interactive defense system. Any alteration in the balance between effector and regulating cells in the immune system will result in changes in the immune responsiveness of the individual [1].

The immunosuppressive action of cytoxic drugs and corticosteroids is more effective in primary than in secondary responses. These drugs do not, however, affect equally all components of the immune system.

This differential effect is well illustrated by the impairment or suppression of the primary immune response after renal allotransplantation by azathioprine and corticosteroids, but these same drugs will not prevent the second set rejection in a presensitized recipient.

The immune response can be divided into an induction phase, during which antigen-responsive cells undergo transformation and replication, and an effector phase, during which the cells produce and secrete their active components. Most immunosuppressive drugs are effective during this induction phase. The drugs are most effective when administered before or immediately after antigenic challenge. There may also be a differential effect on T- and B-lymphocytes, cyclophosphamide having a greater cytotoxic effect on B-lymphocytes and a greater suppression of humoral than cellular responses (table 1–3). Paradoxical effects on immune responsiveness may be noted, and in this the temporal relationship of drug administration to antigenic stimulation is of critical importance. Irradiation or mercaptopurine administration immediately prior to antigen challenge may produce enhanced, rather than depressed, antibody and delayed-type responsiveness. Cyclophosphamide may produce a similar paradoxical increase in cellular responses when administered prior to antigenic stimulation by virtue of its differential cytotoxicity for T-suppressor cells.

Table 1–3. Comparative effect on corticosteroids, cyclophosphamide, azathioprine, and methotrexate on immune responses

	Corticosteroids	Cyclophosphamide	Azathioprine	Methotrexate
Primary antibody response	↓↓	↓↓	↓↓	↓↓
Secondary antibody response	↓↓	↓	(↑↓)	(↑↓)
Graft rejection	↓↓	0	↓↓	0
Second set rejection	0	0	0	0
Delayed type hypersensitivity	0	↓↑	↓	(↓↑)
Mitogenic responses	0	↓↓	0	0
NK-cell function	↓	0	↓↓	0
B-cell numbers	↓↓	↓	0	0

Corticosteroids

Administration for several days is usually associated with a reduction in circulating levels of immunoglobulins. The beneficial effects do not, however, result so much from the reduction in specific antibody titres as from the interference with reticuloendothelial cell function and phagocytosis of antibody-coated cells.

The effect on cellular immunity requires considerably longer administration but can lead to devastating and overwhelming infections, often from microorganisms not normally considered pathogenic. The effects range from inhibition of T-cell migration, reduction in lymphokine secretion, reduction in lymphocyte-monocyte interaction, and reduced target cell lysis.

Corticosteroids inhibit monocyte chemotaxis and interleukin 1 production. Fc and C3 receptors are reduced and bactericidal function suppressed. Both antigenic and mitogenic transformations and proliferation of T-cells are suppressed. In contrast, proliferation and established B-cell responses are relatively resistant to corticosteroid administration. The depression in serum immunoglobulin levels reflects a combination effect of increased catabolism and reduced synthesis and affects IgG and IgA in preference to IgM. IgE levels tend to increase.

The generation of T-suppressor cells appears to be exquisitely sensitive to corticosteroid administration, but, once generated, suppressor cell function appears unimpaired and may even be augmented. The augmentation is brought about by a combination effect of interleukin 2 absorption by the activated suppressor cell and the corticosteroid-induced inhibition of interleukin 1–stimulated interleukin 2 production by macrophages.

Corticosteroids therefore have wide-ranging effects on the immune and inflammatory systems at all levels of therapeutic administration. The precise mechanism of this immunomodulating effect is ill-understood. Whilst the role of intracytoplasmic corticosteroid receptors appears to be integral to their action, the intercompartmental redistribution of macrophages and lymphocytes and membrane stabilisation effect also play their part, particularly in the role of corticosteroid modulation of the allergic and immune complex-mediated tissue-damage reactions [2].

Azathioprine and mercaptopurine

Azathioprine and its parent compound mercaptopurine are phase-specific compounds acting primarily in the S-phase of cell replication. Although cytotoxicity itself may have immuno-suppressive effects, there is evidence that azathioprine can bind to the antigen receptor sites of T-lymphocytes and have a selective inhibiting effect on NK-cells. The inhibiting or cytotoxic effect of azathioprine on the haematopoetic cells also reduces the numbers of circulating neutrophils and monocytes with resultant impairment of phagocytosis potential.

Cyclophosphamide

Cyclophosphamide is a cycle-specific drug that exerts its effect on actively proliferating cells at any stage in the cell cycle. It has a more sustained action on the humoral responses due to a low-dose predilection for B-lymphocytes. The suppression of cellular response is more variable, with some responses being augmented by the differential high-dose toxicity for suppressor T-cells. High doses of cyclophosphamide administered prior to antigenic challenge will augment many cell-mediated and delayed-type hypersensitivity responses, and the T-suppressor cell depletion will also abrogate immune tolerance.

The responses augmented by cyclophosphamide include chemical contact sensitivity, the reaction to tuberculin and other microbial antigens, and the Joness-Motte reaction to soluble protein antigens. This augmenting or potentiating effect depends on the relative cell turnover kinetics of the precursor cells, the maximal effect being exhibited in relation to short-lived and rapidly dividing cells [3].

Similar high-dose immunopotentiating effects may be seen with some other anticancer drugs. Thiotepa, nitrogen mustards, mitomycin-C, and 5-fluoruracil have a more marked potentiating effect than cyclophosphamide. Melphalan, azathioprine, and methotrexate also demonstrate the high-dose immunopotentiating effect, but this effect tends to be rather less marked. In all cases the effect is seen only when drug administration preceeds the antigenic challenge or sensitisation.

Adriamycin

Unlike most other anticancer drugs, adriamycin has a general enhancing effect on the immune system, although the effect can be variable between the different components of the system. There is marked augmentation of macrophage and cytotoxic lymphocyte activity. The effect on the humoral systems and on NK-cell activity is more variable [4] and somewhat less marked due to the increased macrophage production of prostaglandin. The addition of a prostaglandin inhibitor to the therapeutic regimen will obviate this effect and enhance NK-cell activity [5].

Chlorambucil

A cycle-specific drug, chlorambucil generally has effects similar to cyclophosphamide although of slower generation. The immunopotentiating effect is much less marked.

Methotrexate

A potent phase-specific immunosuppressive drug, methotrexate inhibits both B-cells and T-cells. A slightly increased differential effect on T-suppressor cells gives the drug some immunopotentiating effect at high dosage.

Cisplatinum

A potent immunosuppressive drug, cisplatinum has multisite action on the immune system. The precise mode of suppression is uncertain. No augmentation effects are seen at therapeutic dosages.

Cyclosporin A

Cyclosporin A has a selective lymphocytoxic effect without associated myelotoxicity, the primary effect being against T-cells with no effect on the B-cell system. It has no direct effect on macrophage or NK-cell function, although it does reduce the synthesis of T-dependent γinterferon, which is, itself, a positive modulator of NK-cell activity.

The cyclosporin A effect on the T-cell is brought about by inhibition of responsiveness to interleukin 2 (Il–2) and by rendering Il–2 producing T-cells unresponsive to interleukin 1 (Il–1). Reduction in Il–1 synthesis is achieved by inhibition of T-helper cells without affecting its production by macrophages. Once lymphocytes have generated Il–2 receptors, cyclosporin A ceases to have an inhibitory effect. Cyclosporin A prevents mitogenic- and antigenic-induced T-cell proliferation, with the result that T-cell assistance to macrophages in Il–1 production is reduced and of Il–1 receptor formation is inhibited by Il–2 producing cells and by rendering other T-cells unresponsive to Il–2. These distinct but closely interrelated stages are all in the early activation phase of the T-cell immune response, the activated T-cell being relatively resistant or insensitive to the inhibitory and suppressive effect of cyclosporin A [6].

The fact that cyclosporin A binding abrogates the binding of the pan T-cell antiserum OKT-3 suggests that the binding site of both substances is similar if not identical and that cyclosporin A may be binding to the antigen-specific receptor structures on the T-cell membrane. This association helps to explain the inhibiting effect of the agent on all T-cell functions and on the generation of helper, suppressor, and cytotoxic functional subsets.

Whilst the B-cell is not affected directly by cyclosporin A and antibody responses to thymic-independent antigens, such as bacterial endotoxins, are unchanged, there is a marked suppression of thymic-dependent antibody synthesis due to the T-helper cell suppression.

EFFECT OF IRRADIATION ON THE IMMUNE SYSTEM

Irradiation is an immunosuppressive agent with a marked detrimental effect on all the immunological defense systems, both antigen-specific and nonspecific. The increased risk of infection following irradiation is due, in part, to a reduction in number and functional capacity of phagocytic cells and to a reduction in level of some complement components. The effect on the antigen-specific defense mechanisms is a rather more complex affair [7].

Irradiation has long been recognised to abrogate humoral responses more readily than cell-mediated responses, and the depression of the primary antibody response is seen to reflect damage to the inductive rather than the productive phase of antibody synthesis.

Maximal depression of antibody synthesis is seen in antigens administered at or immediately after irradiation. The ability to produce new antibody recovers only two to three months following irradiation. In contrast, the secondary antibody response is relatively radio-resistant.

At the cellular level, irradiation primarily affects the dividing cell. Thus, the numbers of accessory cells are reduced, but their unit functional capacity is relatively unchanged. Lymphocytes are acutely radiosensitive, and lymphopenia is a common sequel to high-dose irradiation. The lymphopenia is induced, not only by a reduction in dividing cells, but also by interphase death. Whilst it is accepted that the unstimulated B-cell is extremely radiosensitive and that the productive B-cell and plasma cell is relatively less so, the radiosensitivity of T-helper and T-suppressor lymphocytes is still a controversial question.

EFFECT OF NUTRITIONAL STATUS ON THE IMMUNE RESPONSE

Adequate nutrition is essential for the maintenance of the functional integrity of the immune system. Malnutrition is a major cause of secondary or acquired immunodeficiency. Protein-calorie malnutrition induces lymphopenia and reduced delayed-type cutaneous hypersensitivity. Mitogenic transformation of lymphocytes is reduced. In the extreme chronic state of marasmus, antibody synthesis and phagocyte function are also reduced.

Vitamin and trace-metal deficiencies also have profound effects on the immune system (table 1–4). T-cell functions are depressed following deficiency of vitamins A, B6, folic acid, zinc, iron, and selenium, whilst B-cell functions are adversely affected by deficiency of vitamins A, B6, biotin, pantothenic acid, folic acid, niacin, and magnesium. Effector cell

Table 1–4. Effect of vitamin and mineral deficiencies on immune function

	T-cell	B-cell	Macrophage	Polymorph
Vitamin A	↓↓	↓↓		
B$_6$	↓↓	↓↓		↓
B$_{12}$	↓			
Niacin		↓		
Biotin		↓↓		
Pantothenic acid		↓↓		
Folic acid	↓	↓↓		
C			↓	↓
D		↓		↓
E	↓	↓	↓	
Minerals:				
Iron	↓↓			↓↓
Copper			↓	↓
Selenium	↓		↓	
Zinc	↓↓			
Magnesium		↓		

functions of macrophages are depressed by lack of vitamins C and E and of copper and selenium, whilst polymorph function is dependent on adequate levels of vitamin B6, C, and D and of iron and copper.

In iron deficiency both specific and nonspecific defense mechanisms are compromised and contribute to the increased incidence of infections. Iron is essential for many enzyme systems and is necessary for maintenance of lymphoid tissues as well as for the bactericidal effect of polymorphs. Cell-mediated immune function is primarily affected with impairment of delayed-type hypersensitivity responses and diminution of lymphokine production.

EFFECT OF AGING ON THE IMMUNE RESPONSE

Thymic involution and a decrease in thymic hormone synthesis with increasing age lead to a generalised reduction in immune capability in the aged population. The reduced thymic mass limits the entry of immature lymphocytes into the thymus and their subsequent differentiation into mature T-cells. This result is reflected in a reduction of E-rosetting cells and a concomitant increase in autorosette-forming cells. This increase tends to mask any age-related fall in functionally active T-cells with the replication potential required for immune competence. The major effect of the reduction in mature T-cells is a reduction in suppressor/cytotoxic T-cells. More subtle changes involve a reduction in interleukin 2 receptors on T-cells and of surface immunoglobulin on B-cells. Many intracellular enzyme systems in lymphocytes are reduced, including the DNA response enzymes, with the result that lymphocytes in the aged patient are more susceptible to damage by irradiation and mitogenic drugs.

Cell-mediated immune function in the elderly is depressed, with a reduction in delayed-type hypersensitivity responses to recall antigens, delayed graft rejection, and reduced mitogenic responsiveness. This latter is due, not to a reduction in lectin- or antigen-binding capacity, but to a reduction in the number of mitogen-responsive cells capable of undergoing proliferation.

Humoral immune mechanisms also show age-related changes. Whilst total serum IgG and IgA increase with age, serum IgM significantly decreases. The lowered IgM levels correlate with the reduction in levels of "natural" antibodies, whilst the increase in IgG and IgA correlates with the increase in autoantibodies and monoclonal gammopathies. In addition to autoantibodies reactive with nuclei and other cellular components, autoanti-idiotype antibodies and autoantibodies to T-suppressor cells have also been demonstrated. The development of these tends to further imbalance the already disordered immune system.

In contrast to the increased frequency of production of autoantibodies, specific antibody production to foreign antigen is reduced. This reduction is thought to be primarily a feature of lowered T-helper cell functions, as the effect is seen more markedly with T-dependent antigens, antibody responses to T-independent antigens being relatively unaffected. This may again relate to the reduced number of interleukin 2 receptors on the cell surface of the T-cell.

An additional factor to further embarrass the already compromised immune system in the elderly is the changing levels of sex steroids. Oestrogens, particularly 16-hydroxylated metabolites, are potent immunostimulants, whereas androgens tend to be immunoregulatory. Whilst the mechanisms of these actions are controversial, the differential effect may partially explain the rather brisker immune response in the young adult female. The marked reduction in oestrogen levels postmenopause may be associated with the increased prevalence of autoantibodies in the elderly female.

REFERENCES

1. Bach JF, Mode of action of immunosuppressive drugs. Amsterdam: North Holland, 1975.
2. Cupps TR, Fanci AS. Corticosteroid immunoregulation. Immunol Rev 65: 133–155, 1982.
3. Turk JL, Parker D. Effect of cyclophosphamide on immunological control mechanisms. Immunol Rev 65: 99–113, 1982.
4. Cohen SA, Ehrke MJ, Mihich E. Selective imbalances of cellular immune responses by adriamycin. In Weber G (ed), Advances in enzyme regulation. New York: Pergamon Press, pp. 335.
5. Ehrke MJ, Cohen SA, Mihich E. Selective effects of adriamycin in murine host defense systems. Immunol Rev 65: 55–78, 1982.
6. Britton S, Palacios R. Cyclosporin A—Usefulness, risks, and mechanisms of action. Immunol Rev 65: 5–22, 1982.
7. Doria G, Agarossi G, Adorini L. Selective effects of ionising radiations in immunoregulatory cells. Immunol Rev 65: 23–54, 1982.

2. ANTITUMOUR LYMPHOCYTE RESPONSES

R.C. REES

S.A. ALI

INTRODUCTION

Despite the considerable achievements in immunology during the past two decades, control of tumour development by effective immunotherapy is still not possible. This situation reflects the complexity of events that occur in response to tumour growth. Other chapters in this book outline the important advances made in the study of macrophage function and the developments in monoclonal antibody production against tumour-associated antigens. In this chapter the role of the lymphocyte in combating tumour development and metastatic spread is considered. Of importance, however, is the understanding that lymphocyte function is influenced by other cell types, hormones, and products released by tumour cells and that much of our current knowledge has stemmed from in vitro experimentation. Caution must be exercised when interpreting the results of laboratory tests and relating these to their in vivo relevance, since it is not possible to mimic the conditions that the in vivo environment imposes on lymphocyte activity.

Clearly, lymphocytes are capable of mediating adaptive and nonadaptive immune responses. That is to say, certain lymphocyte subtypes are capable of recognising foreign antigenic determinants expressed on tumour cells and mounting an effective, tumour-specific immune response toward these determinants, while other cells are capable of recognising abnormal cell types without the requirement of previous encounter with tumour-related antigens. As a basis for discussion, these two elements represent the subdivision of lymphocyte reactivity now recognised.

B.W. Hancock and A.M. Ward (eds.), Immunological Aspects of Cancer. Copyright © 1985, Martinus Nijhoff Publishing, Boston/Dordrecht/Lancaster.

In essence, specific antitumour reactivity is mediated by antigen-sensitised T-lymphocytes, although K-cell-mediated destruction of tumour cells can occur where the specific component is supplied by humoral antibody. An understanding of "tumour antigen(s)" is therefore critical in assessing the significance of specific immune responses, and the nature and expression of these components are discussed below.

It must be realised that the following subdivisions are not absolute. We consider here T-cell-mediated and NK-cell-mediated antitumour reactivity, the in vivo significance of these responses during tumour growth and metastases, modulation of their function by suppressor lymphoid cells and tumour products, and the recent advances in T-cell and NK-cell cloning techniques, which may prove highly relevant to the future immunotherapy of malignant disease.

SPECIFIC ANTITUMOUR IMMUNE RESPONSE

Tumour-associated antigens

Previous authors have highlighted problems associated with the initiation of an effective host response to a developing tumour. The nature of an antigen-specific response, in the main, is determined by the expression, on tumour cells, of antigenic structures, recognised as foreign to the host and capable of initiating cell-mediated or humoral immune responses. It is relevant, therefore, to consider the nature of tumour-associated antigens (TAA) and tumour-associated transplantation antigens (TATA), relative to each other. Thus, whereas tumour cells may express TAAs at the cell surface, these TAAs do not necessarily evoke a tumour rejection response in the host, nor do they necessarily act as target antigens against which rejection takes place. Only tumour-associated antigens capable of functioning to stimulate a tumour rejection response are of significance in specific immunotherapy.

The demonstration of tumour antigens, and assessment of their relevance as targets in transplant rejection, has preoccupied tumour immunologists and has been the subject of much debate during the past two decades. The expression on human tumour cells of antigens recognised as foreign by the host and capable of initiating an effective immune status has recently been questioned, and this point is crucial in determining whether specific immunotherapy is possible. Since the aetiology of most human tumours is unknown, the relevance of many animal models used to study cancer immunology has been questioned. Hewitt [1] has suggested that many of the animal models induced by chemical carcinogens or oncogenic viruses are irrelevant to the study of human tumour immunology, since their immunogenic properties are attributable to an artifactual immunogenicity arising as a result of deliberate induction. It has further been suggested that tumours of spontaneous origin, which are in the main weakly immunogenic, are to be favoured as models for human cancer; however, to draw an analogy between spontaneously arising animal tumours and those of humans is difficult, since there is no adequate way at present of assessing the immunogenic potential of human tumours. The presence of tumour-associated antigens on human tumour cells has been shown using in vitro techniques, but such findings do not fully answer questions as to their in vivo role.

In the light of current knowledge, one cannot dismiss the possibility that many human tumours may be immunogenic and, under suitable conditions, capable of provoking a host immune "rejection" response.

Studies in man have shown that lymphocytes from cancer patients can mediate a specific recognition of autologous tumour cells, as shown by tests demonstrating direct lymphocyte cytotoxicity. These findings support the contention that some human tumours express an antigen capable of inducing a host immune response. Several studies have indicated that freshly isolated blood lymphocytes from cancer patients are weakly reactive against autologous tumour cells [2–5]. However, other studies have further shown that patients' lymphocytes incubated with autologous tumour cells in mixed culture stimulated the development of lymphocytes capable of recognition and lysis of autologous tumour cells; in the majority of individuals this reactivity appeared to be tumour-specific [6–8]. These findings suggest that stimulation with autologous tumour cells expands lymphocyte clones conveying specific recognition of tumour antigen, and together with other studies [9,10] these findings further support the contention that some human tumours express immunologically offensive tumour-associated antigens. Caution must be exercised in the interpretation of these findings because they provide no evidence that this antitumour immune response is functional in vivo.

Since, therefore, under defined experimental conditions specifically reactive lymphocytes can recognise human tumour-associated components expressed at the tumour cell surface, to gain further insight into the mechanism of tumour immunity, it is of interest to consider the antigenic properties of transplantation antigens (TATAs) associated with animal tumours. The expression of TATAs on a variety of experimental tumours has been shown using in vivo transplantation techniques, and certain differences were noted between the different systems. Of the several models available for study, chemically induced and virally induced tumours appear to express the greatest immunogenic potential. Chemically induced tumours, in the main, possess an individually specific tumour rejection antigen that is not cross-reactive with rejection antigens expressed on other tumours induced by the same carcinogen [11–15]. In contrast, tumours induced by DNA viruses express an antigen that is virus-specific (virally determined) and common to all tumours induced by the same virus (see chapter 11).

In considering the ability of TATAs to elicit transplant immunity to tumour challenge, it has been shown that soluble or membrane-associated preparations from tumours are less effective in inducing transplant immunity than intact attenuated tumour cells or tissue [16–18], and in certain instances soluble antigen may induce deviations in the immune response, failing to produce immunity when given in large doses and facilitating enhanced tumour growth rather than inhibition [18,19]. There are, however, exceptions, for example, the Meth-A chemically induced tumour and the CI-4 tumour of BALB/c origin, where the TATAs are immunogenic when solubilized [20]. With some chemically induced tumours a broader specificity of antigenic composition has been demonstrated in cross-protection experiments [21,22]; the precise nature of the antigenic determinants responsible for cross-reactivity has not been fully established, although they may represent reexpressed developmental antigens, which are normally present during foetal development [23,24].

The relationship between TATAs and constituents expressed on normal (nonmalignant) cells has been studied, and evidence has been presented to support the contention that the tumour-associated antigens present on chemically induced tumours may be related to histocompatibility or alloantigens. It has been reported, using murine sarcoma tumours, that alloantigens foreign to the syngeneic host can be demonstrated at the cell membrane of tumour cells [25,26]. Although these antigens may act independently of tumour-specific antigens, immunization against tumour challenge using skin grafts from the appropriate strain, and conversely immunization with tumour followed by implantation of skin grafts, resulted in immunity to challenge and accelerated rejection of skin grafts, respectively [27]. Fujimoto et al. [28] studied a spontaneously arising lymphoma in A/J mice and found the tumour-associated antigen to copurify with the alloantigen components, thus suggesting that the two antigenic determinants resided on the same molecule. Chang et al. [29] also found that the tumour-specific antigen of a murine mammary carcinoma was related to allo-antigens, but was distinct from H2 antigens [30]. Further evidence disassociating tumour-specific from H2 antigens stems from the observation that the gene coding for the tumour-specific antigen is not present on the same chromosome coding for the H2 complex [31,32]. Furthermore, Lennox et al. [33] have separated H2 products from the tumour-specific antigen by affinity chromatography and lectin binding. In the rat hepatoma model [34,35] the D23-hepatoma-specific antigen, which is thought to act as a tumour rejection antigen in this system, is cross-reactive with normal syngeneic tissue antigens. This observation could not be ascribed to reactivity against serologically defined antigens of the major histocompatibility complex or with α-2 microglobulin, inferring a relationship not between the major histocompatibility antigens of the rat but with other, as yet, undefined alloantigen molecules.

The identification and characterization of human tumour-associated antigens are complicated by the number of different antigens reported and the often complex serological assays used to identify these components [36]. The assay of antigens includes organ-specific and organ-nonspecific molecules, oncofetal antigens, and molecular structures present on tumour cells that react with antibodies present in sera from normal individuals (natural antibodies) [36–38]. With the advent of monoclonal antibodies, combined with affinity chromatography techniques, the isolation of human tumour-associated antigens becomes feasible. For example, Natali et al. [39] have reported the production of a monoclonal antibody reactive with, and capable of precipitating out, two human melanoma-specific antigens (antibody not reactive with normal tissue or other tumour tissue) of molecular weight 280,000 and 500,000. Thus, application of hybridoma techniques has increased the degree to which TAA can be purified. However, to draw conclusions as to the in vivo relevance of TAA in human disease is difficult, and these isolated components cannot, as yet, be classified as transplantation antigens.

In only a limited number of experimental tumours has the elucidation of the biochemical nature of TATA been possible, due to the inability of most antigens in soluble form to retain their capacity to elicit transplant resistance in vivo. Amongst the tumours studied, certain virus-induced and chemically induced murine tumours possess a soluble TATA [20,40,41; see chapter 11]. The Meth-A murine sarcoma, for example, expresses a TATA at the cell membrane. Its molecular weight is 60,000, which is identical to antigens that are present in the cytosol fraction of the cells and are capable of inducing transplant immunity [41].

Establishing a clear definition of the expression of TATAs on human and animal tumours represents one of the most important problems facing tumour immunologists, and this question is fundamental to our understanding the nature of tumour immune responses. Since there is evidence that TAAs are expressed on human tumours, albeit restricted to results from in vitro studies, it would be unwise to disregard or ignore animal tumour models that allow us to investigate the properties of TATAs and establish ideas that might have relevance for work on human tumour antigens.

Specific immunity

Complete understanding of the principles associated with the assessment of the specific anti-tumour immune response is hampered by the complexity of the immune pathways involved and our lack of knowledge of many of the elements that contribute to tumour rejection. The main principles associated with specific rejection of a tumour and the framework of immune responses so far documented again have been largely the result of experimental research using animal models. Because of the inadequacy of many of the in vitro techniques in demonstrating the mechanism of cytotoxic rejection of tumour cells, our understanding of the response toward human tumours is sadly lacking. However, as previously empha-sised, the possible existence of tumour rejection antigens cannot be overlooked, and it is pertinent to consider the experimental observations that have led to our current perception of tumour immunology.

The specific antitumour response is directed against tumour antigen (TATAs) expressed at the cell surface of tumour cells; the initiation of immunity is highly complex, requiring the interaction of several cell types. The nature of this response, and the pathways that lead to tumour rejection, may be either humoral—where specific antibody acts in concert with complement to mediate lysis of the tumour cells—cellular—where the interaction between effector cell and target leads to tumour cell lysis—or a combination of a humoral factor, which determines the specific nature of the reaction, and a cellular component, which is triggered into lytic activity following interaction with the specific antibody, itself inter-acting with the tumour cell. This latter mechanism is known as antibody-dependent cellular cytotoxicity (ADCC) and may represent an important element of immunity against some tumours.

Unclear at present is which limb of the immune response plays a dominant role in the development of resistance to tumour growth. Mechanisms that can be demonstrated in vitro may bear little relevance in the intact host; thus, not all in vitro assays have shown correlation with in vivo resistance [42]. One contributing factor in the failure to establish a relationship between in vivo and in vitro tumour cell interaction is that in vitro techniques circumvent the need for immune cells to circulate in order to reach their site of action. In addition, in vitro assays fail to account for the influence of other immunological factors in determining the level of in vivo activity. The Winn assay [43], which has been used widely as an in vivo assay for tumour neutralisation, in many respects is analogous to the in vitro techniques for cytotoxicity, in as much as it entails admixing lymphoid cells with target cells in given ratios prior to inoculation into the intact host. Crumm [44] has recently assessed the capacity of thoracic duct lymph cells from tumour-immune animals to transfer immunity to normal intact rats upon injection intravenously, and this model may prove suitable to study further the cellular components of tumour rejection. In studies using the rat system, it has been shown that the major effector cell is of T-lymphocyte origin, which is in a nonproliferating state when injected into the recipient animal, reactive cells having a life span when transferred of approximately two weeks. The requirement of T-lymphocytes in specific tumour rejection can be readily demonstrated in adoptive transfer, as illustrated in figure 2–1.

In several other studies a correlation has been established between in vitro and in vivo findings. Chauvenet et al. [45] have shown a close association between the tumour-specific killing in vitro and tumour growth inhibition in vivo directed against TATAs expressed on chemically induced murine fibrosarcomas, and similar results have been published by Boon et al. [46] using the P815 mastocytoma. Further studies by Carbone et al. [47] have presented evidence correlating in vitro tumour-cell killing with in vivo transplantation immunity, suggesting immunity to be mediated by T-cells and not through NK-dependent or macrophage-dependent mechanisms. Ting et al. [48] have shown similar findings with the FBL-3 ascites leukaemia; in this system the development of immunity stimulates cytotoxic T-lymphocytes, which are reactive both in vivo and in vitro against homologous tumour cells. In order that cytotoxic T-cells may manifest killing, they require homology between histocompatibility antigens (H2 in the mouse) as well as the specific recognition of the tumour rejection antigen (TATA) on the target cell; this phenomenon is known as genetic restriction. Gooding and Edwards [49] and Carbone et al. [47] have shown this to be necessary for the successful killing of viral-induced and chemically induced murine tumours.

It can be inferred from recent studies that a number of T-lymphocyte subsets are implicated in eliciting an immune response to neoplasia. In the mouse, T-lymphocytes may be subdivided into Lyt-1$^+$ (helper T-cells) or Lyt-2,3$^+$ (T-cytotoxic) populations; this latter phenotype is also associated with suppressor cell activity. In addition, a precursor T-lymphocyte population, which is phenotypically Lyt-1$^+$, Lyt-2,3$^+$, has been implicated in the specific rejection of methylcholanthrene-induced sarcomas [50]. Precursor lymphocytes expressing these surface markers are also associated with delayed hypersensitivity and resistance to microorganisms [51], and allo-transplantation immune reactions against mutants of the class I histocompatibility antigens [52]. A phenotypically similar cell type has also been implicated in the in vivo protection against tumours induced by Rous sarcoma virus [53]. This study concluded that the Lyt-1$^+$, Lyt-2,3$^+$ T-lymphocytes, rather than the conventional cytotoxic lymphocyte, were responsible for transferring tumour immunity, but it is not clear at present whether this precursor cell type further differentiates into a cell possessing either helper T-lymphocyte or cytotoxic cell characteristics. Of interest is that treatment of immune mice with cyclophosphamide, an agent known to subvert the effector function of T-suppressor cells, produces a higher level of immunocompetence than in immune animals not treated with cyclophosphamide. This observation could be interpreted as causing an imbalance in the regulation of the antitumour immune response, and it is important to consider the role of suppressor cells in preventing the development, or function, of an effective antitumour immune response.

The role of T-cell subsets in tumour rejection has been considered in some depth in a recent review by Robbins and Baldwin [54]. It is true to say that the assays available to

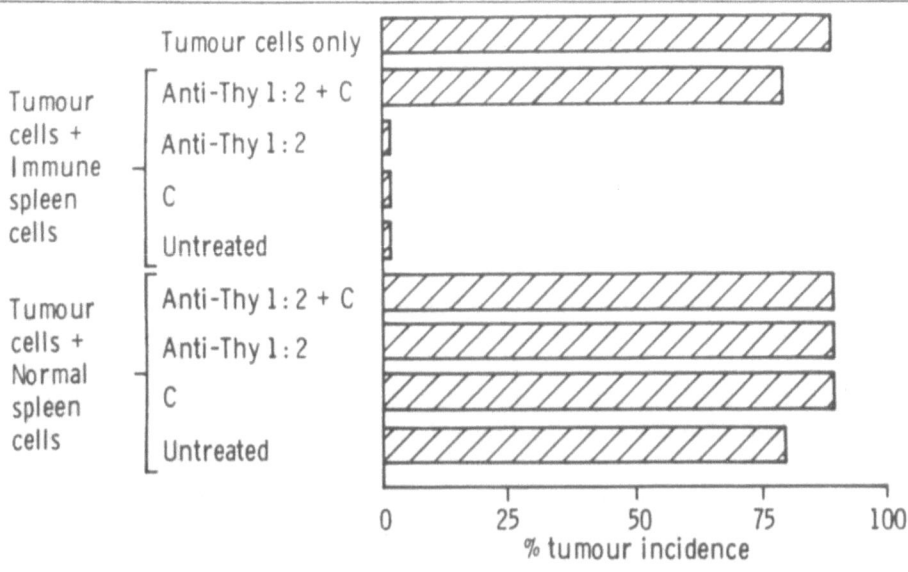

Figure 2-1. Abrogation of adoptive transfer of tumour immunity against a methylcholanthrene-induced C57BL mouse sarcoma-Mc1A by treatment in vitro with anti-Thy 1:2 serum and complement prior to in vivo transfer.

demonstrate cell-mediated destruction of tumour cells in vitro have not clarified the central questions and that difficulties have been encountered in using these techniques and in interpreting the results obtained [55,56]. Indeed, the current assays used to demonstrate cytotoxic activity of specifically sensitised lymphocytes toward tumour cells may not be entirely relevant or aid in establishing the precise nature of the cell responsible for specific antitumour immunity. They also fail to define the role of accessory/helper cells that lack direct cytotoxic activity but may determine the specific nature of the event. Conceivably, therefore, T-lymphocytes may be of paramount importance in graft rejection and determine the specificity of the reaction but lack cytolytic capacity [57,58]. In several experimental tumour systems a lack of correlation has been shown between effective retardation of tumour growth by Winn assay and direct cytolytic activity against syngeneic tumour cells in vitro using tumour immune lymphocytes [42,59].

Several lines of evidence both in tumour and skin graft rejection have shown the importance of Lyt-1+ T-lymphocytes in mediating rejection [57,60–64]. In interpreting these results it must be realised that the expression of markers may not prove exclusive, and they may be expressed on more than one subpopulation of T-lymphocyte. The Lyt-1 T-cell marker, in particular, is subject to variable expression on most mouse T-cells [65]. Confusion in the interpretation of these results may occur since the expression of Lyt-1,2,3 markers may not be representative of T-cell function (help, cytotoxicity, suppression). It can be argued that while the specificity of tumour rejection may be due in certain instances to noncytotoxic specifically sensitised T-lymphocytes, the effector cell responsible for tumour cell destruction and capable of collaborating with the specifically sensitised T-lymphocyte may be of T or non-T (NK or macrophage) origin.

No clear evidence has yet been shown to indicate the precise nature of the cellular inter-actions leading to tumour rejection. One approach used in studies to determine the specificity of the effector phase in vivo in tumour rejection has been to examine whether innocent "bystander" tumour cells are killed as a result of a rejection response mounted against a tumour of different immunogenicity. Thus, it can be determined whether unrelated tumour cells in admixture with cells from the immunising tumour are themselves rejected. In the majority of systems examined, it has been shown that the rejection response mounted against an immunogenic tumour fails to control the growth of "bystander" tumour cells [66,67]. An exception is the guinea pig hepatoma line 1 model, where rejection of "bystander" tumour cells appears to occur [68], although this may not be a consequence of tumour cell killing but of destruction of the tumour due to injury of the common microvasculature [69]. The body of evidence therefore favours the contention that in vivo tumour rejection at the effector cell phase is in the main directed toward a specific antigen-bearing target cell. The further analysis of T-cell subsets using monoclonal antibodies directed against cell surface determinants and their subsequent separation by "fluorescent analytical cell sorting" will help to determine the exact sequence of events in tumour rejection.

To summarise our current ideas relating to the mechanism of specific tumour immunity, it can be said that several mechanisms may operate in vivo, without necessarily showing correlation with in vitro findings. In any event, T-lymphocytes are likely to form a major component of the immune response either operating directly as cytotoxic effectors or regu-lating the function and specificity of other cytolytic effector cells. Correlating in vitro find-ings with in vivo observations is not possible in man, although some evidence shows that specific antitumour immune responses occur in certain human tumours and that in the main these are mediated by T-lymphocytes.

Tumour heterogeneity and immunity

Of considerable importance in assessing the in vivo response to TATAs is the variability of cell types expressing tumour antigens present in the parent/primary tumour cell popula-tion. Tumour cells possessing offensive antigenic determinants, provoking specific host im-mune responses, may be the subject of immunological control, and diversity from this phenotype toward an immunologically inoffensive cell may allow these tumour cells to escape from the host immune defense mechanisms. The heterogeneity of the population present within the primary tumour has therefore been the subject of considerable attention, and studies have shown that tumour cells express heterogeneous characteristics [70,71] with respect to drug susceptibility [72], organ affinity [73], chromosome number [74], biochemical properties [75], and immunogenicity [76–78]. Cells residing within the primary neoplasm may express different metastatic potentials, and certain properties may be ascribed to cells displaying high metastatic ability. Thus, deletion or alteration of a TATA on cells within the primary neoplasm may favour successful tumour metastasis in an environment where they are not readily recognised as foreign by the host's immune system. Given this situation, a cell escaping immunological destruction may have overcome one of the major barriers preventing metastatic disease. Using a hamster tumour induced by *Herpesvirus hominis*, and variant cell lines established from metastatic foci of the original parent tumour, it was found that cell lines displaying increased metastatic potential have a reduced ability to stimulate a tumour rejection response (see chapter 11). This is not to say that TATAs are absent from these tumours, since with some sublines immunization with the related immunologically offensive, parent tumour line induces a state of transplant immunity to tumour challenge with the parent and its metastatic clones. It can be argued that the metastatic variants express sufficient TATAs to be recognised in an appropriately immunised host, but are incapable of stimulating a tumour rejection response (antigenic but not immunogenic). Several explanations can be suggested to account for these findings. First, qualitative or quantitative alterations in the expression of TATAs may fail to establish immunity. Second, altered expression of antigens may occur and provoke the development of suppressor mechanisms, thus altering the balance of host immune competence. Finally, the nature of TATA expression, or the release of nonspecific factors from the tumour, may influence the processing of TATAs by macrophages and subsequently antigen presentation to lymphocytes.

Suppression of tumour immunity

Experimentally, it has been shown that suppressor cells can be activated by tumour cells [79], and cells mediating suppression of the immune response have been isolated from within growing neoplasms [80]. In man, specific [81] and nonspecific [82] suppressor cells can be demonstrated, but whether these regulate the mechanism of tumour rejection has yet to be determined. Conceivably, however, subpopulations of tumour cells of high metastatic potential stimulate suppressor cell activity, thus contributing to the disease process.

Ting et al. [83] have recently shown that tumour cells and tumour cell extracts are capable of suppressing mixed lymphocyte reactivity of spleen cells toward tumour cells, thus preventing the generation of cytotoxic effector T-lymphocytes. This suppression was shown to act mainly at the induction phase of the cytotoxic response and was ineffective in preventing the killing activity of fully generated cytotoxic T-cells. This represents an important mechanism, possibly accounting for the lack of immunogenicity observed in many tumour systems. Frost et al. [84] have recently described an assay for suppressor T-lymphocytes active in down-regulating the generation of cytotoxic responses in vitro against a metastatic tumour line. Tumour-bearer spleen cells were shown to prevent secondary stimulation of immune lymph node cells upon incubation with mitomycin C–treated tumour cells, which would normally allow the generation of functionally active effector lymphocytes. In this model, suppressor T-lymphocytes acted by impairing the precursor, rather than the mature cytotoxic cells. Interestingly, a variant tumour derived from the parent line, which was shown to be highly immunogenic, failed to generate a suppressor cell response. Studies of this nature may give some clue as to the in vivo requirements for the generation of immunoregulatory cell types and of cells possessing the ability to cause tumour rejection.

The nature of suppressor cells operative against cytolytic T-cells is variable depending on the model. In some tumour systems, suppression may be attributed to macrophage activity [85–87] or alternatively, to thymic-derived T-lymphocytes [87–90]. Deutsch et al. [91] have recently reported that suppressor cells can belong to the null cell population, inferring differences between the model systems used and depicting the heterogeneity of suppressor cell types that may be operative.

It has been shown that suppression of cellular proliferation in response to stimulation by tumour-associated antigens can occur following transfer of spleen cells from mice bearing large chemically induced sarcomas [92]. In these studies suppression was mediated by lymphocytes expressing Qa^+ $Thy-1^+$ surface markers. The tumour-bearer host may therefore be influenced by the antigenic load imposed, and antigen released in a soluble form may contribute to the induction of suppressor cells. In some models antigens solubilised by detergent are capable of inducing suppressor cells effective in enhancing the growth of tumours in vivo [93]. The mechanism of operation may require the specific induction of suppressor cells that are capable of mediating their effect against a tumour immune response. Importantly, cells other than lymphocytes are capable of mediating suppression of T-lymphocyte function, and it has been proposed [94,95] that antigen-specific events may lead to the induction of cells capable of mediating nonspecific suppression of a tumour immune response. Clearly, this element of the immune response in neoplasia adds to the complexity of the situation and emphasizes the need for careful analysis of the roles played by effector lymphocytes and their interactions with tumour-mediated suppressor mechanisms.

NONSPECIFIC ANTITUMOUR IMMUNE RESPONSE (NATURAL KILLER CELLS)

Cell-mediated cytotoxicity against tumour cells has generally been thought to be mediated by three types of effector cells [96]: (1) specifically immune mature T-cells, (2) cells mediating antibody-dependent cytotoxicity (ADCC), which bear surface receptors for the Fc portion of IgG molecules and thereby interact with IgG antibodies bound to target cells, and (3) activated macrophages or macrophages armed with specific antibodies. In addition, it was also believed that the in vivo resistance against progressive tumour growth was mainly due to mature T-cells, specifically immune against tumour-associated antigens. This concept of antitumour immune responses to both human and animal tumours was thought applicable until 1972, when it was apparent that the results obtained in vitro in microcytotoxicity tests did not fully justify the conclusion that the antitumour response was of a specific nature [97–100]. The reactivity observed using lymphocytes from normal individuals in assays to detect specific cell-mediated cytotoxicity, and variability of the technical procedures used, led many workers to become sceptical of the published results. At this time also, early reports were appearing suggesting that mice, rats, and humans possessed effector cells capable of mediating natural killing against a variety of leukaemia or lymphoblastoid tissue culture cells [101–105]. It became clear that natural killing (NK) was a phenomenon common to many species, and at this point much attention was focused on the study of natural immune defense mechanisms as opposed to specific immune reactions [106–110]. In the subsequent 10 years up to the present, considerable advances have been made in the understanding of the phenomenon of natural killing, although many questions remain unanswered. It is therefore proper to consider the nature of the effector cells mediating natural cytotoxicity, their specificity, the mechanism of cytolysis, and in vivo relevance.

Identification and characterization of natural killer cells

The reactivity of NK-cells against foetal fibroblasts has been shown, and the morphology of the effector cell has been characterized as being Fc-receptor-positive, E-rosette-negative, displaying either diffuse or granular α-naphthyl-acetate esterase (ANAE) in the cytoplasm [111,112]. Typically, these cells were of large granular lymphocyte morphology and showed many of the characteristics associated with T-lymphocytes. The isolation of NK-effector cells can be achieved either by absorption-elution to NK-sensitive targets [112,113] or by use of discontinuous percoll-density gradients [114,115].

Detection of human NK-cells is largely based on the measurement of in vitro cytotoxic reactivity against certain susceptible target cell lines. Recently, evidence has been presented on the morphological association of human NK-cells with large granular lymphocytes (LGL) (figure 2–2), which show a high cytoplasmic-nuclear ratio and azurophilic granules in their cytoplasm [112,116]. In humans, LGL represent 2 to 6% of the total number of peripheral blood white cells [112,117] and can be enriched up to >90% purity by discontinuous percoll-density gradient centrifugation and subsequent depletion of high-affinity sheep erythrocyte rosette-forming cells present in the NK-cell-enriched low-density percoll fractions [117]. Furthermore, rats have been shown to possess morphologically similar LGL, which can be purified by similar discontinuous density gradient separation [114,118]. However, using morphological characterization and functional properties alone has given no definite answer to the controversy surrounding the lineage of NK-cells.

The production of a monoclonal IgM antibody (HNK–1, Leu–7) that identifies a discrete population of lymphoid cells in humans with NK-cell and K-cell activity has recently been reported [119]. Abo et al. [120] have summarised the characteristics of cells defined by HNK–1 as follows: (1) they are medium-sized lymphocytes possessing azurophilic granules in the cytoplasm; (2) virtually all NK-cell and K-cell function resides in this cell fraction; (3) more than 80% of these cells express Fc receptors for IgG; and (4) they exhibit unique patterns of postnatal expansion as a function of age and sex.

NK-cells and K-cells have also been shown to express two T-cell-associated antigens as defined by xenoantisera [121–123] inferring an association with T-cell lineage. In contrast, certain characteristics of NK-cells and K-cells have also been described that suggest they are of monocyte/macrophage lineage [124–126]. Two different monoclonal antibodies, OKM1 and Mac-1, have been shown to react with NK-cells and macrophages [127–130].

NK-cells have been distinguished from cytotoxic T-cells (Tc) by using a series of monoclonal antibodies; the majority of NK-cells and poly I–C-activated NK-cells are OKM1$^+$ and OKT3$^-$, OKT4$^-$, and OKT8$^-$, whereas Tc cells are OKT3$^+$ and OKT8$^+$ [128]. Abo et al. [120] showed that subpopulations of HNK-1$^+$ cells present in peripheral blood express antigens normally found on mature T-cells (e.g., T1, T3, T4, T8), but not antigens characteristic of immature T-cells (T6, T9). The majority (>60%) of HNK-1$^+$ cells also express a myeloid antigen (M1), whereas a minority (<25%) express HLA-DR antigens. In addition, HNK-1$^+$ cells were separated into HNK-1$^+$ T3$^-$ cells, which exhibit a high level of NK reactivity against K562 target cells and contain many cytoplasmic granules; HNK-1$^+$ T3$^+$ cells have low NK activity and a paucity of cytoplasmic granules. Furthermore, a relationship between T3 and M1 antigen expression and cytotoxicity was also observed. HNK-1$^+$ T3$^-$ M1$^+$ cells appear to be functionally mature in NK assays; this is consistent with other studies showing that treatment with the M1 antibody plus complement eliminates most of the NK-cell activity, whereas treatment with T3 antibody and complement does not [128,131]. Abo et al. [120] also noted that most of the HNK-1$^+$ cells in the bone marrow are of the HNK-1$^+$ T3$^+$ M1$^-$ phenotype, whereas the HNK-1$^+$ T3$^-$ M1$^+$

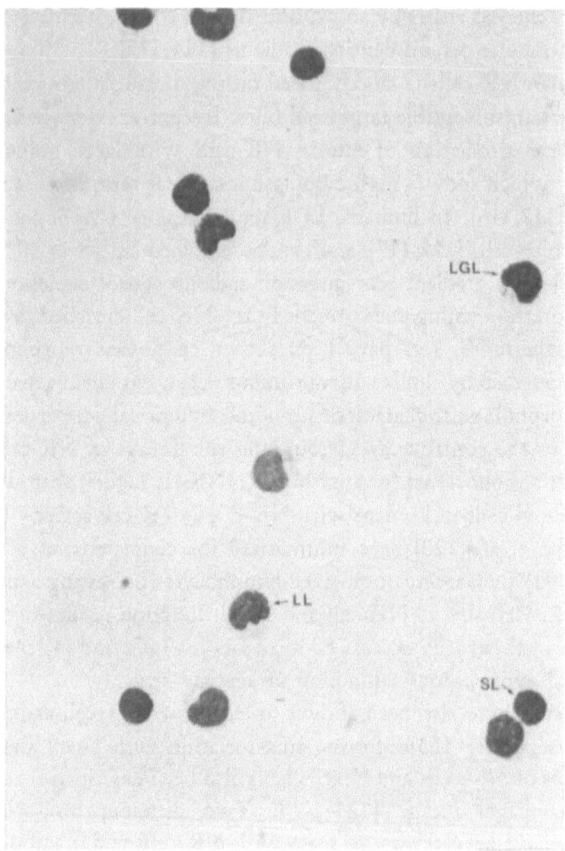

Figure 2-2. Morphology of percoll-separated human peripheral lymphoid cells in Giemsa-stained preparations. LGL = large granular lymphocyte. LL = large lymphocyte. SL = small lymphocyte.

phenotype is prevalent in the circulation; these authors proposed that immature HNK-1+ cells may express T-cell antigens before maturing to HNK-1+ T3-M1+ cells. Further studies by Abo and Balch [132] showed that HNK-1+ cells isolated from human peripheral blood exhibited virtually no response to either mitogens (PHA, con-A, and PWM) or allogenic cells, whereas the HNK-1- cells responded efficiently to these stimuli and acquired potent spontaneous killing activity against 12 different target cells. In addition, Abo et al. [133] showed that the frequency of cells bearing surface HNK-1 antigen was extremely low in the newborn (< 1.0%) and increased progressively through childhood and into adult life. This was correlated with an age-related increase in functional NK-cell and K-cell activities, males having a slightly higher proportion of HNK-1+ cells than females.

No conclusive evidence has been so far obtained demonstrating that LGLs belong to any known haemic lineage [134]. Comparative studies on the surface phenotype of mature and immature LGLs using monoclonal antibodies have shown that whereas the former express preferentially antigenic determinants of monocyte lineage, the latter are characterized by the presence of markers associated with T-suppressor/cytotoxic cells. Thus, the heterogeneity observed for the surface phenotype of LGL could be explained by changes occurring within this lineage during maturation [135]. However, evidence indicates that NK-cells, cultured for some considerable time in vitro, fail to develop either monocyte or T-cell activity, and such cells maintain their characteristic morphology and function; this would not be expected if one were dealing with precursor cells [130,136]. Because of the high degree of phenotypic overlap with T-cells and monocytes and because of the atypical expression of other markers, the possibility that NK-cells are of a third lineage should be considered a realistic alternative. The production of further NK-specific monoclonal antibodies may help in establishing more precisely their affinity to other lymphoid cells.

Specificity and mechanism of NK cytotoxicity

As with other cell-mediated cytotoxic systems, the molecular mechanisms by which target cell lysis is achieved through NK-effector cells remain unknown, and it is not clear whether different effector cell populations induce lysis by distinct or related mechanisms. Much information is available relating to the biochemical process required for lysis by cytotoxic T-lymphocytes (CTL) and has permitted the lytic event to be analysed in terms of definable phases [137–139]: (1) specific recognition and binding to cell targets, (2) the lethal hit step, during which the target cells become irreversibly programmed for lysis, and (3) the lytic step, which is independent of the presence of CTL. Although, it is believed that NK-cells show clear specificity in their activity, unlike T-cell mediated lysis, NK activity is not genetically restricted [140,141]. Initial studies with murine lymphomas suggested that NK cytolysis was directed against C-type virus-associated cell surface antigens [109,108,142,143]. Using ''cold target competition'' experiments [108], it was concluded that NK-cells recognised several antigenic specificities associated with C-type viruses. Also cell lines releasing exogenous, C-type viral antigens were shown to be good NK-cell targets [141]. In contrast, Becker and Klein [140] found no correlation between NK sensitivity and the presence on targets of type-specific or group-specific antigens of murine C-type viral proteins. It was shown that human cell lines superinfected with xenotropic mouse C-type viruses expressed surface MuLV antigens, but showed no difference in their sensitivity to NK activity compared to uninfected lines [144].

Natural cytotoxicity in rodents has been detected against a variety of tumour types, including lymphomas, fibrosarcomas, and carcinomas [108,109,141,145,146]. Transformed fibroblasts are also susceptible targets for natural killing [147]. Natural cell-mediated cytotoxicity (CMC) in humans also demonstrates a similar broad range of sensitive target cells [148], and studies in both humans and mice suggest that T-cell leukaemias often prove to be highly susceptible targets [149–151]. However, some nonhuman primate and chicken T-lymphoblastoid cell lines are only weakly susceptible to lysis by natural CMC [147]. Cross-reactivity between species has been observed by many investigators [152–154], demonstrating that mouse NK-effector cells can kill human target cell lines. The xenogeneic determinants were not C-type virus-determinants, and spontaneous CMC was not influenced by the source of bovine serum used [155]. It has also been shown that certain glycoproteins isolated from the surface of target cells bind selectively to the surface of NK-cells and specifically prevent subsequent recognition of the homologous intact target [156,

157]. In addition, Roder [158] suggested that NK-cells mature during ontogeny to higher avidity binding, whereas the decline in NK function during senescence can be attributed solely to a decrease in population size. In comparative studies of high (CBA) and low (A/Sn) NK reactive mouse strains, it was observed that NK-cells from low responders possessed the following properties: (1) the absolute NK frequency was decreased, (2) the relative adsorption of individual NK-cells was low, and (3) the relative avidity of NK-cells was identical to that in the high responder strains. It was concluded that the NK receptor to the target cells used may be of restricted heterogeneity, although no strong evidence favours extensive polyclonality in NK-cells. Other investigators have argued, from essentially the same premise, that there are several subsets of NK-cells, each of which is directed against a different "specificity" [159]. Interestingly, recent studies involving NK-cell clones also failed to reveal evidence for a clonal expression of specificity.

The discoveries that mouse NK-cells can be activated by interferon [160,161] and interferon-inducing agents [162,163] have increased the complexity of the process of NK-cell recognition and specificity. These activated NK-cells lyse target cells normally resistant to endogenous NK-cell-mediated lysis, including cells of various morphologies and cells from different species [164–167]. In fact, cells from nearly every continuous cell line and most normal tissues are sensitive to lysis by activated NK-cells. However, so far no evidence has been presented showing activated mouse NK-cells to bind to target cells more avidly than endogenous NK-cells, although it has been shown that activated NK-cells may be more adherent than endogenous cells to nylon and plastic surfaces [168,169]. Although it has been reported that endogenous NK-cells bind to the cell line L-929, which is resistant to endogenous NK-cell-mediated lysis, the cytotoxic effect of bound NK-cells is manifested only when the target cells are poisoned with metabolic inhibitors or when the effector cells are activated by interferon [170]. In studies conducted in our department, staphylococcal protein A was found to induce interferon and to augment NK activity; interferon present in the supernatants from effector cells cultured with protein A was characterized as γ-interferon. Using the single-cell cytotoxicity assay, protein A did not appear to increase the frequency of binding, since the percentages of binding cells of protein A treated and nontreated populations were similar (table 2–1). The frequency of killer cells among target-binding protein A treated or nontreated lymphocytes was determined by assessment of target death of 100 or more conjugates at each time point. The lytic binders were detected within 30 minutes, where the percentages of killers among binders were 29 and 13 for protein A treated and nontreated effectors, respectively. This clearly shows that augmentation of cytotoxicity is manifested by an increase in the kinetics of killing.

Recently, Hiserodt et al. [171] have summarised the cellular events operative during NK-mediated cytotoxicity: (1) the effector NK-cell recognises and binds to its target—binding is rapid, temperature-insensitive, and requires the divalent cation Mg^{++}; (2) the NK-cell undergoes a series of steps (sensitive to the effects of various pharmacologic agents) collectively known as activation. During this phase the NK-cell modifies the surface of the target cell such that the target becomes programmed to lyse. Activation is Ca^{++} dependent and occurs optimally at 37°C. Subsequent to these lymphocyte-dependent events, the

Table 2-1. Frequency of killer cells among target-binding cells in single-cell cytotoxicity assays

Exp. No.	Time in mins.	% Killer cells among binding cells		% binding cells	
		− Protein A	+ Protein A	− Protein A	+ Protein A
	30	13	29		
	90	19	40		
1				14	15
	180	19	57		
	240	26	54		
	30	10	32		
	90	17	35		
2				16	15
	180	19	35		
	240	28	39		

Note: Results from two independent experiments testing for the percentage of conjugated K562 cells lysed as a function of time.
− Protein A = Nontreated effector cells (control).
+ Protein A = Effector cells (5×10^6/ml) pretreated with 50 μg/ml of staphylococcal protein A for 18 hr.

NK-cell can detach from the target and cytolysis will proceed during the killer cell independent phase of the reaction (killer cell independent lysis).

More recently, Quan et al. [172] demonstrated that the initiation of postbinding cytolysis was Ca^{++} dependent and appeared to be blocked by various protease inhibitors. These events were inhibited by verapamil, lidocaine, cAMP, and EGTA (ethyleneguanyltetraacetic acid), and also by PGE_2 and 2-ME (2-mercaptoethanol), which is a reducing agent [171]. These authors found these inhibitors to block the Ca^{++}-dependent programming events without affecting the frequency of NK target-binding cells. The observation that Ca^{++} flux may initiate the early events of NK programming lends strong support to the stimulus-secretion model as the mechanism of cytolysis. Timonen et al. [117] demonstrated that NK-cells are LGL and contain a system of intracellular granules. Mobilization of such granules to the plasma membrane with subsequent release of their cytolytic content may be a requisite step for cytolysis during programming. In addition, the recent observation that $SrCl_2$ induction of LGL degranulation inhibits subsequent NK lytic activity without inhibition of target cell binding also supports such a process in NK cytolysis [173]. Other agents, such as monensin and colchicine, are known to block classic secretory processes and also inhibit NK cytolysis [174,175]. However, release of LGL cytoplasmic granules can account for only a portion of the complete lytic mechanism, since components present on the NK-cell plasma membrane also participate in the lytic event [171,176]. It is apparent that NK cytolysis occurs via a two-step process involving both membrane and cytoplasmic components. Furthermore, soluble cytotoxic factors, which may be derived from intracytoplasmic granules, have been shown to be effective in causing lysis of target cells in both human and murine systems [177–179].

Evidence supports the involvement of various biochemical pathways during the cytotoxic process. With phospholipid metabolism, two aspects have been associated with human NK activity [180]. Upon contact of human peripheral blood mononuclear cells

(PBMC) with an NK susceptible target cell, increased phospholipid methylation has been detected [180]. In contrast, no such increase in methylation was seen upon incubation of the effector cells with a resistant target cell. The widely used procedure for inhibition of phospholipid methylation, with deazo-adenosine (DZA) plus homocysteine, was found to inhibit NK activity [180]. There is also increasing evidence for a role of proteases as mediators of NK activity, especially in relation to human NK-cells. As described by Goldfarb et al. [181], purified preparations of LGL have been shown to have detectable protease activity, with the enzyme having the general features of a plasminogen activator. However, there is no indication whether such an enzyme is in fact involved in the lytic process. A more direct indication of the role of protease(s) in natural cytotoxicity has come from observations that inhibitors of proteases, particularly those with chymotryptic characteristics, strongly inhibit NK activity [182,183]. It is not clear whether these enzymes are themselves the lytic molecules, or whether they lead to activation of some other processes more directly associated with lysis.

Enhancement and regulation of natural killer cells

A variety of agents have been shown to augment natural killer cytotoxicity [160], and most of these are capable of augmenting NK-cell cytotoxicity through the induction of interferon both in vivo [161,184] and in vitro [185,186]. It is clear from these and subsequent studies that interferon is a major component in determining in vivo NK status, although interferon-independent enhancement of NK activity has also been reported [187]. There are now three discrete classes of interferon (IFN), namely, α (leukocyte IFN), β (fibroblast IFN), and γ ("immune" IFN), which are subdivided further on differences in molecular structure. All three types of IFN augment NK and antibody-dependent cellular cytotoxicity (ADCC) of peripheral blood mononuclear cells. Certain reagents also selectively stimulate production of a subtype of IFN; for example, *Staphylococcus enterotoxin A* and OKT3 monoclonal antibody stimulate γ-IFN from human PBMC [188]. Moreover, Lee et al. [189] have shown that one of several human leukocyte interferon subtypes A (LeIF-A), obtained in purified form from a gene cloned in *E.coli*, stimulated human NK-cell activity, whereas another human leukocyte interferon subtype D (LeIF-D) had no effect on NK-cell killing of K562 target cells. But using Daudi cells as targets, both LeIF-A and LeIF-D augmented NK-cell killing. Although the exact pathway by which NK-cell activation occurs is still unclear, both alterations of the cell surface and activation of steps in the lytic machinery have been described [190]. Djeu et al. [191] and Ortaldo et al. [192] have demonstrated that the effect of IFN is dependent on both de novo mRNA and protein synthesis during the actual killing process. More recently, Gustafsson et al. [193] have shown that interferon (IFN-α or -β as well as E.coli-produced IFN-α_2) induced the rapid formation of several proteins in human effector lymphocyte populations, and a good correlation was found between the ability of actinomycin D to inhibit the formation of new proteins and prevent the augmentation of natural killer activity.

Ortaldo et al. [194] have recently divided 10 species of human interferon into high- and low-level boosters of NK activity. Up to a 100-fold difference was noted in the ability of some species to enhance NK-cell cytotoxicity, and this may be important in respect to the use of IFN for clinical trials, since stimulation of lymphocyte reactivity may be important in mediating restriction of tumour development. The importance of recognising the NK phenotype of patients receiving interferon or other biological response modifiers as therapy must be considered. In this regard, Lotzova et al. [195] divided cancer and noncancer subjects into NK high, medium, and low reactive groups and showed that only the medium and low reactive groups responded to IFN, suggesting that high reactors had already reached maximum cytolytic activity. Carter [196] has recently outlined some important principles regarding assessing the influence of biological response modifiers in cancer patients. The question, as yet unanswered, is whether NK low reactors are more susceptible to cancer. If NK cells are proved to be important in tumour surveillance, then NK deficiency could result in an increased risk of malignant conditions. Another key issue is whether low NK activity in treated cancer patients could be indicative of residual or recurrent disease and be of prognostic value. At present the evidence is too scant to answer these questions clearly, although Lotzova et al. [195] have indicated that NK cytotoxicity declines several weeks prior to relapse in leukaemia patients.

The role played by IFN in regulating NK-cell, monocyte/macrophage, and T-cell responses may represent one of the most important control mechanisms of the immune defense system. Other factors that are involved and of importance include interleukin (IL) 1 and 2, prostaglandins, colony-stimulating factor, and lysozyme. Thus, one of the main consequences of IFN therapy would be to alter the balance of immune responses. Our understanding of the regulation of lymphocyte function is increasing, thus allowing a more precise evaluation of their in vivo influence.

The initiation of clinical trials with human leukocyte IFN has been based largely on the results obtained from animal studies, and the development of a system for the large-scale production of IFN from human leukocytes has proved possible [197,198]. In addition, the implication of an interferon inducer for cancer therapy stems from early results using viruses and synthetic interferon inducers [199–202]. In some patients with different types of malignant tumours, interferon has been found to exert an antitumour effect. These include multiple myeloma [203], malignant lymphoma [204], acute leukaemia [205], mammary carcinoma [203], and ovarian carcinoma [206]. The mechanisms behind these effects are not known. One possibility is a direct multiplication-inhibitory effect on the tumour cells [207], another being that IFN acts by augmenting possible antitumour activities of the immune system [208]. Since IFN has been shown to enhance natural killer activity [185], it has been suggested that enhanced NK activity is a mechanism by which IFN exerts its antitumour effect. However, Einhorn et al. [206] have shown that in patients with multiple myeloma, no correlation could be observed between the response of the tumours to IFN therapy and pretreatment levels of NK activity, IFN-induced enhancement of NK activity in vitro, or IFN-induced enhancement of NK activity in vivo. Whether elevated NK activity contributes to the therapeutic effects of IFN in other malignancies has yet to be established.

It was thought that interferon might be the sole positive signal for NK activity, with other augmenting agents mediating their effects by their ability to induce interferon. However, several augmenting agents or treatments appear to act independently of interferon. Antibodies specific for the major histocompatibility complex haplotype and other antigens associated with the surface of effector cells cause enhancement of NK activity against xenogeneic targets [209–211]. Lectins reactive with NK cells have been shown to augment NK activity, effects that appear to be interferon-independent, since inhibitors of protein synthesis do not interfere with augmentation [210]. More recently, Goldfarb and Herberman [212] have shown that retinoic acid, which generally inhibits interferon production [213], was able to augment both mouse and human NK activity. Treatment of mouse [214] and human [215] NK-cells with IL-2 has also been shown to augment NK activity; however, it has not yet been determined whether the IL-2 acts by stimulating the production of gamma interferon. Furthermore, Goldfarb et al. [181] have found that addition of low concentration of various enzymes (trypsin, chymotrypsin, or phospholipase A_2) during the NK assay leads to augmented cytotoxicity. Roder et al. [216] have also reported that stimulation of cyclic GMP levels in mouse NK-cells caused moderate elevations in NK activity. However, Herberman [187] has failed to confirm such observations with either mouse or human NK-cells.

Negative regulation of the NK system

Some biologic response modifiers have been shown to have an inhibitory effect on a variety of specific immune responses and to down-regulate NK-cell activity. Reversible inhibition of NK activity can be produced by a variety of agents that are not themselves directly toxic to the cells. There are numerous situations in which murine NK activity is depressed following injection of a number of immunomodulating agents—for example, hydrocortisone, carrageenan, silica, or glucan—that can substantially reduce NK activity [184,217–219]. The effect of prostaglandins (PG) on murine NK-cell activity was examined by Brunda et al. [220], who showed that the addition of PGE_1, PGE_2, PGA_1, or PGA_2 to the cytotoxicity assay resulted in a marked depression of NK activity, whereas addition of PGB_1, PGB_2, PGF_1, or PGF_2 resulted in little or no inhibition. Administration of inhibitors of prostaglandins (indomethacin and aspirin) to tumour-bearing mice can cause the complete or partial restoration of NK activity; this could be due to in vivo suppression of increased production of PG in these mice, thus reducing the regulatory effect of PG on the NK system. Droller et al. [221] have also reported the inhibitory effects of PGs on human NK activity in vitro. In addition, c-AMP-elevating agents such as PGE_1, theophylline, and histamine markedly suppress NK cytotoxic activity in a dose- and rate-dependent manner [222]. In contrast to this, dibutryl c-GMP, and the cGMP-inducing cholinergic agonist, carbamylcholine, causes a small but significant increase in NK cytolysis, whereas the frequency of target-binding cells is not affected. Thus, it would appear that the cAMP-cGMP ratio is important in determining the threshold for triggering NK-cells subsequent to target cell contact. Yanagihara and Adler [223] have shown that cyclosporin A (an antifungal agent) caused rapid inhibition of mouse NK activity both in vitro and in vivo; the inhibition, which was dose-dependent, did not require the presence of T-cells, B-cells or macrophages. This study also complements the recent finding of suppressed NK activity among cultures of human peripheral blood lymphocytes treated with cyclosporin A in vitro [224]. Although administration of cyclosporin A to mice did not totally inhibit splenic NK activity, the rate of inhibition was similar to results obtained in studies measuring levels of suppression of NK activity by PGs [220] and adriamycin [225]. In contrast to findings with mouse spleen cells, cyclosporin A added to human lymphocyte cultures during the four-hour ^{51}Cr-release assay had no effect on NK cytolytic activity; a 20-hour exposure of human lymphocytes to the agent was required to produce the effect. The reasons for these discrepancies are unclear [223,224].

More recently, Goldfarb and Herberman [212] have demonstrated that PMA (phorbol-12-myristate-13-acetate), the potent tumour promoter, inhibits both mouse and human NK activity. In these studies PMA consistently inhibited both spontaneous and IFN-augmented NK activity of mouse effector cells. In contrast, PMA had more variable effects on human effector cells, causing either of two patterns of inhibitory effects on NK activity: (1) both spontaneous and IFN-augmented NK reactivity were inhibited, (2) only IFN-boosted natural cytotoxicity was diminished. In addition, these authors have also observed the inhibition of spontaneous and IFN-enhanced NK activity by cholera toxin (an agent known to stimulate adenylyl cyclase activity) [226]. The depression by cholera toxin was quite profound, regardless of the sequence of addition of IFN or other stimulators to the effector cells. In contrast to cholera toxin, cholera toxin subunit A (which is responsible for adenylyl cyclase stimulation) or cholera toxin subunit B (which binds to the GM1 ganglioside) alone was shown not to inhibit NK activity. The cholera toxin inhibitory effect on NK activity has also been confirmed by Fuse et al. [227] and in our own laboratory [Ali and Rees, unpublished results].

Sulica et al. [228] have presented evidence for a new mechanism for negative regulation of human NK activity, by cytophilic IgG in a monomeric form (mIgG). The expression of Fc receptors for mIgG has been reported recently by Merrill et al. [229]. As suggested by these authors, attachment of IgG to the specific binding sites on NK-cells provides a negative regulatory signal that seems to be mediated through elevation of cyclic AMP. Furthermore, the reversible inhibition of the cytolytic activity induced by the binding of mIgG to human PBMC was not blocked by indomethacin, an inhibitor of prostaglandin synthesis; this suggests that the inhibitory effect of cytophilic IgG is carried out by a novel mechanism for the negative regulation of NK activity, an effect distinct from the inhibitory effects of prostaglandins [220].

The existence of cells regulating NK activity has been suggested from a number of observations: NK activity of normal mouse spleen cells can be suppressed in vitro by spleen cells of mice exhibiting low cytotoxic activity as the result of age or by experimental treatment [217,218,230,231]. This regulatory mechanism of NK activity has been shown to be due to the presence of suppressor cells in the spleens of mice that were *Corynebacterium parvum*-injected, bone-marrow-tolerant, infant, carrogeenan-treated, or hydrocortisone-treated. In humans, nonspecific suppressor cells have been shown to explain the impaired mitogenic response of patients with advanced cancer [232–234], but little is known about suppressor cells of NK activity in humans [235]. However, macrophages from human neoplastic pleural effusions can inhibit NK activity, the expression of suppression requiring high suppressor-effector ratios (1:1) and overnight interaction with effector cells [236]. Studies by Bordignon et al. [237] have also shown that alveolar macrophages are potent inhibitors of the expression of NK function.

In a recent study [Griffith, Rees, Rogers, unpublished data] of patients with digestive tract carcinoma, natural killing against K562 target cells was assessed in blood taken from

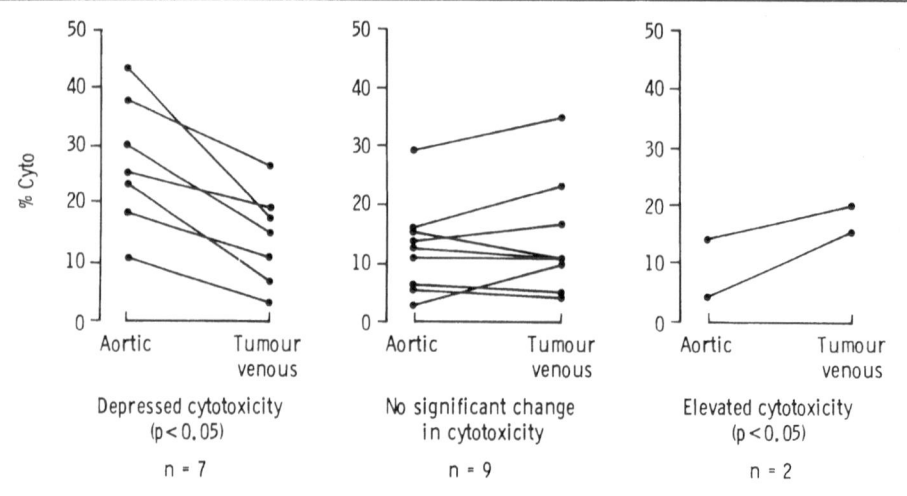

Figure 2-3. Comparison of natural cytotoxicity in blood supplying (aortic) and draining (tumour venous) human colon carcinomas (18 patients).

the peripheral venous blood, aortic supply, tumour-draining blood, and blood-draining adjacent normal colonic/stomach tissue. Approximately a third of patients showed depressed NK function in the blood draining the tumour, compared with other blood samples. In addition, plasma separated from the tumour venous blood was shown to be capable of abrogating natural cytotoxicity in vitro, thus inferring that tumour or host cell products can modulate NK function (figure 2-3). Further studies are in progress to determine the exact mechanism of this effect and whether other limbs of the immune response are influenced in a similar way.

Influence of tumour burden on NK activity

Modification of NK status may be an important consequence of tumour development, and many studies have been initiated to assess the effect of tumour burden on spontaneous cytotoxicity. The relative importance of NK-cells in vivo is outlined later in the chapter, but several lines of evidence suggest that depressed NK-cell function may give rise to progressive tumour growth and metastatic disease. The influence of the tumour on NK-cell cytotoxicity has been studied in experimental and human systems. For example, a decrease in peripheral blood and splenic NK-cell activity has been shown in mice bearing tumours induced by Moloney sarcoma virus [108,238], although the natural cytotoxic (NC) cell activity of spleen cells from tumour-bearer mice remains functionally intact [239].

A substantial body of evidence now shows that cancer patients have depressed NK-cell activity, although the precise cause has not been fully established [240–243]. However not all patients, especially those in the early stages of the disease, show reduced NK function [243,244].

NK activity has been shown to be low or undetectable in 50% of patients with advanced disease [245], although in vitro treatment of peripheral blood lymphocytes (PBL) with interferon restored normal NK function in half the patients exhibiting low NK activity. Interferon induction from PBL also appeared to be normal in these studies. Similar results have been obtained in a group of patients with malignant lymphoma [243], of whom only a proportion exhibiting low NK levels responded upon exposure to human IFN. There was no apparent correlation between low spontaneous NK activity and the ability to respond to IFN treatment, and many patients with seemingly normal spontaneous killing activity failed to show augmentation of NK function upon IFN exposure. In other studies (Ali et al., in press), reduced natural cytotoxicity was observed with splenic effector cells from eight patients with abdominal carcinoma compared with six noncancer patients undergoing major surgery for other disorders. These results are comparable with those obtained with peripheral venous blood of patients with digestive tract carcinoma or benign conditions (table 2–2).

Experiments in animal systems have shown that NK activity is apparent within the tumour, at least in the case of virally and chemically induced tumours, and are functionally active against NK-sensitive K562 target cells [238,246]. In contrast, other studies have generally shown that the human lymphoid cells infiltrating tumour sites have little or no NK activity [247–249]. Our own studies in human colonic carcinoma would support the view that functionally active NK-cells are present at the tumour site, but their cytolytic capacity is impaired.

Niitsuma et al. [250] have reported that tumour-infiltrating lymphocytes (TIL) from human pulmonary tumours have decreased proportions of T-cells that show decreased activity in T-cell function assays, including alloantigen-induced proliferation and generation of cytotoxic T-cells; low NK activity against K562 targets was also observed. In addition, these authors showed that removal of residual tumour cells did not result in increased NK activity, indicating that the low NK activity was not due to cold target competition by residual tumour cells. The defective NK activity of TIL, as suggested by Introna et al. [251], could in principle be accounted for by the presence either of suppressor cells or factors or by a low number of relevant effector cells (LGL). Preliminary evidence for the presence in situ of cells inhibiting NK activity was obtained in three peritoneal effusions from ovarian cancer [252], two breast carcinomas [253], and in pleural carcinomatous effusions [236]. The nature of the suppressor cells was determined to be of monocyte-macrophage origin. In contrast, Moore and Vose [254] found no evidence for suppressive activity in lymphoid cells from lung tumours; however, in other studies Vose et al. [249] have shown that adherent cells from peripheral blood of cancer patients, but not tumour-infiltrating lymphocytes, possessed suppressor function against NK-cells.

More recently, Golub et al. [255], using the single-cell assay, found equivalent numbers of target binding cells among TIL to those among PBMC from the same patients (with pulmonary tumours), and the proportion of those binding cells actually mediating cytolysis was similar among the two cell populations. These authors suggested that the low activity observed in ^{51}Cr-release assays was probably not due to a lack of NK-cells among the TIL but to a functional impairment of these cells, which was most likely a defect in the recycling ability of the NK effectors. In agreement with the above hypothesis are the results showing that TIL cannot be activated to further NK activity with interferon, an agent that promotes the recycling of NK cells [249,256]. TIL obtained from tumours injected with intralesional BCG two weeks prior to surgery exhibited a higher level of NK activity than did TIL from

Table 2-2. Natural cytotoxicity of peripheral venous blood (whole blood cytotoxicity) and spleen cells from patients with digestive tract carcinoma or benign conditions

Effector cells from:	Patients with:-	Mean % cytotoxicity* dilution of blood		
		1/2	1/4	1/8
Peripheral blood (whole blood)	Carcinoma (advanced disease) (n = 5)	7.4**	5.1**	3.4
	Carcinoma (Local disease) (n = 15)	12.6	8.3	4.4
	Benign conditions (n = 14)	17.9	9.7	4.6
		Mean % cytotoxicity* spleen cell:target cell ratio		
		100:1	50:1	25:1
Spleen (cells)	Carcinoma (4 local, 4 advanced disease)	23.0***	15.0***	10.6***
	Benign conditions (n = 6)	62.2	48.5	32.6

*K562 targets: 4-hr ^{51}Cr-release assay.
**p = <0.01.
***p = < 0.001 by students 't' test.

uninjected tumours [257]. BCG is an agent known to stimulate interferon production and augment NK activity in humans [202]. Furthermore, Golub et al. [255] were able to obtain TIL from BCG-injected and uninjected tumours from the same patients possessing multiple pulmonary metastases. They found that the NK activity of unstimulated TIL remained low while the NK activity of TIL from the adjacent BCG-injected tumour was high. They further suggested that the induction of augmented NK activity at one tumour site, even in combination with augmented systemic NK activity among PBMC and lymph node lymphocytes, does not necessarily ensure the delivery of active NK-cells into other tumour deposits.

Natural killer cells: Effect on in vivo tumour growth and metastasis

In humans the role of NK-cells in resistance to tumour growth, or other in vivo phenomena, is difficult to define, and most of the information accumulated in the field has come from studies in experimental animals. Resistance of F1 hybrid mice to some parental tumours correlates closely with high levels of NK-cell activity [109,142,258–260]. Tumour resistance in mice is strongest at the time of peak levels of NK activity and wanes concurrently with spontaneous CMC in older animals [142,259]. In addition, in vivo resistance to lymphoma and sarcoma growth [261,262] can be adoptively transferred in neutralisation assays using normal spleen cells, the active effector cells most likely being NK [110]. T-cell-deficient (congenitally athymic Nu^+/Nu^+) mice have the same or higher levels of NK-cells than do their thymic counterparts and display a high degree of in vivo resistance to the growth of certain tumours [110,263], inferring mature T-lymphocytes to be ineffective in mediating growth restriction.

Studies in the Beige mouse model and in mice rendered deficient in NK function by administration of cyclophosphamide, β-oestradiol, or antiserum specific for NK-cell determinants offer important systems for determining the in vivo role of NK cells. In addition, enhancement of NK activity by administration of immune adjuvants such as BCG and C. parvum serves to increase host resistance to tumour transplantation [264,265]. It would appear that agents that induce interferon, as well as interferon itself, promote in vivo resistance to tumour growth [259,266]. The Beige (Bg) mutation in C57BL mice had been shown to be a particularly relevant system for studying the role of NK-cells [267]. Comparison of the growth of leukaemic cells in C57BL Bg/Bg homologous and +/Bg heterozygous littermates revealed increased growth ability in Bg/Bg compared with +/Bg animals. 125-IUdR-labeled leukaemia cells were also eliminated at a faster rate in +/Bg mice. Since Bg/Bg mice show a considerable impairment of NK function, these results suggest a central role for NK-effector cells in vivo.

Other model systems have been utilised to assess the functional significance of NK cells. Recently, convincing evidence has been documented that in vivo treatment of mice with anti-NK serum reduced splenic NK activity toward YAC-1 target in vitro, with a concomitant reduction in the ability of intact mice to eliminate 125-IUdR-labeled lymphoma cells in vivo [268], thus providing direct evidence for a role for NK-cells in the elimination of circulating tumour cells in vivo. Although the growing weight of evidence is strongly in favour of NK-cell participation in natural resistance, the correlations between tumour survival and host levels of NK activity, or tumour sensitivity to NK-cells, are not totally consistent with this hypothesis [267], suggesting that natural resistance may be a heterogeneous phenomenon. A number of other natural effector mechanisms, including natural antibody [269,270] and macrophages [271], have been proposed as antitumour mechanisms that may contribute to tumour resistance.

The process of metastasis is a multistep phenomenon involving dissemination from the primary tumour, passage via the blood and/or lymphatics to target organs, traversion of the endothelial lining of blood vessels, and establishment of progressively developing tumour foci. Not all transformed cells are capable of spontaneous metastasis, which is the outcome of interplay between intrinsic cell properties and host factors influencing cell survival and growth. Cloned cell lines from lung foci [272] possess an increased metastatic ability compared with the parent tumour cells. Using a hamster tumour model, these cells proved to be less susceptible to lysis by hamster NK-cells [273,274], while cells from the parent line were shown to be as susceptible to NK-cell lysis as K562 targets. Interestingly, a recent study demonstrated the possible relevance of a tumour cell factor in depressing host natural resistance [275]. Cell lines producing "resistance depressing factor" proved to be the most highly metastatic. It must be realised that surviving the natural resistance mechanism of the host may not account fully for the metastatic behaviour of all cancer cells, but this process may be a necessary prerequisite for tumour cells to form metastases. The multifactorial nature of the metastatic process must therefore be appreciated to assess, in perspective, the merits of NK-cells in preventing tumour spread.

It is relevant to consider whether benefit could be gained by modulation of natural cytotoxicity, as part of a treatment programme for malignant disease, and whether biological response modifiers such as interferon may prove important for future therapy. In studies using nude (Nu+/Nu+) mice, tumour metastasis is rarely seen unless newborn or immunosuppressed adult mice are used, in which the NK activity is low [276,277]. An inverse correlation has been reported between NK status and metastases [278–280], and boosting NK activity with IFN results in a decrease in tumour metastases [278]. Convincing evidence suggesting the NK-cell as an effector cell capable of acting to prevent metastases has been shown in studies using murine tumour models. Anti-Asialo-GM1 antiserum, reactive toward murine NK-cells, selectively inhibits the cytotoxic activity of NK-cells [281], producing accelerated tumour growth [282] and metastases in vivo [283]. Recently, it has been shown that NK-deficient rats are susceptible to tumour metastases but can be rendered resistant to metastases by selective transfer of LGL [Reynolds and Herbermann, personal communication]. This work provides, perhaps, the most direct evidence suggesting a role in vivo for NK-cells.

LYMPHOCYTE GROWTH IN CULTURE

It is becoming increasingly apparent that the control of the immune response is governed by the complex interaction between different cell types and the products they release. Certain molecules, for example, interleukin 1 (IL-1) and interleukin 2 (IL-2), have been studied in great detail and have proved of considerable value in furthering the technological advances in immunology. The discovery of IL-2 (T-cell growth factor) has allowed workers to establish the continual expansion of normal and neoplastic T-cells in culture. IL-2 is released from subsets of mature T-lymphocytes following lectin/antigen reaction and acts on other antigen-reactive T-lymphocytes possessing receptors for IL-2. IL-1 (lymphocyte activating factor or LAF) plays a crucial role in the production of IL-2. This factor is a macrophage-derived product capable of promoting thymocyte proliferation and enhancing lectin-initiated proliferation of T-lymphocytes [284,285]. Although IL-1 has been shown to affect and enhance the production of IL-2 from antigen reactive cells, it is not obligatory for IL-2 release.

Certain important functions can be ascribed to IL-2, namely, (1) stimulation of long-term proliferation of antigen-specific T-lymphocytes, (2) enhancement of thymocyte mitogenesis, and (3) induction of cytotoxic T-lymphocyte reactivity and plaque-forming cells in cultures of lymphocytes taken from the spleens of congenitally athymic (Nu^+/Nu^+) nude mice [286–289]. In the absence of IL-2, lymphocytes become arrested in the G1-phase of the cell cycle; however, continued growth and entry into the S-phase can be achieved by further addition of IL-2 [290]. Hence, the discovery of IL-2 and its application to the study of lymphocyte function is of prime significance, allowing investigators to study the expansion of polyclonal-activated or antigen-specific T-lymphocytes in culture under defined laboratory conditions and to derive lymphocyte clones from single-cell progeny, many of which have been shown to retain their antigen-specific reactivity. Recent evidence would suggest that several effector functions can be studied in vitro using lymphocytes driven by IL-2, and interesting observations have been made that are of significance in studying the antitumour lymphocyte response against neoplastic disease.

There would appear to be three main sources of IL-2. First, lymphocytes obtained from peripheral blood or lymphoid organs such as the spleen or tonsils can be stimulated in vitro with mitogen and the supernatant harvested 72 hours following culture; production may also be enhanced by pooling lymphocytes from several donors, thus initiating mixed lymphocyte reactions (MLR) in addition to mitogen response. IL-1, produced by macrophages, acts as a differentiation signal together with antigen or mitogen and leads to the subsequent activation of resting T-lymphocytes, driving them into an activated state [291,292]. Activated T-lymphocytes subsequently produce IL-2 [292,293], which supports the continuous growth of factor-dependent antigen-stimulated cytotoxic T-lymphocytes (CTL) [294,295], as well as other varieties of T-lymphocyte subsets including suppressor cells [296]. Alvarez et al. [297] have described the optimum conditions for the production of IL-2 by mitogen activation. Bonnard et al. [298] provided evidence that individuals can be either high or low producers of IL-2 and that the presence of adherent monocytes was suppressive to IL-2 production. Enhanced IL-2 release from con-A stimulated T-cells could be achieved by the addition of phorbol myristate acetate, causing a 5- to 20-fold increase in production levels.

A second major source of IL-2 is from in vitro cultured T-cell lines following stimulation with the mitogens con-A or PHA [299]. A third source of IL-2 comes from cell lines that spontaneously release the factor without the requirement for mitogen stimulation. Recently, Rabin et al. [300] have reported the spontaneous release of IL-2 from a T-cell line of gibbon origin (a lymphosarcoma, designated MLA144). This offers a distinct advantage over the lectin-produced IL-2, where it may be difficult to achieve the complete removal of mitogen. Figure 2–4 illustrates the influence of the IL-2 on polyclonal-activated human

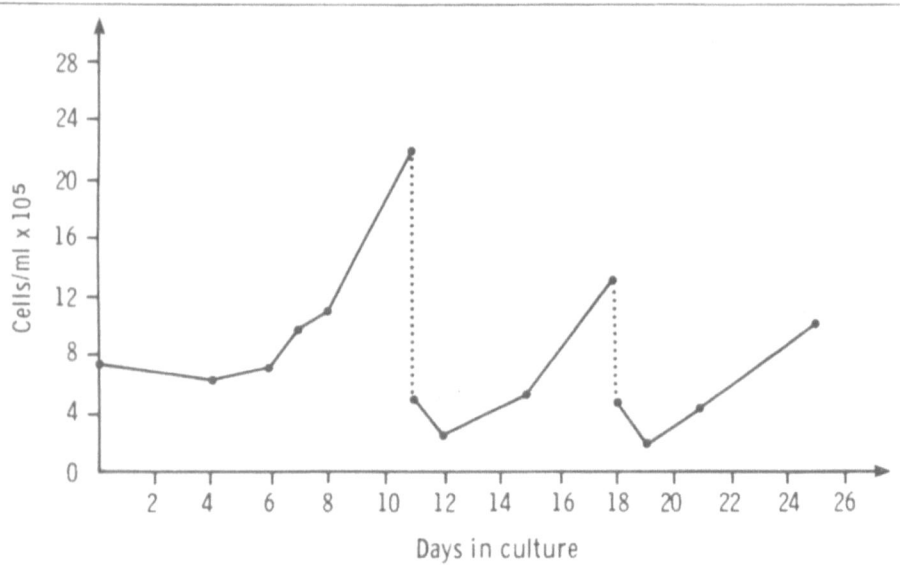

Figure 2–4. In vitro growth (expansion) of PHA-stimulated human T-lymphocytes in medium supplemented with interluekin 2. Cultures split to 5×10^5 cells per ml on days 11 and 18.

T-lymphocytes. Culture supernatant derived from MLA144 cell cultures appears to be a rich source of IL-2, and its production is a stable characteristic of this cell line.

Recently, Meuer et al. [301] provided some evidence for the selective production of IL-2 by T-lymphocyte subsets. It has been reported that whereas lymphocytes expressing the T4 (helper/inducer) cell marker as well as the subpopulation expressing the T8 (suppressor/cyto-toxic) cell surface marker were both capable of producing IL-2 following mitogen activation, only cells expressing the T4 surface component produced IL-2 on allogeneic stimulation. It was suggested that although both major subsets of T-lymphocytes were capable of producing IL-2, the expression of receptor sites leading to molecular interactions may differ between the subsets, and thus the triggering necessary for IL-2 production may vary.

Although it is possible to derive antigen-specific T-lymphocyte clones under the influ-ence of IL-2, other cell types mediating nonspecific reactivity appear also to possess recep-tors for IL-2 and to grow continuously in culture. Using mouse or human lymphocytes, several workers have reported the IL-2-dependent expansion of cells mediating natural killing; these effector cells may be related to NK-cells, although they possess some distinct charac-teristics. Kedar et al. [302] were successful in culturing mouse spleen cells prepared from normal and tumour-bearer mice in crude and lectin-depleted IL-2, and derived clones either by limiting dilution experiments or growth in soft agar. The lines established appeared to possess a wide degree of nonspecific cytolytic activity toward mouse, rat, and human cell targets, and of the clones analysed for surface marker profile all appeared to be positive for Thy-1.2 (T-cell marker), T200, and Asialo-GM1 (marker for NK-cells); some were also positive for the Lyt-2 antigen (cytotoxic/suppressor T-cell marker). It was not firmly established whether these clones were of characteristic NK-cell morphology, but they did appear to possess certain properties ascribed to NK-cells, such as activation following treatment with exogenous interferon. Whether these cells represent activated T-lymphocytes or cells closely aligned with NK lineage is not yet clear.

Other workers have also reported NK-like killing from clones derived by growth of lymphocytes in IL-2 [303,304]. Hercend et al. [305], by a process of negative selection of NK-cells, depleting monocytes, B-lymphocytes, and T-lymphocytes, were able to demonstrate IL-2-dependent proliferation of the remaining cell population. The cells exhibiting natural cytotoxicity proved difficult to maintain in long-term culture, although these authors reported in detail the marker profile and characteristics of a long-term clone designated JTI. Krensky et al. [306] generated NK-like cell lines that were negative for the T3 (T-cell) marker, but expressed receptors for sheep red blood cells (SRBC). These cell lines, when repeatedly stimulated with Daudi cells, could be maintained for a considerable time in culture. It is becoming clear that the surface marker profile of cells cultured in vitro under the infuence of IL-2 may be somewhat bizarre, and expression of cell surface marker determinants may not be relied upon to give an accurate classification of the cell type involved. In a recent study by Timonen et al. [307] cultures of large granular lymphocytes (LGL) and T-cells could be readily established and showed variable specificity of natural killing. LGL-enriched and T-cell-enriched subpopulations underwent prolific growth in PHA-conditioned medium; although LGL cultures could be easily initiated in lectin-free IL-2, seven to ten days following initiation of culture, they were shown to express surface markers characteristic of T-cells. Indeed, much work is required to establish more precisely the characteristics of cells grown in IL-2 and to differentiate between the specificity of killing of NK, LGL-like cells, nonspecifically activated T-lymphocytes, and lymphocytes possessing antigen-specific reactivity.

Clearly, T-cell growth in vitro presents important implications for the future developments in tumour immunology, and it is important to address the following questions. First, is it possible to generate in vitro specifically reactive T-lymphocytes that mediate tumour cell destruction, and that have in vivo relevance both in terms of abating primary tumour growth and/or preventing tumour dissemination and metastases? Second, are lymphocytes driven in vitro under the influence of IL-2, and mediating either specific reactivity toward a tumour antigen or nonspecific natural killing, capable of conveying tumour cell destruction in vivo, thus proving to be of therapeutic significance?

To date relatively few reports concern the specific or nonspecific antitumour reactivity of cultured lymphocytes in vivo. In a recent study by Mule et al. [308], tumour-infiltrating lymphocytes were separated by cell sorting, and Thy-1 positive cells cultured in IL-2. Distinct differences were apparent between T-lymphocytes cultured from small tumours and those cultured from larger tumour masses. In the former, cultured lymphocytes were capable of specifically inhibiting the growth of tumour cells when adoptively transferred into normal mice, and expressed the cell surface markers Lyt-1^+2^+. Lymphocytes derived from larger tumours, and cultured in IL-2, were shown to be phenotypically Lyt-1^-2^+ and to enhance the growth of tumours in adoptive transfer in admixture with tumour cells. This study would suggest a distinct shift in cell populations present within a tumour or, alternatively, an altered responsiveness of different cell populations in vivo to IL-2. The in vivo reactivity of IL-2-driven T-lymphocytes may not always correlate with their in vitro cytotoxic potential, suggesting that other factors may be required for the full expression of immunity in vivo.

In a recent study, peripheral blood lymphocytes from melanoma patients were expanded in partially purified supernatants containing IL-2, and this resulted in the generation of cytotoxic cells possessing activity against autologous melanoma targets and nonmelanoma cells lines [309]. The study inferred that melanoma-reactive lymphocytes could be induced into culture in the presence of IL-2 alone without the requirement of tumour cell stimulation. Apparently, however, under the experimental conditions of these tests, lymphocytes with nonspecific reactivity as opposed to antigen-specific lymphocytes were generated and the possibility cannot be ignored that polyclonal activation of killer T-lymphocytes was initiated due to the presence of small amounts of residual PHA in the conditioned media. Further work is required to establish the specificity of reactivity and the therapeutic potential of lymphocytes derived from individual patients. Results pertinent to this approach to human therapy come from studies by Vanky et al. [310]. These authors showed that peripheral blood lymphocytes obtained from human cancer patients, when cultured in the presence of autologous tumour cells or incubated in mixed lymphocyte culture, were able to generate lymphocytes with different spectrums of killing activity. Whereas MLC-reactive lymphocytes gave a broad spectrum of activity, causing lysis of numerous target cells, culture of lymphocytes with autologous tumour cells generated populations of lymphocytes specifically reactive against the stimulating cell type; this killing pattern was maintained when cells were grown and expanded in IL-2. The results indicated that nonspecifically activated (MLC) lymphocytes lysed third-party target cells due to recognition of alloantigens, and not cross-reactive tumour associated antigens, and that these cells were distinct from the autologous reactive lymphocytes. Further studies in other systems will help establish the significance of cultured lymphocytes and their therapeutic value.

REFERENCES

1. Hewitt HB. Animal tumour models and their relevance to human tumour immunology. J Biol Resp Modif 1: 107–119, 1982.
2. Vose BM, Vanky F, Klein E. Lymphocyte cytotoxicity against autologous tumour biopsy cells in humans. Int J Cancer 20: 512–519, 1977.
3. Vose BM, Vanky F, Fopp M, Klein E. Restricted autologous lymphocytotoxicity in lung neoplasia. Brit J Cancer 38: 375–387, 1978.
4. Vanky F, Vose BM, Fopp M, Klein E. Human tumour lymphocyte interaction in vitro. VI. Specificity of primary and secondary autologous lymphocyte mediated cytotoxicity. J Nat Cancer Inst 62: 1407–1413, 1979.
5. Vose, BM. Specific T-cell-mediated killing of autologous lung tumour cells. Cell Immunol 55: 12–19, 1980.
6. Vose BM, Vanky F, Fopp M, Klein E. In vitro generation of secondary cytotoxic response against autologous human tumour biopsy cells. Int J Cancer 21: 588–593, 1978.
7. Vanky F, Vose BM, Fopp M, Klein E., Stjernsward J. Human tumour-lymphocyte interaction in vitro. IV. Comparison of the results with autologous tumour stimulation (ATS) and lymphocytotoxicity (ALC). In Flad HD, Erfarth Ch, Betzler M (eds.), Immunodiagnosis and immunotherapy of malignant tumours—Relevance to surgery? Berlin: Springer Verlag, 1979, pp. 143–152.
8. Vanky F, Klein E. Specificity of auto-tumour cytotoxicity exerted by fresh, activated and propagated human T-lymphocytes. Int J Cancer 29: 547–553, 1982.
9. Vose BM, Bonnard GD. Specific cytotoxicity against autologous tumour and proliferative responses of human lymphocytes grown in interleukin 2. Int J Cancer 29: 33–39, 1982.
10. Troye M, Vilien M, Pape GR, Perlmann P. Cytotoxicity in vitro of blood lymphocytes from bladder cancer patients and controls to allogeneic or autologous tumour cells derived from established cell lines or short-term cultures. Int J. Cancer 25: 33–43, 1980.

11. Law LW. Changes in tumour-specific antigen expression during passage in vitro and in vivo of newly derived methylcholanthrene induced sarcomas of BALB/c mice. Int J Cancer 25: 251–259, 1980.
12. Forbes JT, Yoshinobu N, Smith RT. Tumour-specific immunity to chemically induced tumours. J Exp Med 141: 1187–1200, 1975.
13. Foley RT. Antigen properties of methylcholanthrene-induced tumours in mice of the strain of origin. Cancer Res 13: 835–837, 1957.
14. Prehn RT, Maine JM. Immunity to methylcholanthrene-induced sarcoma. J Nat Cancer Inst 18: 769–778, 1957.
15. Bosombrio MA. Search for common antigenicites among 25 sarcomas induced by methylcholanthrene. Cancer Res 30: 2458–2452, 1970.
16. Pellis NR, Kahan BD. Tumour specific immunity induced with soluble materials: Restricted range of antigen dose and of challenge tumour load for immunoprotection. J Immunol 115: 1717–1722, 1975.
17. McCollester DL. Isolation of Meth-A cell surface membranes possessing tumour-specific transplantation antigen activity. Cancer Res 30: 2872–2880, 1970.
18. Bubenik J, Indrova M, Nemeckova S, Malkovsky M, Von Broen B, Palek V, Anderlikova J. Solubilised tumour-associated antigens of methylcholanthrene-induced mouse sarcomas. Comparative studies by in vitro sensitisation of lymph node cells, macrophage electrophoretic mobility assay and transplantation tests. Int J Cancer 21: 348–355, 1978.
19. Yamagishi H, Pellis NR, Kahan BG. Tumour protective and facilitating antigens from 3MKCL-solubilised tumour extracts. J Surg Res 4: 392–398, 1979.
20. Roger MJ, Law LW. Some immunogenic and biochemical properties of tumour-associated transplantation antigens (TATA) obtained in soluble form or solubilized from 2-methylcholanthrene-induced sarcomas Meth-A and Cl-4. Int J Cancer 27: 789–796, 1981.
21. Leffell MS, Coggin JH. Common transplantation antigens of methylcholanthrene-induced murine sarcomas detected by three assays of tumour rejection. Cancer Res 37: 4112–4119, 1977.
22. Economou GC, Takeidu N, Boone CW. Common tumour rejection antigens in methylcholanthrene-induced squamous cell carcinomas of mice detected by tumour protection and radioisotopic foot-pad assay. Cancer Res 37: 37–41, 1977.
23. Rees RC, Price MR, Baldwin RW. Oncodevelopment antigen expression in chemical carcinogenesis. Methods Cancer Res 18: 99–133, 1979.
24. Coggin JH, Ambrose KR. Embryonic and foetal determinants on viral and chemically-induced tumours. Methods Cancer Res 18: 371–389, 1979.
25. Parmiani G, Invernizzi G. Alien histocompatibility determinants on the cell surface of sarcomas induced by methylcholanthrene. I. in vivo studies. Int J Cancer 16: 756–767, 1975.
26. Invernizzi G, Parmiani G. Tumour-associated transplantation antigens of chemically-induced sarcomata cross-reacting with allogeneic histocompatibility antigens. Nature 254: 713–714, 1975.
27. Meschini A, Invernizzi G, Parmiani G. Expression of alien H-2 specificity on a chemically-induced BALB/c fibrosarcoma. Int J Cancer 20: 271–283, 1977.
28. Fujimoto S, Chen CH, Sabbadini E, Sehon AH. Association of tumour and histocompatibility antigens in sera of lymphoma bearing mice. J Immunol 111: 1093–1100, 1973.
29. Chang S, Nowinski RC, Nowinski K, Irie RF. Immunological studies on a mouse mammary tumour. A further characterisation of a mammary tumour antigen and its distribution in lymphatic cells of allogeneic mice. Int J Cancer 9: 409–416, 1972.
30. Kubota K, Takizawa K, Yamamoto T. Detection of H-2 antigens or H-2-like molecules on LFM3A2 hybrid cells by immunoprecipitation with specific anti-TASA serum. Jap J Exp Med 46: 325–328, 1976.
31. Klein G, Klein E. Are methylcholanthrene-induced sarcoma-associated rejection-induced (TSTA) antigens modified forms of H-2 or linked determinants? Int J Cancer 15: 879–887, 1975.
32. Klein G. Tumour associated antigens in H-2 hemizygous isoantigenic variants of a somatic cell-hybrid derived from the fusion of a 3-methylcholanthrene induced sarcoma and a mammary carcinoma. J Nat Cancer Inst 58: 383–386, 1977.
33. Lennox E, Sikora K, Koch G. The tumour specific-transplantation antigens of methylcholanthrene-induced murine sarcomas. In Ferrone S, Herberman RB, Reisfeld RA, Gorini L (eds.), Current trends in tumour immunology. New York: Garland Publishing, 1979.
34. Bowen JG, Baldwin RW. Tumour antigens and alloantigens. I. Relation of a rat tumour-specific antigen with normal alloantigens of the host strain. Int J Cancer 23: 826–832, 1979.
35. Bowen JG, Baldwin RW. Tumour antigens and alloantigens. II. Lack of association of rat hepatoma-D 23-specific antigen with Beta-2 microglobulin. Int J Cancer 23: 833–839, 1979.
36. Rosenberg SA (ed.). Serological analysis of human cancer antigens. New York: Academic Press, 1980.
37. Shimano T, Loor RM, Papsidero LD, Kuriyama M, Vincent RG, Nemoto T, Holyoke ED, et al. Isolation, characterization and clinical evaluation of pancreas cancer-associated antigen. Cancer 47: 1602–1613, 1981.

38. Banwo O, Versey J, Hobbs JR. New oncofetal antigen for human pancreas. Lancet 1: 643–645, 1974.
39. Natali PG, Imai K, Wilson BS, Bigotti A, Cavaliere R, Pellegrino MA, Ferrone S. Structural properties and tissue distribution of the antigen recognized by the monoclonal antibody 653.405 to human melanoma cells. J Natl Cancer Inst 67: 591–601, 1981.
40. Rees RC, Potter CW. In vivo studies of cell-mediated and humoral immune response to adenovirus 12-induced tumour cells. Arch ges Virusforsch 41: 116–126, 1973.
41. Dubois G, Appella E, Law LW, Deleo AB, Old LJ. Immunogenic properties of soluble cytosol fractions of Meth-A sarcoma cells. Cancer Res 40: 4204–4208, 1980.
42. Howell SB, Dean JH, Esber EC, Law LW. Cell interactions in adoptive immune rejection of a syngeneic tumour. Int J Cancer 14: 662–674, 1974.
43. Winn HJ. Immune mechanisms in homotransplantation. II. Quantitative assay of the immunologic activity of lymphoid cells stimulated by tumour homograft. J Immunol 86: 228–239, 1961.
44. Crumm ED. Lymphocytes that mediate systemic resistance to in vivo growth of carcinogenic/induced syngeneic tumour. Int J Cancer 26: 53–60, 1980.
45. Chauvenet PH, McArthur CP, Smith RT. Demonstration in vitro of cytotoxic T-cell with apparent specificity toward tumour-transplantation antigens on chemically induced tumours. J Immunol 123: 2575–2581, 1979.
46. Boon T, Van Snick J, Van Pel A, Uyttenhove C, Marchand M. Immunogenic variants obtained by mutagenesis of mouse mastocytoma P815. II. T-lymphocyte-mediated cytolysis. J Exp Med 152: 1184–1193, 1980.
47. Carbone G, Colombo MP, Sensim L, Cernuschi A, Parmiani G. In vitro detection of cell-mediated immunity to individual tumour-specific antigens of chemically induced BALB/c fibrosarcomas. Int J Cancer 31: 483–489, 1983.
48. Ting CC, Rodrigues D, Nordan R. Studies on the mechanism for the induction of in vivo tumour immunity. VI. Induction of specific and non-specific cell-mediated immunity in tumour bearing host and its correlation with transplantation tumour immunity. Cellular Immunol 66: 45–58, 1982.
49. Gooding LR, Edwards CB. H-2 antigen requirement in the in vitro induction of SV40-specific cytotoxic T-lymphocytes. J Immunol 124: 1258–1262, 1980.
50. Shimizu K, Shen FW. Role of different T-cell subsets in the rejection of syngeneic chemically-induced tumours. J Immunol 122: 1162–1165, 1979.
51. Kaufmann SHE, Simon MM, Hahan H. Specific Lyt-1,2,3 T-cells are involved in protection against Listeria monocytogenes and in delayed-type hypersensitivity to listerial antigens. J Exp Med 150: 1033–1038, 1979.
52. Wettstein PJ, Bailey DW, Mobraaten LE, Klein J, Frelinger JA. T-lymphocyte response to H-2 mutants: Cytotoxic effectors are Lyt-1$^+$2$^+$. Proc Natl Acad Sci 76: 3455–3459, 1979.
53. Prat M, DiRenzo MP, Comoglio PM. Characterisation of T-lymphocytes mediating in vivo protection against RSV-induced murine sarcomas. Int J Cancer 31: 757–764, 1983.
54. Robbins RA, Baldwin RW. Role of T-lymphocyte subsets in tumour rejection. Implications for developing biological response modifiers and monitoring tumour-host interactions during tumour development. J Biol Resp Mod 2: 101–109, 1983.
55. Baldwin RW. In vitro assays of cell-mediated immunity to human solid tumours: Problems of quantitation, specificity and interpretation. J Natl Cancer Inst 55: 745–748, 1975.
56. Herberman RB, Oldham RK. Problems associated with study of cell mediated immunity to human tumors by microcytotoxicity assays. J Natl Cancer Inst 55: 749–753, 1975.
57. Loveland BE, McKenzie IFC. Which T-cells cause graft rejection? Transplantation 33: 217–221, 1982.
58. Dallman MJ, Mason DW. Role of thymus derived and thymus independent cells in murine skin allograft rejection. Transplantation 33: 221–223, 1982.
59. Wang KC, Berczi I, Sehon AH. Effector and enhancing lymphoid cells in plasmacytoma-bearing mice. I. Methodological studies on the Winn assay. Int J Cancer 25: 487–492, 1980.
60. Bhan AK, Perry LL, Cantor H, McCluskey RT, Benacerraf B, Greene MI. The role of T-cell sets in the rejection of a methylcholanthrene induced sarcoma (S1509a) in syngeneic mice. Am J Pathol 102: 20–27, 1981.
61. Nelson M, Nelson DS, McKenzie IFC, Blanden RV. Thy and Ly markers on lymphocytes initiating tumour rejection. Cell Immunol 60: 34–42, 1981.
62. Loveland BE, McKenzie IFC. Cells mediating graft rejection in the mouse. IV. The Lyt-5,6 and 7 effector cell phenotype. Transplantation 33: 411–413, 1982.
63. Loveland BE, McKenzie IFC. Cells mediating graft rejection in the mouse. I. Lyt-1 cells mediate skin graft rejection. J Exp Med 153: 1044–1057, 1981.
64. Loveland BE, McKenzie IFC. Cells mediating graft rejection in the mouse. II. The Lyt phenotype of cells producing tumor allograft rejection. Transplantation 33: 174–180, 1982.

65. Ledbetter JA, Rouse RV, Micklem HS, Herzenberg LA. T-cell subsets defined by expression of Lyt-1,2,3 and Thy-1 antigens. Two parameter immunofluorescence and cytotoxicity analysis with monoclonal antibodies modifies current views. J Exp Med 152: 280–295, 1980.

66. Klein E, Klein G. Specificity of the homograft rejection in vivo, assessed by inoculation of artificially mixed compatible and incompatible tumor cells. Cell Immunol 5: 201–208, 1972.

67. Weissman IL. Tumor immunity in vivo: Evidence that immune destruction of tumor leaves "bystander" cells intact. J Natl Cancer Inst 51: 443–448, 1973.

68. Bast RC, Zbar B, Rapp HJ. Local antitumor activity of a primary and an anamnestic response to a syngeneic guinea pig hepatoma. J Natl Cancer Inst 55: 989–994, 1975.

69. Galli SJ, Bast RC, Bast BS, et al. Bystander suppression of tumor growth: Evidence that specific targets and bystanders are damaged by injury to a common microvasculature. J Immunol 129: 890–899, 1982.

70. Fidler IJ, Hart IR. The origin of metastatic heterogeneity in tumours. Europ J Cancer 17: 487–494, 1981.

71. Di-Renzo MF, Bretti S. Characterization of stable spontaneous metastatic variant lines of RSV-transformed mouse fibroblast. Int J Cancer 30: 751–757, 1982.

72. Trope C. Different sensitivity to cytostatic drugs of primary tumour and metastasis of the Lewis lung carcinoma. Neoplasma 22: 171–180, 1975.

73. Fidler IJ, Nicolson GL. Organ selectivity for implantation survival and growth of B16 melanoma variant tumour lines. J Natl Cancer Inst 57: 1199–1202, 1976.

74. Rabotti G. Ploidy of primary and metastatic human tumours. Nature 183: 1276–1277, 1959.

75. Chatterjee SK, Kim O. Fucosyl transferase activity in metastasizing and non-metastasizing rat mammary carcinomas. J Natl Cancer Inst 61: 151–162, 1978.

76. Schirrmacher V, Bosslet K, Shantz G, Glawer K, Hubsch D. Tumour metastases and cell mediated immunity in a model system in DBA/2 mice. IV. Antigenic differences between a metastasizing variant and the parental tumour line revealed by cytotoxic T-lymphocytes. Int J Cancer 23: 245–252, 1979.

77. Kerbel RS. Immunological studies of membrane mutants of a highly metastatic murine tumour. Am J Path 97: 609–622, 1979.

78. Marganski JL. Immunogenic variants obtained by mutagenesis of mouse mastocytoma P815. II. Occasional escape from host rejection due to antigen-loss secondary variants. Int J Cancer 31: 119–123, 1983.

79. Broder S, Mool L, Waldmann TA. Suppressor cells in neoplastic disease. J Natl Cancer Inst 61: 5–11, 1978.

80. Holden HT, Haskill JS, Kirchner H, et al. Two functionally distinct anti-tumour effector cells isolated from primary murine sarcoma virus-induced tumours. J Immunol 117: 440–446, 1976.

81. Yu A, Watts M, Jaffe N, Parkman R. Concomitant presence of tumour-specific cytotoxic and inhibitor lymphocytes in patients with osteogenic sarcoma. N Engl J Med 297: 121–127, 1977.

82. Goodwin JS, Messner RP, Bankurst AD, Peak GT, Saike JM, Williams RC. Prostaglandin producing suppressor cells in Hodgkin's disease. N Engl J Med 297: 963–968, 1977.

83. Ting CC, Rodrigues D, Ting RC, Wyvel N, Collins MJ. Suppression of T-cell mediated immunity by tumour cells: Immunogenicity versus immunosuppression and preliminary characterisation of the suppressor factors. Int J Cancer 24: 644–655, 1979.

84. Frost P, Prete P, Kerbel R. Abrogation of the in vitro generation of the cytotoxic T-cell response to a murine tumour: The role of suppressor cells. Int J Cancer 30: 211–217, 1982.

85. Pope BL, Whitney RB, Levy JG, Kilburn DG. Suppressor cells in the spleen of tumour-bearing mice: Enrichment by centrifugation on highpaque-ficoll and characterisation of the suppressor population. J Immunol 116: 1342–1346, 1976.

86. Veit BC, Feldman JD. Altered lymphocyte functions in rats bearing syngeneic Moloney sarcoma tumours. II. Suppressor cells. J Immunol 117: 655–660, 1976.

87. Yamagishi H, Pellis NR, Margalit B, Mokyr MB, Kahn BD. Specific and non-specific immunologic mechanisms of tumour growth facilitation. Cancer 45: 2929–2933, 1980.

88. Treves AS, Carnaud C, Trainin N, Feldman M, Cohen IR. Enhancing T-lymphocytes from tumour-bearing mice suppressed host resistance to a syngeneic tumour. New Look J Immunol 4: 722–727, 1974.

89. Fujimoto S, Greene MI, Sehon AH. Regulation of the immune response to tumour antigens. I. Immunosuppressor cells in tumour bearer hosts. J Immunol 116: 791–799, 1976.

90. Fujimoto S, Greene MI, Sehon MH. Regulation of the immune response to tumour antigens. II. The nature of immune-suppressor cells in tumour-bearing hosts. J Immunol 116: 800–806, 1976.

91. Deutsch O, Devens B, Naor D. Immune responses to weakly immunogenic murine leukaemia-virus induced tumours. VIII. Characterisation of suppressor cells. Isr J Med Sci 16: 538–544, 1980.

92. Mule JJ, Stanton TH, Helstrom I, Helstrom KE. Suppressor pathways in tumour immunity: A requirement for Qa-1$^+$ tumour-bearer spleen T-cells in suppression of the afferent immune response to tumour antigens. Int J Cancer 28: 353–359, 1981.

93. Mianami A, Mizushimi Y, Takeichi N, Hosokawa M, Kobayashi H. Dissociation of antitumour immune responses in rats immunised with soluble tumour associated antigens from methyl-cholanthrene-induced fibrosarcomas. Int J Cancer 23: 358–365, 1979.
94. Hellstrom KE, Hellstrom I. Cell mediated suppression of tumour immunity has a non-specific component. I. Evidence from transplantation tests. Int J Cancer 27: 487–485, 1981.
95. Hellstrom I, Hellstrom KE. Cell-mediated suppression of tumour immunity has a non-specific component. II. Evidence from cell culture experiments. Int J Cancer 27: 487–491, 1981.
96. Cerottini JC, Brunner KT. Cell-mediated cytotoxicity, allograft rejection, and tumour immunity. Adv Immunol 18: 67–132, 1974.
97. Hellstrom I, Hellstrom KE, Pierce GE, Yang JPS. Cellular and humoral immunity to different types of human neoplasms. Nature 220: 1352–1354, 1968.
98. Hellstrom I, Hellstrom KE, Sjogren HO. Demonstration of cell-mediated immunity to human neoplasms of various histological types. Int J Cancer 7: 1–16, 1971.
99. O'Toole C, Perlmann P, Unsgaard B, et al. Lymphocyte cytotoxicity in bladder cancer. No requirement for thymus-derived effector cells. Lancet 1: 1085–1088, 1973.
100. Herberman RB. Cell mediated immunity to tumour cells. Adv Cancer Res 19: 207–263, 1974.
101. Oldham RK, Siwarski D, McCoy JL, Plata EJ, Herberman RB. Evaluation of a cell-mediated cytotoxicity assay utilizing 125 iododeoxyuridine-labelled tissue culture target cells. Natl Cancer Inst Monogr 37: 49–58, 1973.
102. Takasugi M, Mickey MR, Terasaki PI, Reactivity of lymphocytes from normal persons on cultured tumour cells. Cancer Res 33: 2892–2902, 1973.
103. Herberman RB, Nunn ME, Lavrin DH, Asofsky R. Effect of antibody to theta antigen on cell-mediated immunity induced in syngeneic mice by murine sarcoma virus. J Natl Cancer Inst 51: 1509–1512, 1973.
104. Oldham RK, Herberman RB. Evaluation of cell-mediated cytotoxic reactivity against tumour associated antigens with 125I-iododeoxyuridine labelled target cells. J Immunol 111: 862–871, 1973.
105. Le Mevel BP, Wells SA Jr. A microassay for the quantitation of cytotoxic antitumour antibody: Use of 125-I-iododeoxyuridine as a tumour cell label. J Natl Cancer Inst 50: 803–806, 1973.
106. De Vries JE, Cornain S, Rumke P. Cytotoxicity of non-T versus T-lymphocytes from melanoma patients and healthy donors on short- and long-term cultured melanoma cells. Int J Cancer 14: 427–434, 1974.
107. Herberman RB, Nunn ME, Lavrin DH. Natural cytotoxic reactivity of mouse lymphoid cells against syngeneic and allogeneic tumours. I. Distribution of reactivity and specificity. Int J Cancer 16: 216–229, 1975.
108. Herberman RB, Nunn ME, Holden HT, et al. Natural cytotoxic reactivity of mouse lymphoid cells against syngeneic and allogeneic tumours. II. Characterization of effector cells. Int J Cancer 16: 230–239, 1975.
109. Kiessling R, Klein E, Wigzell H. Natural killer cells in the mouse. I. Cytotoxic cells with specificity for mouse Moloney leukaemia cells. Specificity and distribution according to genotype. Eur J Immunol 5: 112–117, 1975.
110. Kiessling R, Petranyi G, Klein G. Wigzell H. Non T-cell-resistance against a mouse Moloney lymphoma. Int J Cancer 17: 275–281, 1976.
111. Saksela E, Timonen T, Ranki A, Hayry P. Morphological and functional characterization of isolated effector cells responsible for human natural killer activity to fetal fibroblasts and to cultured cell line targets. Immunol Rev 44: 77–123, 1979.
112. Timonen T, Saksela E, Ranki A, Hayry P. Fractionation, morphological and functional chacterization of effector cells responsible for human natural killer activity against cell-line targets. Cell Immunol 48: 133–148, 1979.
113. Timonen T, Ranki A, Saksela E, Hayry P. Human natural cell-mediated cytotoxicity against fetal fibroblasts. III. Morphological and functional characterization of the effector cells. Cell Immunol 48, 121–132, 1979.
114. Timonen T, Reynolds CW, Ortaldo JR, Herberman RB. Isolation of human and rat natural killer cells. J Immunol Methods 51: 269–277, 1982.
115. Kurnick JT, Ostberg L, Stegagno M, Kimura AK, Orn A, Sjoberg O. A rapid method for the separation of functional lymphoid cell populations of human and animal origin on PVP-silica (Percoll) density gradients. Scand J Immunol 10: 563–573, 1979.
116. Timonen T, Saksela E. Isolation of human NK cells by density gradient centrifugation. J Immunol Methods 36: 285–291, 1980.
117. Timonen T, Ortaldo JR, Herberman RB. Characteristics of human large granular lymphocytes and relationship to natural killer and K-cells. J Exp Med 153: 569–582, 1981.
118. Reynolds CW, Timonen T, Herberman RB. Natural killer (NK) cell activity in the rat. I. Isolation and characterisation of the effector cells. J Immunol 127: 282–287, 1981.

119. Abo T, Balch CM. Differentiation antigen of human NK and K cells identified by a monoclonal antibody (HNK-1). J Immunol 127: 1024–1029, 1981.
120. Abo T, Cooper MD, Balch CM. Characterization of HNK-1⁺ (Leu-7) human lymphocytes. I. Two distinct phenotypes of human NK cells with different cytotoxic capacity. J Immunol 129: 1752–1757, 1982.
121. Balch CM, Ades EW, Loken MR, Shore SL. Human "null" cells mediating antibody-dependent cellular cytotoxicity express T-lymphocyte differentiation antigens. J Immunol 124: 1845–1851, 1980.
122. Kaplan J, Callwaert DM, Peterson WD. Expression of human T-lymphocyte antigens by killer cells. J Immunol 121: 1366–1369, 1978.
123. Kaplan J, Callewaert DM. Expression of human T-lymphocyte antigens by natural killer cells. J Natl Cancer Inst 60: 961–964, 1978.
124. Lohmann-Matthes ML, Domzing W, Roder JC. Promonocytes have the functional characteristics of natural killer cells. J Immunol 123: 1883–1886, 1979.
125. Lohmann-Matthes ML, Domzing W, Taskov H. Antibody-dependent cellular cytotoxicity against tumour cells. I. Cultivated bone marrow-derived macrophages kill tumour targets. Eur J Immunol 9: 261–266, 1979.
126. Domzing W, Lohmann-Matthes ML. Antibody dependent cellular cytotoxicity against tumour cells. II. The promonocyte identified as effector cell. Eur J Immunol 9: 267–272, 1979.
127. Breard J, Reinherz EL, Kung PC, Goldstein G, Schlossman SF. A monoclonal antibody reactive with human peripheral blood monocytes. J Immunol 124: 1943–1948, 1980.
128. Zarling JM, Kung PC. Monoclonal antibodies which distinguish between human NK cells and cytotoxic T-lymphocytes. Nature 288: 394–396, 1980.
129. Ault KA, Springer TA. Cross-section of a rat-anti-mouse phagocyte-specific monoclonal antibody (anti-Mac-1) with human monocytes and natural killer cells. J Immunol 126: 359–364, 1981.
130. Ortaldo JR, Sharrow SO, Timonen T, Herberman RB. Determination of surface antigens on highly purified human NK cells by flow cytometry with monoclonal antibodies. J Immunol 127: 2401–2409, 1981.
131. Kay HD, Horwitz DA. A monoclonal antibody reactive with human peripheral blood monocytes. J Immunol 124: 1943–1948, 1980.
132. Abo T, Balch CM. Characterization of HNK-1⁺ (Leu-7) human lymphocytes. II. Distinguishing phenotypic and functional properties of natural killer cells from activated NK-like cells. J Immunol 129: 1758–1761, 1982.
133. Abo T, Cooper MD, Balch CM. Postnatal expansion of the natural killer and killer cell population in humans. Identified by the monoclonal HNK-1 antibody. J Exp Med 155: 321–326, 1982.
134. Herberman RB. In Herberman RB (ed.), Natural cell-mediated immunity against tumours. New York: Academic Press, 1980.
135. Ferrarini M, Romagnani S, Montesoro E, Zicca A, Del Preto GF, Nocera A, Maggi E, Leprini A, Grossi CE. Lymphoproliferative disorder of the large granular lymphocytes with natural killer activity. J Clin Immunol 3: 30–41, 1983.
136. Dennert G, Yogeeswaran G, Yamagata S. Cloned cell lines with natural killer activity specificity, function, and cell surface markers. J Exp Med 153: 545–556, 1981.
137. Henney CS, Lichtenstein LM, Gillespie E, Roley RT. In vivo suppression of immune response to alloantigen by cholera toxin. J Clin Invest 52: 2853–2857, 1973.
138. Golstein P, Smith ET. The lethal hit stage of mouse T and non-T-cell-mediated cytolysis: Differences in cation requirements and characterization of an analytical "cation pulse" method. Eur J Immunol 6: 31–37, 1976.
139. Martz E. Mechanism of specific tumour-cell lysis by alloimmune T-lymphocytes: Resolution and characterization of discrete steps in the cellular interaction. Contemp Top Immunobiol 7: 301–361, 1977.
140. Becker FF, Klein E. Decreased "natural killer" effect in tumour bearer mice and its relation to the immunity against oncornavirus-determined cell surface antigens. Eur J Immunol 6: 892–898, 1976.
141. Shellam GR, Hogg N. Cross-virus-induced lymphoma in the rat. IV. Cytotoxic cells in normal rats. Int J Cancer 19: 212–224, 1977.
142. Sendo F, Aoki T, Boyse EA, Buofo CK. Natural occurrence of lymphocytes showing cytotoxic activity to BALB/c radiation-induced leukaemia RL male 1 cells. J Natl Cancer Inst 55: 603–609, 1975.
143. Zarling JM, Nowinski N, Bach FH. Lysis of leukaemia cells by spleen cells of normal mice. Proc Natl Acad Sci USA 72: 2780–2784, 1975.
144. Kiessling R, Haller O. Natural killer cells in the mouse: An alternative immune surveillance mechanism. Contemp Top Immunobiol 8: 171–201, 1978.
145. Nunn ME, Herberman RB, Holden HT. Natural cell-mediated cytotoxicity in mice against non-lymphoid tumour cells and some normal cells. Int J Cancer 20: 381–387, 1977.
146. Stutman T, Paige CJ, Figarella FE. Natural cytotoxic cells against solid tumours in mice. I. Strain and age distribution and target cell susceptibility. J Immunol 121: 1819–1826, 1978.

147. Hansson M, Karre K, Bakacs T, Kiessling R, Klein G. Intra- and interspecies reactivity of human and mouse natural killer (NK) cells. J Immunol 121: 6–12, 1978.
148. Herberman RB, Holden HT. Natural cell-mediated immunity. Adv Cancer Res 27: 305–377, 1978.
149. Ojo E, Haller O, Kimura A, Wigzell H. An analysis of conditions allowing *Corynebacterium parvum* to cause either augmentation or inhibition of natural killer cell activity against tumour cells in mice. Int J Cancer 21: 444–452, 1978.
150. Haller O, Kiessling R, Örn A, Karre K, Nilsson K, Wigzell H. Natural cytotoxicity to human leukaemias mediated by mouse non-T cells. Int J Cancer 20: 93–103, 1977.
151. Callwaert DM, Kaplan J, Peterson WD Jr, Lightbody JJ. Spontaneous cytotoxicity of human lymphoblast cell lines mediated by normal peripheral blood lymphocytes. I. Differential susceptiblility of T-versus B-cell lines. Cell Immunol 33: 11–19, 1977.
152. Pross HF, Jondal M. Cytotoxic lymphocytes from normal donors. A functional marker of human non-T lymphocytes. Clin Exp Immunol 21: 226–235, 1975.
153. Petranyi GG, Benczur M, Onody CE, Holland SR. HLA 3,7 and lymphocyte cytotoxic activity. Lancet 1: 736, 1974.
154. Santoli D, Trinchieri G, Zmijewski CM, Koprowski H. HLA-related control of spontaneous and antibody-dependent cell mediated cytotoxic activity in humans. J Immunol 117: 765–770, 1976.
155. Haller O, Gidlund M, Kurnick JT, Wigzell H. In vivo generation of mouse natural killer cells: Role of the spleen and thymus. Scand J Immunol 8: 207–213, 1978.
156. Roder JC, Ahrlund-Richter L, Jondal M. Target-effector interaction in the human and murine natural killer system. Specificity and xenogeneic reactivity of the solubilized natural killer target structure complex and its loss in a somatic cell hybrid. J Exp Med 150: 471–487, 1979.
157. Roder JC, Rosen A, Fenjo EM, Troy FA. Target-effector interaction in the natural killer cell system: Isolation of target structures. Proc Natl Acad Sci USA 76: 1405–1409, 1979.
158. Roder JC. Target-effector interaction in the natural killer (NK) cell system. VI. The influence of age and genotype on NK binding characteristics. Immunology 41: 483–489, 1980.
159. Nunn ME, Herberman RB. Natural cytotoxicity of mouse, rat, and human lymphocytes against heterologous target cells. J Natl Cancer Inst 62: 765–771, 1979.
160. Welsh RM. Mouse natural killer cells: Induction, specificity, and function. J Immunol 121: 1631–1635, 1978.
161. Gidlund M, Orn A, Wigzell A, Gresser I. Enhanced NK activity in mice injected with interferon and interferon inducers. Nature 273: 759–761, 1978.
162. Wolfe SA, Tracey DE, Henney CS. Induction of "natural killer" cells by BCG. Nature 262: 1584–1586, 1976.
163. Herberman RB, Nunn ME, Holden HT, Staals S, Djeu JY. Augmentation of natural cytotoxicity against syngeneic and allogeneic target cells. Int J Cancer 19: 555–564, 1977.
164. Welsh RM, Zinkernagel RM. Heterospecific cytotoxic cell-activity induced during the first three days of acute lymphocytic choriomeningitis virus infection in mice. Nature 268: 646–648, 1977.
165. MacFarlan RI, Burns WH, While DO. Two cytotoxic cells in the peritoneal cavity of virus-infected mice: Antibody dependent macrophages and non-specific killer cells. J Immunol 119: 1569–1574, 1977.
166. Tracey DE, Wolfe SA, Durdik JM, Henney CS. BCG-induced murine effector cells. I. Cytolytic activity in peritoneal exudates: An early response to BCG. J Immunol 119: 1145–1151, 1977.
167. Welsh RM, Zinkernagel RM, Hallenbeck LA. Cytotoxic cells induced during lymphocytic choriomeningitis virus infection of mice. II. Specificities of the natural killer cells. J Immunol 122: 475–481, 1979.
168. Kiessling R, Eriksson E, Hallenbeck LA, Welsh RM. A comparative analysis of the cell surface properties of activated versus endogenous mouse natural killer cells. J Immunol 125: 1551–1557, 1980.
169. Welsh RM, Doe WF. Cytotoxic cells induced lymphocytic choriomeningitis virus infection of mice. III. Natural killer activity in cultured spleen leukocytes concomitant with T-cell-dependent immune IFN production. Infect Immun 30: 473–483, 1980.
170. Kunkel LA, Welsh RM. Metabolic inhibitors render "resistant" target cells sensitive to natural killer cell-mediated lysis. Int J Cancer 27: 73–79, 1981.
171. Hiserodt JC, Britvan J, Targan S. Differential effects of various pharmacologic agents on the cytotoxic reaction mechanism of the human natural killer lymphocyte: Further resolution of programming for lysis and KCIL into discrete stages. J Immunol 129: 2266–2270, 1982.
172. Quan PC, Ishizaka T, Bloom BR. Studies on the mechanism of NK cell lysis. J Immunol 128: 1786–1791, 1982.
173. Neighbour PS, Huberman HS. Sr^{++}-induced inhibition of human natural killer (NK) cell-mediated cytotoxicity. J Immunol 128: 1236–1240, 1982.

174. Roder JC, Halliotis T. A comparative analysis of the NK cytolytic mechanism and regulatory genes. In Herberman RB (ed.), Natural cell-mediated immunity against tumours. New York: Academic Press, 1980, pp. 379–389.

175. Carpen O, Virtanen I, Saksela E. The cytotoxic activity of human natural killer cells requires an intact secretory apparatus. Cell Immunol 58: 97–106, 1981.

176. Neville ME, Hiserodt JC. Inhibition of human antibody-dependent cellular cytotoxicity, cell mediated cytotoxicity, and natural killing by xenogeneic antiserum prepared against "activated" autoimmune human lymphocytes. J Immunol 128: 1246–1251, 1982.

177. Yamamoto RS, Hiserodt JC, Granger GA. The human LT system: V. A comparison of the relative lytic effectiveness of various MW human LT classes on ^{51}Cr-labelled allogeneic target cells in vitro: Enhanced lysis by LT complexes associated with Ig-like receptor(s). Cell Immunol 45: 261–275, 1979.

178. Wright S, Bonavida B. Selective lysis of NK-sensitive target cells by a soluble mediator released from murine spleen cells and human peripheral blood lymphocytes. J Immunol 126: 1516–1521, 1981.

179. Farram E, Targan SR. Identification of human natural killer soluble cytotoxic factor(s) (NKCF) derived from NK-enriched lymphocyte populations: Specificity of generation and killing. J Immunol 130: 1252–1256, 1983.

180. Hoffman T, Hirata F, Bougnoux P, Fraser BA, Goldfarb RH, Herberman RB. Phospholipid methylation and phospholipase A2 activation in cytotoxicity by human natural killer cells. Proc Natl Acad Sci 78: 3839–3843, 1981.

181. Goldfarb RH, Timonen T, Herberman RB. Mechanism of tumour cell lysis by natural killer cells. Adv Exp Med Biol 146: 403–421, 1982.

182. Hudig D, Haverly T, Fucher C, Redelman D, Mendelsohn J. Inhibition of human natural cytotoxicity by macromolecular antiproteases. J Immunol 126: 1569–1574, 1981.

183. Lavie G, Weiss H, Pick A, Franklin EC. The role of surface associated proteases in lymphocyte spontaneous cytotoxic activity. Fourth Congress of Immunology Abstracts 11.4, 30, 1980.

184. Djeu JY, Heinbough JA, Viera WD, Holden HT, Herberman RB. The effect of immunopharmacologic agents on mouse natural cell-mediated cytotoxicity and its augmentation by poly I- C. Immunopharmacology 1: 231–244, 1979.

185. Trinchieri G, Santoli D, Dee RR, Knowles BB. Anti-viral activity induced by culturing lymphocytes with tumour-derived or virus-transformed cells. J Exp Med 147: 1299–1313, 1978.

186. Einhorn S, Blomgren H, Strander H. Interferon and spontaneous cytotoxicity in man. I. Enhancement of the spontaneous cytotoxicity of peripheral lymphocytes by human leukocyte interferon. Int J Cancer 22: 405–412, 1978.

187. Herberman RB. Overview on NK cells and possible mechanisms for their cytotoxic activity. Adv Exp Med Biol 146: 337–351, 1982.

188. Platsoucas CD. Analysis of human natural killer cells by monoclonal antibodies. In Herberman RB (ed.), NK cells and other natural effector cells. New York: Academic Press, 1982, pp. 67–72.

189. Lee SH, Kelley S, Chin H, Stebbing N. Stimulation of natural killer cell activity and inhibition of proliferation of various leukemic cells by purified human leukocyte interferon subtypes. Cancer Res 42: 1312–1316, 1982.

190. Gustafsson A, Lundgren E. Augmentation of natural killer cells involves both enhancement of lytic machinery and expression of new receptors. Cell Immunol 62: 367–376, 1981.

191. Djeu JY, Stocks N, Varesio L, Holden HT, Herberman RB. Metabolic requirements for the in vitro augmentation of mouse natural killer activity by interferon. Cell Immunol 58: 49–60, 1981.

192. Ortaldo JR, Phillips W, Wasserman K, Herberman RB. The effect of metabolic inhibitors on spontaneous and IFN boosted human natural killer cell activity. J Immunol 125: 1839–1844, 1980.

193. Gustafsson A, Sundstrom S, Ny T, Lundgren E. Rapid induction of seven proteins in human lymphocytes by interferon, correlation to natural killer cell activity. J Immunol 129: 1952–1959, 1982.

194. Ortaldo JR, Mantovani A, Hobbs D, Robinstein M, Pestka S, Herberman RB. Effects of several species of human leukocyte interferon on cytolytic activity of NK cells and monocytes. Int J Cancer 31: 285–289, 1983.

195. Lotzova E, Savary CA, Gutterman JU, Hersh EM. Modulation of natural killer cell-mediated cytotoxicity by partially purified and cloned interferon-alpha. Cancer Res 42: 2480–2488, 1982.

196. Carter SK. The clinical trial evaluation strategy for interferons and other biological response modifiers— Not a simple task. J Biol Resp Modif 1: 101–105, 1982.

197. Strander H, Cantell K. Production of interferon by human leukocytes in vitro. Ann Med Expl Biol Fenn 44: 265–273, 1966.

198. Mogensen KE, Cantell K. Production and preparation of human leukocyte interferon. Pharm Ther C 1: 369–383, 1977.

199. Southam CM. Present status of oncolytic virus studies. Trans NY Acad Sci 83: 551–572, 1960.
200. Southam CM, Moore AE. Clinical studies of viruses as antineoplastic agents with particular reference to Egypt 101 virus. Cancer 5: 1025–1030, 1952.
201. Mathé G, Amiel L, Schwarzenberg L, Schneider M, Hayat M, DeVassal F, Jasmin C, Rosenfeld C, Choay J. Remission induction with poly IC in patients with acute lymphatic leukemia. Europ J Clin Biol Res 15: 671–684, 1970.
202. Thatcher N, Swindell R, Crowther D. Effect of repeated Corynebacterium parvum and BCG therapy on immune parameters: A weekly sequential study of melanoma patients. 1. Changes in non-specific (NK, K, and T cell) lymphocytotoxicity, peripheral blood counts and delayed hypersensitivity reactions. Clin Exp Immunol 36: 227–236, 1979.
203. Gutterman JU, Blumenschein GR, Alexanian R, Hwee-Yong Y, Buzdar AU, Cambanillar F, Hortobagy GN, Hash EM, et al. Leukocyte interferon-induced tumour regression in human metastatic breast cancer, multiple myeloma, and malignant lymphoma. Ann Intern Med 93: 399–406, 1980.
204. Blomgren H, Cantell K, Johansson B, Lagergren C, Ringborg U, Strander H. Interferon therapy in Hodgkin's disease. A case report. Acta Med Scand 199: 527–532, 1976.
205. Hil NO, Pardue A, Kahn A, Aleman D, Hill JM. High-dose human leukocyte interferon trials in leukemia and cancer. Med Pediatr Oncol 9: 82–89, 1981.
206. Einhorn N, Cantell K, Einhorn S, Strander H. Human leukocyte interferon therapy for advanced ovarian carcinoma. Cancer Clin Trials 5: 167–172, 1982.
207. Paucker G, Cantell K, Henle W. Quantitative studies on viral interference in suspended L-cells. III. Effect of interfering viruses and interferon on the growth rate of cells. Virology 17: 324–334, 1962.
208. Epstein LB. The interferon system. Tex Rep Biol Med 36: 42–56, 1978.
209. Saxena RK, Alder WH, Nordin AA. Modulation of natural cytotoxicity by alloantibodies. IV. A comparative study of the activation of mouse spleen cell cytotoxicity by anti-H2 antisera, interferon, and mitogens. Cell Immunol 63: 28–41, 1981.
210. Brunda MT, Herberman RB, Holden HT. Interferon-independent activation of murine natural killer cell activity. In Herberman RB (ed.), Natural cell-mediated immunity against tumours. New York: Academic Press, 1980, pp. 525–536.
211. Brunda MJ, Herberman RB, Holden HT. Antibody-induced augmentation of murine natural killer cell activity. Int J Cancer 27: 205–212, 1981.
212. Goldfarb RH, Herberman RB. Natural killer cell reactivity: Regulatory interactions among phorbol ester, interferon, cholera toxin and retinoic acid. J Immunol 126: 2129–2135, 1981.
213. Blalock JE. Inhibition of interferon production by RA (vitamin A acid). Tex Rep Biol Med 35: 69–73, 1977.
214. Kuribayashi K, Gillis S, Kern DE, Henney CS. Murine NK cell cultures: Effects of interleukin 2 and interferon on cell growth and cytotoxic reactivity. J Immunol 126: 2321–2327, 1981.
215. Domzing W, Stadler BM. The relation between human natural killer cells and interleukin 2. In Herberman RB (ed.), NK cells and other natural effector cells. New York: Academic Press, 1982, pp. 409–415.
216. Roder JC, Argov S, Klein NM, Peterson C, Kiessling R, Anderson R, Anderson K, and Hansson M. Target-effector interaction in the natural killer cell system. V. Energy requirement, membrane integrity, and the possible involvement of lysosomal enzymes. Immunology 40: 107–116, 1980.
217. Hochman PS, Cudkowicz G. Suppression of natural cytotoxicity by spleen cells of hydrocortisone-treated mice. J Immunol 123: 968–971, 1979.
218. Cudowicz G, Hochman PS. Do natural killer cells engage in regulated reactions against self to ensure homeostasis? Immunol Rev 44: 13–41, 1979.
219. Lotzova E, Gutterman JU. Effect of glucan on NK cells: Further comparison between NK cell and bone marrow effector cell activities. J Immunol 123: 607–611, 1979.
220. Brunda MJ, Herberman RB, Holden HT. Inhibition of murine natural killer cell activity by prostaglandins. J Immunol 124: 2682–2687, 1980.
221. Droller JJ, Schneider MU, Perlmann P. A possible role of prostaglandins in the inhibition of natural and antibody-dependent cell-mediated cytotoxicity against tumour cells. Cell Immunol 39: 165–177, 1978.
222. Roder JC, Klein M. Target-effector interaction in the natural killer cell system. IV. Modulation by cyclic nucleotides. J Immunol 123: 2785–2790, 1979.
223. Yanagihara RH, Alder WH. Inhibition of mouse natural killer activity by cyclosporin A. Immunology 45: 325–332, 1982.
224. Introna M, Allavena P, Spreafico F, Mantovani A: Inhibition of human natural killer activity by cyclosporin A. Transplantation 31: 113–316, 1981.
225. Santoni A, Riccardi C, Sorci V, Herberman RB. Effects of adriamycin on the activity of mouse natural killer cells. J Immunol 124: 2329–2335, 1980.

226. Sharp GWG, Hynie S. Stimulation of intestinal adenyl cyclase by cholera toxin. Nature 229: 226–229, 1971.

227. Fuse A, Sato T, Kuwata T. Inhibitory effect of cholera toxin on human natural cell-mediated cytotoxicity and its augmentation by interferon. Br J Cancer 27: 29–36, 1981.

228. Sulica A, Cherman M, Galaliuc C, Maciulea M, Herberman RB. Negative regulation of human NK activity by monomeric IgG. In Herberman RB (ed.), NK cells and other natural effector cells. New York: Academic Press, 1982, pp. 621–629.

229. Merrill JE, Ullberg M, Jondal M. Influence of IgG and IgM receptor triggering on human natural killer cell cytotoxicity measured on the level of the single effector cell. Eur J Immunol 11: 536–541, 1981.

230. Hochman PS, Cudkowicz G, Dausset J. Decline of natural killer cell activity in sublethally irradiated mice. J Natl Cancer Inst 61: 265–268, 1978.

231. Santoni A, Riccardi C, Barlozzari T, Herberman RB. Suppression of activity of mouse natural killer (NK) cells by activated macrophages from mice treated with Pyran copolymer. Int J Cancer 26: 837–843, 1980.

232. Uchida A, Hoshino T. Clinical studies on cell-mediated immunity in patients with malignant disease. II. Suppressor cells in patients with cancer. Cancer Immunol Immunother 9: 153–158, 1980.

233. Zembala M, Mytar O, Popiela T, Asherson GL. Depressed in vitro peripheral blood lymphocyte response to mitogens in cancer patients: The role of suppressor cells. Int J Cancer 19: 605–613, 1977.

234. Vose BM, Moore M. Suppressor cell activity of lymphocytes infiltrating human lung and breast tumours. Int J Cancer 24: 579–585, 1979.

235. Allavena PM, Introna C, Mangioni C, Mantovani A. Inhibition of natural killer activity by tumour-associated lymphoid cells from ascitic ovarian carcinomas. J Natl Cancer Inst 67: 319–325, 1981.

236. Uchida A, Micksche M. Suppressor cells for natural killer activity in carcinomatous pleural effusions of cancer patients. Cancer Immunol Immunother 11: 255–263, 1981.

237. Bordignon C, Villa F, Vecchi A, Giavazzi R, Introna M, Avallone R, Mantovani A. Natural cytotoxic activity in human lungs. Clin Exp Immunol 47: 437–444, 1982.

238. Becker S, Klein E. Decreased ''natural killer''-NK effect in tumour bearing mice and its relation to the immunity against oncornavirus determined cell surface antigens. Eur J Immunol 6: 892–898, 1976.

239. Stutman O, Dien P, Wisun RE, Lattime EC. Natural cytotoxic cells against solid tumours in mice: Blocking of cytotoxicity by D-mannose. Proc Natl Acad Sci 77: 2895–2898, 1980.

240. Forbes JT, Greco FA, Oldham RK. Natural cell-mediated cytotoxicity in human tumour patients. In Herberman RB (ed.), Natural cell-mediated immunity against tumours. New York: Academic Press, 1980, pp. 1031–1045.

241. Pross HF, Baines MG. Studies of human natural killer cells. I. In vivo parameters affecting normal cytotoxic function. Int J Cancer 18: 593, 1976.

242. Platsoucas CD, Gupta S, Good RA, Fernandes G. T and non-T-cell-mediated NK and ADCC. Augmentation of T-cell-mediated NK and ADCC by interferon treatment in vitro. Fed Proc 39: 932, 1980.

243. Hawrylowicz CM, Rees RC, Hancock BW, Potter CW. Depressed spontaneous natural killing and interferon augmentation in patients with malignant lymphoma. Eur J Cancer 18: 1081–1088, 1982.

244. Zeigler HW, Kay NE, Zarling JM. Deficiency of natural killer cell activity in patients with chronic lymphatic leukemia. Int J Cancer 27: 321–327, 1981.

245. Kadish AS, Doyle AT, Steinhauer EH, Ghossein NA. Natural cytotoxicity and interferon production in human cancer: Deficient natural killer activity and normal interferon production in patients with advanced disease. J Immunol 127: 1817–1822, 1981).

246. Moore K, Moore M. Systemic and in situ NK activity in tumour-bearing rats. Br J Cancer 39: 636–647, 1979.

247. Moore M, Vose BM: Natural cytotoxic effectors in human tumours and tumour draining nodes. In Herberman RB (ed.), NK cells and other natural effector cells. New York: Academic Press, 1982, pp. 1127–1132.

248. Totterman TH, Hayny P, Saksela P, Timonen T, Eklund B. Cytological and functional analysis of inflammatory infiltrates in human malignant tumours. II. Functional investigation of the infiltrating inflammatory cells. Eur J Immunol 8: 872–875, 1978.

249. Vose BM, Vanky F, Argov S, Klein E. Natural cytotoxicity in man: Activity of lymph node and tumour infiltrating lymphocytes. Eur J Immunol 7: 353–357, 1977.

250. Niitsuma M, Golub SH, Edelstein R, Holmes EC. Lymphoid cells infiltrating human pulmonary tumors: Effect of intralesional BCG injections. J Natl Cancer Inst 67: 997–1003, 1981.

251. Introna M, Allavena P, Acero R, Colombo N, Molina P, Mantovani A. Natural killer activity in human ovarian tumours. In Herberman RB (ed.), NK cells and other natural effector cells. New York: Academic Press, 1982, pp. 1119–1126.

252. Mantovani A, Allavena P, Sessa C, Bolis G, Mangioni C. Natural killer activity of lymphoid cells isolated from human ascitic ovarian tumours. Int J Cancer 25: 573–582, 1980.

253. Eremin O. NK cell activity in the blood, tumour-draining lymph nodes and primary tumours of women with mammary carcinoma. In Herberman RB (ed.), Natural cell-mediated immunity against tumours. New York: Academic Press, 1980, pp. 1011–1029.

254. Moore M, Vose BM. Extravascular natural cytotoxicity in man: Anti-K562 activity of lymph node and tumour-infiltrating lymphocytes. Int J Cancer 27: 265–272, 1981.

255. Golub SH, Niitsuma M, Kawate N, Cochran AJ, Holmes EC. NK activity of tumour infiltrating and lymph node lymphocytes in human pulmonary tumours. In Herberman RB (ed.), NK cells and other natural effector cells. New York: Academic Press, 1982, pp. 1113–1118.

256. Vose BM, Moore M. Natural cytotoxic effectors in human tumours and tumour draining nodes. In Herberman RB (ed.), NK cells and other natural effector cells. New York: Academic Press, 1982, pp. 1127–1132.

257. Holmes EC, Ramming KP, Bein ME, Coulson WF, Callery CD. Intralesional BCG immunotherapy of pulmonary tumours. J Thor Cardiovasc Surg 77: 362–368, 1979.

258. Petranyi G, Kiessling R, Klein G. Genetic control of natural killer lymphocytes in the mouse. Immunogenetics 2: 53–651, 1975.

259. Haller O, Hanson M, Kiessling R, Wigzell H. Generation of natural killer cells: An autonomous function of the bone marrow. J Exp Med 145: 1411–1416, 1977.

260. Harmon RC, Clark EA, O'Toole C, Wicker LS. Resistance of H-2 heterozygous mice to prenatal tumours. Hybride resistance and natural cytotoxicity to EL-4 are controlled by the H-2D-Hh-I region. Immunogenetics 4: 601–607, 1977.

261. Shellam GR. Cross-virus-induced lymphoma in the rat. V. Natural cytotoxic cells are non-T cells. Int J Cancer 19: 225–235, 1977.

262. Harmon RC, Clark EA, Reddy AL, Hildermann WH, Mullen YS. Immunity to MCA-induced rat sarcomas: Analysis of in vivo and in vitro results. Int J Cancer 20: 748–758, 1977.

263. Warner NL, Woodruff MFA, Burton RC. Inhibition of the growth of lymphoid tumours in syngeneic athymic (nude) mice. Int J Cancer 20: 146–155, 1977.

264. Ojo E. Positive correlation between the levels of natural killer cells and in vivo resistance to syngeneic tumour transplants as influenced by various routes of administration of Corynebacterium parvum bacteria. Cell Immunol 45: 182–187, 1979.

265. Henney CS, Tracey DE, Wolfe SA. BCG-induced natural killer cells: Immunotherapeutic implications. Isr J Med Sci 14: 75–88, 1978.

266. Riccardi C, Santoni A, Barlozzuri T, Puccetti P, Herberman RB. In vivo natural reactivity of mice against tumour cells. Int J Cancer 15: 475–486, 1980.

267. Karre KK, Kiesling R, Klein G, Roder J. Low natural in vivo resistance to syngeneic leukemias in natural killer-deficient mice. Nature 284: 624, 1980.

268. Pollack SB, Hallenbeck LA. In vivo reduction of NK activity with anti-NK1 serum: Direct evaluation of NK cells in tumour clearance. Int J Cancer 15: 203–207, 1982.

269. Menard S, Colnaghi MI, Porta GD. Natural anti-tumour serum reactivity in BALB/c mice. I. Characterization and interference with tumour growth. Int J Cancer 19: 267–274, 1977.

270. Chow DA, Wolosin LB, Greenberg AH. Murine natural anti-tumour antibodies. II. The contribution of natural antibodies to tumour surveillance. Int J Cancer 27: 459–469, 1981.

271. Carlson GA, Melnychuk D, Meeker MJ. H-2 associated resistance to leukemia transplantation: Natural killing in vivo. Int J Cancer 25: 111–122, 1980.

272. Walker JR, Rees RC, Teale DM, Potter CW. Properties of a herpes virus transformed hamster cell line. I. Growth and culture characteristics of sublines of high and low metastatic potential. Eur J Cancer Clin Oncol 18: 1017–1026, 1982.

273. Teale DM, Rees RC, Clark A, Walker JR, Potter CW. Reduced susceptibility to natural killer cell lysis of hamster tumours exhibiting high levels of spontaneous metastasis. Cancer Lett 19: 221–229, 1983.

274. Teale DM, Rees RC, Clark A, Potter CW. Detection and characterization of natural killer cells in Syrian golden hamsters. Eur J Cancer Clin Oncol 19: 537–545, 1983.

275. Reichman GI, Kluchareva TE, Kashkina LM, Matveera VA, Vendrov EL, Zemtsova VI. Correlation between the metastasizing activity of in vitro spontaneously transformed hamster cells and their natural resistance-depressing activity. Int J Cancer 30: 349–353, 1982.

276. Sordat B, Merenda C, Carrel S. Invasive growth and dissemination of human solid tumours and malignant cell lines grafted subcutaneously to newborn nude mice. In Nomura T, Ohsawa N, Tamaoki N, Fujiware K (eds.), Proceeding of the Second International Workshop on Nude Mice. Tokyo: University of Tokyo Press, 1977, pp. 313–326.

277. Reid LM, Holland J, Jones C, Wolf B, Sato G. Some of the variables affecting the success of transplantation of human tumours into the athymic nude mice. In Houchens DP, Ovejera AA (eds.), Proceeding of the Symposium on the Use of Athymic (nude) Mice in Cancer Research. New York: Gustav Fischer Verlag, 1978, pp. 107–121.

278. Hanna A, Fidler IJ. Role of natural killer cells in the destruction of circulating tumour emboli. J Natl Cancer Inst 65: 801–809, 1980.

279. Hanna N, Fidler IJ. Expression of metastatic potential of allogenic and xenogeneic neoplasms in young nude mice. Cancer Res 41: 438–444, 1981.

280. Talmage JE, Meyers KM, Prieur DJ, Starkey JR. Role of NK cells in tumour growth and metastasis in beige mice. Nature 284: 622–624, 1980.

281. Kasai M, Yoneda T, Habu S, Maryama Y, Okumura K, Tokunaga T. In vivo effect of anti-asialo GM1 antibody on natural killer activity. Nature 291: 334–335, 1980.

282. Habu S, Fukui H, Shimamura K, Kasai M, Nagai Y, Okumura K, Tamaoki N. In vivo effects of anti-asialo GM1. I. Reduction of NK activity and enhancement of transplanted tumour growth in nude mice. J Immunol 127: 34–38, 1981.

283. Gorelik E, Witrout RH, Okumura K, Habu S, Herberman RB. Role of NK cells in the control of metastatic spread and growth of tumour cells in mice. Int J Cancer 309: 107–112, 1982.

284. Smith KA, Lachman LB, Oppenheim JJ, Favata MF. The functional relationship of the interleukins. J Exp Med 151: 1551–1556, 1980.

285. Gillis S, Watson J. Biochemical and biological characterisation of lymphocyte regulatory molecules. J Exp Med 152: 1709–1719, 1980.

286. Watson J, Gillis S, Marbrook J, Mochizuki D, Smith KA. Biochemical and biological characterization of lymphocyte regulatory molecules. J Exp Med 150: 849–861, 1979.

287. Gillis S, Smith K, Watson J. Biochemical characterization of lymphocyte regulatory molecules. II. Purification of a class of rate and human lymphokines. J Immunol 124: 1954–1962, 1980.

288. Farrar WL, Elgert KD. Suppressor cell activity in tumour-bearing mice. II. Inhibition of DNA synthesis and DNA polymerases by TBH splenic suppressor cells. J Immunol 120: 1354–1361, 1978.

289. Shaw J, Monticone V, Mills G, Paetkan V. Effects of constimulator on immune responses in vitro. J Immunol 120: 1974–1980, 1978.

290. Sekaly RP, Macdonald HR, Zaech P, Nabholz M. Cell cycle regulation of cloned cytolytic T cells by T cell growth factor: Analysis by flow microfluorometry. J Immunol 129: 1407–1415, 1982.

291. Farrar WL, Mizel SB, Farrar JJ. Participation of lymphocyte activating factor (interleukin 1) in the induction of cytotoxic T cell response. J Immunol 124: 1371–1377, 1980.

292. Larsson EL, Iscove NN, Coutinho A. Two distinct factors are required for induction of T-cell growth. Nature 283: 664–666, 1980.

293. Wagner HM, Rollinghoff M, Pfizenmaier K, Hardt C, Johnscher G. T-T cell interactions during in vitro cytotoxic T lymphocyte (CTL) response. II. Helper factor from activated Lyt 1$^+$T cells is rate limiting (i) in T cell response to non immunogenic alloantigen, (ii) in thymocyte responses to allogeneic stimulator cells, and (iii) recruits allo- or H-2-restricted CTL precursors from the Lyt 123$^+$T subset. J Immunol 124: 1058–1067, 1980.

294. Dennert G. Cytolytic and proliferative activity of a permanent T killer cell line. Nature 227: 476–477, 1979.

295. Baker PC, Gillis S, Smith KA. Monoclonal cytotoxic T-cell lines. J Exp Med 149: 273–278, 1979.

296. Pawelec G, Rehbein A, Muller C, Sonneborn HH, Wernet P. Human T lymphocytes grown in T-cell growth factor: Functional attributes in MLC, CML, PLT and allogeneic suppression. Immunology 42: 529–540, 1981.

297. Alvarez JM, Silva A, De Laudazuri MO. Human T cell growth factor. I. Optimal conditions for its production. J Immunol 123: 977–983, 1979.

298. Bonnard GD, Yasaka K, Maca RD. Continued growth of functional human T lymphocytes: production of human T-cell growth factor. Cell Immunol 51: 390–401, 1980.

299. Gillis S, Scheid M, Watson J. Biochemical and biological characterization of lymphocyte regulatory molecules. III. The isolation and phenotypic characterization of interleukin-2 producing T cell lymphomas. J Immunol 125: 2570–2578, 1980.

300. Rabin H, Hopkins RF, Francis W, Neubauer RH, Brown RL, Kawakami TG. Spontaneous release of a factor with properties of T cell growth factor from a continuous line of primate tumour T cells. J Immunol 127: 1852–1856, 1981.

301. Meuer SC, Hussey RE, Penta AC, Fitzgerald KA, Stadler BM, Schlossman SF, Reinherz EL. Cellular origin of interleukin 2 (IL2) in man: Evidence for stimulus-restricted IL2 production by T4$^+$ and T8$^+$ T lymphocytes. J Immunol 129: 1076–1079, 1982.

302. Kedar E, Ikejiri B, Sredni B, Bonavida B, Herberman RB. Propagation of mouse cytotoxic clones with characteristics of natural killer (NK) cells. Cell Immunol 69: 305–329, 1982.

303. Dennert G. Cloned lines of natural killer cells. Nature 287: 47–49, 1980.

304. Dennert G. Yogeeswaran G, Yamagata S. Cloned cell lines with natural killer activity. Specificity, function, and cell surface markers. J Exp Med 153: 545–556, 1981.

305. Hercend T, Meuer S, Reinerz E, Schlossman S, Ritz J. Generation of a cloned NK cell line derived from the

306. Krensky AM, Ault KA, Reiss CS, Strominger JL, Burakoff SJ. Generation of long-term human cytolytic cell clones with persistent natural killer activity. J Immunol 129: 1748–1751, 1982.

307. Timonen T, Ortaldo JR, Stadler BM, Bonnard GD, Sharrow SO, Herberman RB. Cultures of purified human natural killer cells: Growth in the presence of interleukin 2. Cell Immunol 72: 178–185, 1982.

308. Mule JJ, Hellstrom I, Hellstrom KE. Cell surface phenotypes of radiolabelled immune long-lived lymphocytes that selectively localize in syngeneic tumours. Am J Pathol 107: 142–149, 1982.

309. Hersey P, Bindon C, Edwards A, Murray E, Phillips G, McCarthy WH. Induction of cytotoxic activity in human lymphocytes against autologous and allogeneic melanoma cells in vitro by culture with interleukin 2. Int J Cancer 28: 695–703, 1981.

310. Vanky F, Gorsky T, Gorsky Y, Masucci M, Klein E. Lysis of tumour biopsy cells by autologous T lymphocytes activated in mixed cultures and propogated with T cell growth factor. J Exp Med 155: 83–95, 1982.

3. THE MACROPHAGE AND CANCER

A. CLARK

INTRODUCTION

The characterization of the immune response to tumours is a scientific development in oncology that has run an extremely uncertain course over approximately the last 30 years. The basic concept and potential of the immune system to respond to tumours has been appreciated for some time, but it is only recently that relatively solid scientific information has been established about the role of the immune system in the control of tumours. It is now accepted, although poorly understood, that as well as being directly tumouricidal the immune system may be anergic in the tumour-bearing host. This lack of immune reactivity may actually allow the initiation, growth, and spread of a tumour and also account for the increased susceptibility to infection that cancer patients experience. In addition, once established, the tumour cells and their products may exert a local or systemic depressive effect upon the immune system that could produce a further reduction in immune responsiveness to the tumour and to unrelated antigens.

The monocyte/macrophage or mononuclear phagocyte is now recognized as a cell that is very important not only as a phagocytic effector cell but also as a cell that is vital in the initiation of an adequate immune response to a specific antigen. Indirect evidence for a role for macrophages in tumour immunity is provided by the fact that these cells are usually prominent in the stroma of many tumours and are frequently observed in very close relation to tumour cells that appear to be undergoing lysis. Besides exerting a cytotoxic but, as yet, poorly characterized effector function against tumour cells, the role of the macrophage in the induction of an immune response to a tumour must be a critical factor in tumour immunity. Although most tumours possess demonstrable foreign tumour antigens on their plasma membranes, these antigens usually fail to induce an immune response. Effects of tumour cells and their products on macrophage immunoinduction of the immune response have been postulated as being a factor that may partially account for the lack of a specific immune response to most tumours and the subsequent ease of tumour establishment.

Despite the obvious potential role of macrophages in tumour immunology, their position remains ill-defined and poorly characterized. This is largely accounted for by the difficulties encountered in studying these cells in vivo and in vitro and also by the now-recognized heterogeneity of the functionally mature cells of the monocyte/macrophage series. Many of the current and postulated immunostimulatory compounds that may have a place in future cancer immunotherapy are known to have stimulatory effects on macrophages. There is limited in vivo experimental evidence that these immunostimulatory compounds have a direct effect on tumour immunity via their interaction with macrophages; further study of such compounds on macrophage function is an area of tumour immunology that should be an important step in their development as therapeutic agents.

This chapter first covers the basic characteristics and functions of cells of the monocyte/macrophage series, an essential introduction to the latter section about the relationship of this cell to cancer. Recently, a number of reviews [1–5], books [6], and symposia reports [7–11] have described studies of basic macrophage function [6,7] and the relationships of macrophages to cancer [1–5,8–11]. The recent developments in the field of the macrophage and cancer amply justify this further review, especially in the rapidly developing area of the effect of tumours upon macrophage immunomodulatory capacity.

THE BASIC CHARACTERISTICS OF MACROPHAGES

The morphological and functional heterogeneity of this cell has led a number of workers [16] to suggest that the cell line, in all its manifestations, should most appropriately be termed the mononuclear phagocyte. This would obviously encompass cells that are well established in this lineage, such as the blood monocyte, tissue macrophage, and Kupffer cells, as well as a tentative designation of other cells about which there is still some dispute. However, despite the logic of the use of the generic term *mononuclear phagocyte*, it has not been widely adopted and we are still faced with the broad nomenclature of monocyte/macrophage cell types, which may all be of the same basic lineage. This section is designed to provide a brief summary of the cells that are of the monocyte/macrophage series and also to describe their basic characteristics.

Characterisation of macrophages

Cells may be identified on a morphological basis, the major factor in determining that the vast number of fixed and free macrophages in the body are all of the same lineage. However, other criteria must be applied; cytoplasmic enzyme and secretory product markers, plasma membrane markers, and functional characteristics are all parameters now regularly applied in the identification of any cell type. In addition, fine antigenic differences between relatively closely related cell types such as those of the monocyte/macrophage series can now be resolved using monoclonal antibodies.

Enzymatic markers

Macrophages exhibit specific markers when examined using enzyme histochemistry. The most reliable marker for the identification of macrophages of human and nonhuman origin is nonspecific esterase [12]. This enzyme is a good general marker but varies in staining intensity between species and depends on the stage of cell maturation.

Lysozyme is another good marker for macrophages and can be demonstrated using a variety of techniques [13,14], although the intensity of immunohistochemical staining varies. Peroxidase has also been used to identify macrophages and staining for this enzyme reveals interesting differences depending upon the type of macrophage: immature and mature monocytes as well as exudate macrophage are positive whereas resident macrophages such as Kupffer cells are negative [15]. Another enzyme, 5'-nucleotidase, that identifies macrophages is additionally useful in that it helps to differentiate activated from resting macrophages, as the former have much lower activity [16].

Many components of the complement cascade are synthesised by macrophages, and this fact may be applied to the identification of macrophages using the appropriate antisera in immunohistochemical techniques.

Plasma membrane markers

The two best documented membrane markers are the receptors for the Fc portion of IgG (γFcR) and the activated by-product of complement activation C3b [17]. Another membrane marker is the dense display of immune-associated (Ia) antigens [18], which are functionally important in the induction of the specific immune response. These three markers are not unique to macrophages; yet the γFc and C3b receptors have important functions in that they can act as receptors for opsonized particles and Ia antigens assist in the induction of the specific immune response, although there may be a subpopulation that does not display Ia antigens.

Functional markers

The functional markers, which include adhesion, pinocytosis, and phagocytosis, are too unreliable and time-consuming to be used for identification purposes. However, these properties are extremely important in terms of function, perturbations of which are considered in subsequent sections.

Monoclonal antibodies

These reagents have recently created a minor revolution in immunology because they allow the recognition of very fine antigenic differences between cells. Monoclonal antibodies directed against macrophages are now commercially available and are becoming widely used for the rapid and precise identification of macrophages in tissue sections and in cell suspensions. Monoclonal antibodies are homogeneous and specific for one antigenic determinant. Thus, these reagents are invaluable in the study of functional membrane receptors of macrophages and enable the detailed study of binding kinetics of immune reactants.

The cells of the macrophage series

The classification of the macrophage series is subject to widely varying ideas and opinions. This author considers that the cells comprising the series are best classified functionally in three groups: (1) the blood monocyte and its immature precursors in the bone marrow, (2) the resident recruited macrophages, which are normally present in many tissues of the body, and (3) the macrophages present in exudates and chronic inflammatory infiltrates.

The blood monocyte

The circulating blood monocyte is almost certainly the source of both the resident macrophage and the exudate/infiltrate macrophage and may have limited ability to divide. It is derived from rapidly dividing precursors in the bone marrow, where monoblasts proliferate to produce promonocytes, which, in turn, mature into monocytes and enter the circulation. Monocytes enter tissues and become recruited resident or infiltrating macrophages.

Recruited resident macrophages in normal tissues

Cells of the macrophage series are extremely numerous in many tissues, where they fulfill essential physiological roles. Such cells include normal connective tissue histiocytes; Kupffer cells in the liver; sinusoidal lining cells in the spleen and lymph nodes; microglial cells; Langerhans's cells in skin; osteoclasts; Paneth cells of the small intestine; and alveolar, pleural, and peritoneal macrophages. The lineage and origin of these resident macrophages has prompted considerable debate, which has been based mainly upon their diverse ultrastructural and cytochemical properties [16,19]. However, the weight of evidence now supports the circulating blood monocyte as the source of all these tissue-recruited macrophages despite their morphological and cytochemical differences.

Connective tissue histiocytes are ubiquitous and play an essential role in the presentation of antigens to the specific immune system [17,20,21]. Kupffer cells of the liver function as the prime antigen-binding and processing cells for material presented to the host via the alimentary tract. Kupffer cells do not divide [22] and are constantly recruited from blood monocytes, which may also be the case for other resident macrophages. Paneth cells of the small intestine are now considered to be of the macrophage series [23], and they may play an important role in the processing and presentation of antigens encountered in the gut. Sinusoidal lining macrophages of the spleen and lymph nodes also trap antigens and initiate specific immune responses at these sites through efective presentation of antigens to lymphocytes. However, the dendritic reticulum cells in these two organs may also function as antigen-presenting cells, but they are not considered to be of the macrophage series [16]. Alveolar and, to a lesser extent, pleural and peritoneal macrophages act chiefly as scavengers of their respective sites but can also act as antigen-presenting cells. Langerhans cells, with their characteristic cytoplasmic Birbeck granules, are of macrophage lineage and of bone marrow origin [24]. Osteoclasts are important cells in bone physiology and calcium homeostasis; they are derived by the fusion of monocytes, and imbalance of osteoclast activity may be an important aspect of the establishment of bone metastases from primary tumours.

Exudate and chronic infiltratory macrophages

The number of tissue macrophages increases in an inflammatory response, particularly in chronic inflammation, but the macrophage numbers depend upon the nature and duration of the stimulus and the character of the tissues involved. Blood monocytes are the source of infiltrating macrophages [25], and sometimes morphologically transitional forms between monocytes and resident macrophages have been observed [26]. Epithelioid cells and multinucleate giant cells are established descriptions of macrophages present in chronic inflammatory infiltrates. Epithelioid cells have reduced phagocytic activity, which may be increased by the products of activated lymphocytes. Multinucleate giant cells are formed by the fusion of macrophages and are present in various histological forms, which may be determined to a degree by the nature of the tissue [16].

THE BASIC FUNCTION OF MACROPHAGES

This section concentrates on fundamental immunological aspects of macrophage function that are most relevant to tumour immunology. These aspects are the role of macrophages as effective antigen presenters in the induction of the specific immune response and their role as efficient effector cells whose function is improved by active specific immunity. The direct roles of these functions in relation to cancer are covered later in this chapter. As described earlier, macrophages are not only morphologically but also functionally heterogeneous.

Macrophages and the induction of the immune response

Macrophage presentation of antigen to lymphocytes is now appreciated to be a vital part of the induction of the specific immune response [17,20].

The site of antigen presentation

Normally, the body first encounters antigens in the skin or in the mucous membranes lining the gastrointestinal and respiratory tracts. Macrophages may present antigen to lymphocytes at these sites, where a specific response may be initiated. This response is probably uncommon, especially in the primary immune response where there are few antigen-specific lymphocytes. The chance of initiating a primary immune response is greatly increased if the antigen is transported from the superficial epithelial sites to local lymphoid tissue such as lymph nodes, gut, and bronchial-associated lymphoid tissue, where there is a continuous recirculation of lymphocytes. Transport of antigens from epithelia to local lymphoid tissue is mediated by macrophages that trap antigens (they may or may not phagocytose them) and then migrate to the local lymphoid tissue. This is best illustrated by Langerhans cells in the skin [27], which trap antigens and then migrate through dermal lymphatics where they are termed a veiled cell to the local lymph node where they are described as interdigitating cells. Similar mechanisms may operate in the mucous membranes, although the local lymphoid tissue is very closely associated with the epithelia. Systemic presentation of antigens will result in trapping by resident recruited macrophages lining the sinusoids of the spleen and liver. In chronic inflammatory responses, infiltrating macrophages can trap and present antigen locally to lymphocytes or transport the antigen to local lymphoid tissue. This will be modified by factors such as the tissue involved and the duration and extent of the inflammatory response.

Macrophage presentation of antigen and the induction of the specific immune response

Although the importance of macrophage presentation of antigens to lymphocytes for an effective immune response has been recognised for some time, only relatively recently have the mechanisms become elucidated, yet further further work is required.

Large antigens such as tumour cells and bacteria may be phagocytosed and partly broken down by macrophages, prior to regurgitation and display on the cell's plasma membrane for recognition by appropriate lymphocytes, whereas small antigen molecules may merely be trapped on the macrophage surface. T-cells circulate more than B-cells and are therefore more likely to encounter macrophage-presented antigen for which the lymphocyte has a receptor. This is important because appropriate activation of antigen-specific T-helper (T_H) cells and T-suppressor (T_S) cells is an essential part of normal immune reactions in that, following an adequate effective immune response, specific immunological homeostatic mechanisms turn it off. Imbalance of T_H and T_S activity may be an important pathogenic mechanism in conditions that have an underlying immune disorder such as autoimmunity, hypersensitivity, and possibly some forms of cancer. The activation of an antigen-specific T-cell is augmented by macrophages in several ways; later sections of this chapter will describe how this may fail in the tumour-bearing host and thus may be a major factor in the growth and spread of a tumour.

Efficient macrophage presentation of antigen and activation of specific T-cells can occur only if the two cell types share the same type-2 major histocompatibility (MHC) antigens. Most macrophages are rich in these type-2 MHC antigens, which are often referred to as immune-associated (Ia) antigens and are represented by products of the HLA-D locus in man. Complementarity of "self" may seem to be an obvious component of the normal immune response, but, rather than simple matching, this self-recognition, coupled with antigen recognition, is an essential part in the induction of a normal immune response. Lymphocytes that have a receptor for an antigen presented by a macrophage are triggered to respond only if they also recognize their own Ia antigen type on the macrophage plasma membrane. Therefore, we have at last a rational role for this component of the MHC complex, and functional roles for the human type-1 MHC antigens in T-cell cytotoxicity are well established; the MHC system was not designed purely to thwart transplantation surgeons.

A number of immunologically relevant low-molecular-weight products of activated macrophages and lymphocytes have been given the respective labels of monokines and lymphokines. The synthesis of these molecules probably depends upon antigen stimulation in the case of lymphokines, but the effect is antigen nonspecific, and these molecules can act as nonspecific immunological mediators. An important monokine is lymphocyte-activating factor (LAF), which is now designated interleukin 1 (IL-1). IL-1 is synthesized by activated macrophages and activates T-helper and T-suppressor cells in the induction and control of specific immunity. The IL-1 synthesizing macrophage and the responsive T-cell have to be activated at the same time—the macrophage nonspecifically or through lymphokines and the T-cell specifically through antigen presentation.

Macrophages are the main source of most of the major complement components, which play an indirect but important function as immunodulators. Complement may lyse susceptible antibody-coated cells, but its most important function is the mediation of inflammation and thus it may play an important role in the response to neoplastic processes.

It has been suggested that two distinct subpopulations of macrophage exist that exert helper and suppressor effects in the induction of the immune response [28,29]. A distinct subpopulation of suppressor macrophages that synthesize prostaglandins, particularly of the E series (PGE$_2$) [30], has been postulated to inhibit human T-cell mitogenesis [31]. Therefore, antigen presentation by suppressor macrophages could profoundly depress a specific immune response. However, the evidence for suppressor macrophages is indirect and the reported subpopulations may be merely maturational variants. The evidence for suppressor macrophages rests mainly on the results of experiments where crude mononuclear cell populations have been depleted of adherent macrophages or, on the blocking of PGE$_2$ synthesis by putative suppressor macrophages using indomethacin. This modified population is then assessed for its ability to modulate a mitogen or a mixed lymphocyte response (MLR) in a separate "responder" lymphocyte population in vitro. However, all "responder" lymphocyte subpopulations would themselves be contaminated with a variable number of monocyte/macrophages that could interfere with these assays. In addition, the results of the use of indomethacin blocking to inhibit and thus identify suppressor PGE$_2$ synthesizing macrophages must be interpreted cautiously because indomethacin, especially at high doses, inhibits the synthesis of other inflammatory modulators, particularly the leukotrienes. Despite uncertainty about macrophage subpopulations, there is a differential requirement for macrophages in the induction of T$_H$ and T$_H$-induced B-cell proliferation [32] that applies to stimulation by any antigen—including tumour cells.

Macrophages as effector cells

The specific role of macrophages as potential killers of tumour cells will be covered later. The following is a brief summary of how macrophages mediate the elimination of foreign antigens where the mechanisms are essentially similar for any chronic inflammatory response irrespective of whether the antigen is a mismatched tissue graft, chronic bacterial infection, or tumour cell. Effector function of macrophages is best considered logically in terms of maturation, migration, phagocytosis, and extracellullar and intracellular killing. Clearly, in comparison to immune inducer function, the different cells of this heterogeneous series do not all function as effector cells in the same way—especially in relation to tumours.

Maturation of macrophages

As described earlier in this chapter, there is now considerable evidence that both exudate and recruited macrophages are derived from the blood monocyte. In turn, this cell is derived from bone marrow stem cells that differentiate into monocytes via monoblasts and promonocytes. Therefore, as recruited macrophages probably do not divide, the bone marrow is a crucial source of all types of macrophages, and bone marrow failure could produce dramatic loss of cells of the monocyte/macrophage series with ensuing loss of both immune inducer and effector function.

Migration of macrophages

The establishment of a blood monocyte as a recruited resident macrophage is a very different process to the migration of monocytes into tissues as exudate/infiltrating macrophages [33], where the monocyte must first marginate against a capillary wall, squeeze between endothelial cells into the tissue space, and then move toward the chronic inflammatory stimulus. Therefore, the natural random locomotion of the macrophages has to be guided, a result that is achieved in a number of ways and is given the collective term *chemotaxis*. This description is not strictly accurate, as some stimuli merely enhance macrophage locomotion-chemokinesis but are not truly tactic. Macrophage locomotion is based upon an actin microfilament system [34] that is calcium and magnesium dependent [33], partly controlled by calmodulin and fueled by ATP [34]. The cell, therefore, must also rely upon a ready two-way flux of these divalent cations across the plasma membrane, and macrophages may be activated or inactivated by substances that show an affinity for the hydrophobic inner cell membrane and thus penetrate the membrane and increase the permeability to ions. Lipids have such properties, which may partially account for the predominant macrophage response to mycobacterial infections and also for the immunoadjuventicity of BCG and *Corynebacterium parvum*.

Chemotactic stimuli are varied in origin and nature and include products of tissue damage, bacterial metabolism and breakdown, products of activated lymphocytes, and by-products of complement activation. Therefore, some chemotactic stimuli may be nonspecific products of tissue damage, but some may be the direct or indirect result of activation of the specific immune response. However, this may not always be true chemotaxis but rather chemokinesis, which would augment the effect of a true chemotactic agent.

Probably the most potent chemotactic factors are the products of complement cleavage that may be initiated by the classical pathway through the interaction of antigen and specific antibody, by the alternative pathway through activation by bacterial endotoxins or aggregated immunoglobulin, or, by the nonspecific action of proteases that may be abundant in sites of chronic inflammation. The complement cleavage fragments that are most chemotactic for macrophages are C3a and C5a, whilst the C567 trimolecular complex is chemotactic for neutrophils but probably not for macrophages [35]. An important point is that macrophages synthesize the native C3 and C5 along with most other complement components [36] and may thus augment local effects of complement activation due to the high concentration of these components at the site. In addition, factors that activate the alternative pathway of complement, and are chemotactic, are elaborated by many microorganisms and possibly also by mammalian cells [37]. These factors are frequently small heterogeneous peptides with blocked amino groups, especially small formylmethionyl peptides [38].

A number of macrophage chemotactic factors produced by antigen- and mitogen-activated lymphocytes have been demonstrated in vitro and are given the generic abbreviation (a habit beloved of immunologists) of LDCF (lymphocyte derived chemotactic factor) [39]. In common with other lymphokines, LDCF is synthesized by activated lymphocytes early in the cell cycle prior to blastogenesis before demonstrable DNA replication [40]. LDCF production is a property of both T-cells and B-cells [41] and has been roughly characterized as of approximately 12,500 molecular weight [42]. B-cells can also be activated to produce LDCF by immune complexes or aggregated immunoglobulin [43], presumably acting directly through the B-cell γFc receptor. Interestingly, there is evidence that LDCF cannot be produced by lymphocytes unless macrophages are also present [44], a fact that may represent a homeostatic-controlling mechanism.

These described studies of monocyte/macrophage chemotactic factors are largely based on in vitro work, and any extrapolation as to their role, or even existence, in vivo must be cautious. Techniques for the in vitro study of chemotaxis rest with migration through agarose or a membrane using a modified Boyden chamber, whereas in vivo studies utilize various skin window techniques. Clearly, there is a need to equate these in vitro and in vivo techniques in order to evaluate the significance of the results of some of these studies.

Phagocytosis by macrophages

Macrophages live up to their name in that they are capable of endocytosing enormous quantities of material. The cell's plasma membrane is in a state of constant activity, and an unstimulated murine macrophage can interiorize an area of plasma membrane equivalent to its total surface area of plasma membrane every 35 minutes [45], and this rate of interiorization is considerably increased in a stimulated cell [46]. The plasticity of the macrophage plasma membrane is evident when the cells are observed phagocytosing; this also emphasizes the fusion of the pseudopodial process around particles being interiorized rather than adhesion to surrounding cells of the same nature. The phagocytic process is enhanced by opsonins for which the macrophage has plasma membrane receptors. The density of such receptors on the macrophage plasma membrane influences the efficiency and rate of uptake of particles. The most important macrophage plasma membrane receptors are for the Fc portion of IgG (γFcR) and the cleaved third component of complement, C3b.

Macrophage γFc membrane receptors probably constitute a heterogeneous population [47,48] with certain IgG class restrictions [49,50]. These receptors may theoretically be saturated by normal serum IgG, which may thus block the phagocytosis of IgG-opsonized particles. However, IgG-coated particles and immune complexes appear to be phagocytosed preferentially, and this may indicate that concentrated IgG, either aggregated or cell bound, is more readily phagocytosed than soluble monomeric IgG. This is an important point in relation to how immune complexes may block the phagocytosis of tumour cells. However, the heterogeneity of the IgG subclass responses to most antigens would mean that macrophage subclass Fc receptor specificity would not normally exert an important influence on macrophage function. Macrophages do not have membrane receptors for the Fc portion of IgM and IgA, which cannot therefore act as opsonic immunoglobulins for this cell line.

The second important membrane receptor is that for the cleaved third component of complement, C3b. This component may be deposited on a target particle either because it was first coated with complement-fixing antibody or because the particle or one of its products could activate the alternative pathway of complement. The effective function of the C3b receptor appears to vary depending on the state of stimulation of the macrophage, as it enhances particle binding but not phagocytosis by resting cells, whereas stimulated macrophages readily ingest complement-coated red cells [51]. Although the γFc and C3b receptors mediate similar functions, they are not coupled to each other, and signals generated by binding to one receptor are not transmitted to the other [52].

Irrespective of which receptors are involved, the phagocytosis of a particle appears to be a local event, with the activation of the pseudopodial and contractile aspects of the cytoskeleton being restricted to the area closely related to a membrane-attached particle [52]. This principle has led to the development of a "zipper" model for the phagocytosis of a particle [53,55,64], whereby the engulfing movement of the macrophage is governed by the sequential and circumferential interaction of plasma membrane receptors with complementary ligands on the particle surface. This implies that there must be even and relatively equal distribution of plasma membrane receptors and particle-bound ligands for effective phagocytosis to occur; unequal distribution would result in binding but not subsequent ingestion of the particle. However, the binding of a particle without ensuing ingestion does not prohibit the macrophage from phagocytosing different particles at other membrane sites where the receptor/ligand distribution is more even or equal [34]. Engulfment and subsequent interiorization of the particle is mediated by the ordered assembly and activation of actin filaments, which is controlled by the mechanisms outlined earlier. The actual linkage of the membrane receptor to the contractile cytoskeleton is mediated by an actin-binding protein that is released from the macrophage plasma membrane during phagocytosis [56]. This protein binds stoichiometrically to actin and helps to localize the assembly of contractile proteins to within a restricted zone of the macrophage cytoplasm.

Besides the membrane receptors already described, other compounds have been proposed as being able to enhance phagocytosis nonspecifically. In particular, fibronectin, a membrane-bound protein closely related to serum "cold insoluble globulin," is reported to be an opsonic protein [57]; any foreign cell that was relatively deficient in this ubiquitous protein would be less readily phagocytosed than a cell rich in fibronectin.

The process of phagocytosis initiates the changes in the macrophage's biochemistry that are required to mediate killing either intra- or extracellularly. Thus the cytotoxic and cytolytic mechanisms are activated almost before the foreign particle such as a bacterium or tumour cell is in a suitable position to be assailed by the macrophage's battery of toxic agents.

Intracellular killing by macrophages

Following phagocytosis the ingested particle is held within the macrophage in a vacuole bound by everted plasma membrane—the phagosome. The particle is then exposed to a battery of toxic agents that may be formed rapidly following phagocytosis or may have been previously synthesized and stored within lysosomes, which must first fuse with the phagosome before their contents can reach the ingested particle. The basic killing mechanisms either are oxygen dependent and consist of the highly reactive radicals resulting from the partial reduction of oxygen or they are oxygen independent and consist of cytotoxic compounds such as lactoferrin, lysozyme, cationic proteins, and changes to an acidic pH [58]. Both mechanisms apply to polymorphonuclear neutrophils (PMN) and macrophages, although there are some qualitative differences and considerable quantitative differences that vary depending upon the type of macrophage.

In the oxygen-dependent mechanism, the partial reduction of oxygen generates free radicals and oxygen derivatives that are highly reactive and toxic and probably represent the most important intracellular killing mechanism of macrophages [58]. The triggering of the reaction is principally controlled by the respiratory burst that is initiated by phagocytosis. Part of the oxygen consumed is converted into singlet oxygen through the increased activation of the hexose monophosphate shunt pathway following phagocytosis [59]. When molecular oxygen (O_2) accepts a single electron, it is converted into the superoxide anion (O_2^-), which may act as a reductant (e.g., of nitroblue tetrazolium, in the NBT test), or as an oxidant when it is reduced to hydrogen peroxide (H_2O_2) spontaneously, or under the catalytic effect of superoxide dismutase, with the release of native oxygen. Oxygen itself may be reduced directly to H_2O_2 by enzymes such as glucose oxidase. Further reduction of H_2O_2 results in the formation of the highly reactive hydroxyl radical ($OH\cdot$), which, again, releases more native O_2. Singlet oxygen ($^1O_2$) may be produced in a variety of ways from O_2^- and also from the interaction of hypochlorite ions with H_2O. Macrophages contain lysosomal and free peroxidase [60], although the quantity is considerably less than in PMNs and varies considerably between the different types of macrophage, with active infiltrating and exudate cells containing more than resident macrophages [15]. Through the peroxidase system, H_2O_2 and halides produce toxic compounds such as hypochlorite ions, which in turn react with H_2O to form more singlet oxygen. Thus, the partial reduction of oxygen results in the generation of a number of potent toxic agents. Although the superoxide anion is not particularly toxic, the hydrogen peroxide, hydroxyl radical, singlet oxygen, and halide derivatives are, and there is a built-in amplification mechanism in that the products of one reaction can be used as substrates for another. Table 3-1 summarizes the generation of toxic oxygen species by macrophages. The plasma membrane is the site for the control of the generation of toxic oxygen species; that is to say, although the effect of these potent oxygen derivatives is best documented in relation to intracellular killing, they could be equally effective in extracellular tumour cell killing [60].

Table 3–1. Macrophage metabolic pathways that generate toxic oxygen species

Pathway			Toxic Product
Hexose monophosphate shunt activation			
$\rightarrow$ NADPH + O_2	Oxidase $\blacktriangleright$	$NADP^+ + O_2^-$	Superoxide anion
$2O_2^- + 2H^+$	Superoxide Dismutase $\blacktriangleright$	$H_2O_2 + O_2$	Hydrogen peroxide
$2O_2^- + 2H^+$	Spontaneous $\blacktriangleright$	$H_2O_2 + {}^1O_2$	Hydrogen peroxide Singlet oxygen
$H_2O_2 + Cl^-$	Peroxidase $\blacktriangleright$	$OCl^- + H_2O$	Hypochlorite ion
$OCl^- + H_2O$	$\blacktriangleright$	${}^1O_2 + Cl^- + H_2O$	Singlet oxygen
$O_2^- + H_2O_2$	$\blacktriangleright$	$OH\cdot + OH + {}^1O_2$	Hydroxyl radical Singlet oxygen

O_2 = Superoxide anion.
$^1O_2$ = Singlet oxygen.
$OH\cdot$ = Hydroxyl radical.
OCl^- = Hypochlorite ion.

Studies of oxygen-independent killing mechanisms have concentrated on PMNs, yet the same systems can operate in macrophages. Lysozyme is an enzyme that can lyse a restricted range of bacteria on its own, but this property is extended to a wide range of bacteria and foreign mammalian cells if they are also coated with antibody and complement. In the macrophage, in contrast to the PMN, not all the lysozyme is lysosome bound and relatively large proportions are constantly secreted [61], which is relevant to the malignant state. Lactoferrin is a potent antimicrobial agent because as an iron-binding protein when not fully saturated, it chelates iron from bacteria and inhibits their metabolism. Cationic proteins with antibacterial properties are probably present in macrophages comparable with those isolated from PMN lysosomes [62]. A heterogeneous group of proteins that are bactericidal in vitro, they have been detected in the phagosome, by cytochemical techniques, bound to ingested organisms, although their mode of action is not clear. The function of these last two systems against ingested nonbacterial particles is uncertain.

MACROPHAGES AND TUMOUR IMMUNITY

So far this chapter has reviewed the basic characteristics and function of the cells of the macrophage series, with occasional reference to cancer. This section initially considers the role of the macrophage as an inducer cell in the specific immune response to a tumour and later as a cytotoxic effector cell that may be spontaneous, or "natural," or under the control of a specific immune response. Many experimental animal tumour models exhibit strong tumour-specific antigens that elicit a brisk immune response. In contrast, little success has been achieved in detecting comparable tumour-specific immunogenic antigens on human tumours. However, the techniques employed are still relatively crude, and fine immunological differences must exist between the neoplastic cell and the normal cell from which it was derived. Macrophages are crucial in the initiation of a specific response to a tumour cell and their dysfunction may contribute to the relative nonimmunogenicity of human cancers.

Macrophages and the induction of immune responses to tumours

Little work has been done on the actual functional role of macrophages in the initiation of specific immune responses to tumours, and most approaches have been oriented toward the study of the effect of tumour cells on the induction potential of macrophages described below. An important aspect is the available number of monocytes and their precursors and also the degree of natural and inducible maturation of the cells, which has been reported to be reduced in a number of malignancies [4]. In this context, large numbers of macrophages in the stroma of a tumour are reported to correlate with a good prognosis and reduced metastatic potential [63]. It has also been suggested that a reduction in the numbers of resident macrophages may predispose to malignancy [64].

Monocyte/macrophage numbers and maturity

A lack of macrophages could be an important factor in enhancing the chance of tumour development because of the importance of this cell in the induction and effector arms of the immune response. Reduction in macrophage numbers may result from a lack of monocytes and their precursors such as may occur in malignant disease involving the bone marrow [4,65], and occasionally following drug-induced marrow toxicity and irradiation damage. In addition to reduced numbers of macrophages in skin window exudates in patients with Hodgkin's disease [65], a general increase in immature forms of macrophages in such exudates has been reported in patients with malignant lymphoma [66]. In these patients a much higher proportion of macrophages with a ridged or ruffled membrane morphology was found, compared with normal subjects in whom the predominant cells had a mature microvillous appearance. In vitro culture studies have also demonstrated an immaturity of blood monocytes in a wide range of malignancies [67–72], including squamous cell carcinoma of the lung [67], malignant melanoma [68,70], colonic carcinoma [70], renal carcinoma [71], and breast cancer [72]. These in vitro studies suggest that, in malignancy, there may be an in vivo depression of maturation of the cells of the monocyte/macrophage series, which may correlate with the inability to respond to a tumour or may be the direct result of tumour growth on macrophage maturation. Depression of macrophage maturation has been reported to correlate with an increased tumour load in experimental animals [73] and is associated with a poor prognosis in humans [74,75].

So far, this section has covered only the suggestion that immaturity of blood monocytes and tissue macrophages and reduced numbers of tissue macrophages might facilitate the emergence and growth of neoplastic cells. In contrast, there are reports that blood monocyte numbers are normal or raised in a number of lymphoid and nonlymphoreticular malignant states [76,77]. However, the number of blood monocytes in tumour-bearing experimental animals and patients does not provide information about the functional status of these cells. The results of the maturation studies indicate that although blood monocyte numbers are normal in some malignant states, the increased proportion of morphologically immature forms may reflect a depressed functional capacity of the cells both as inducers and effectors of the specific immune response. The monocytosis reported in a number of malignant states has lead to the concept that the monocytosis may consist predominantly of "suppressor" monocytes that could exert a depressive effect on the specific immune response [28].

Recently, attention has been drawn to the relationship of resident macrophage numbers in certain organs and malignant disease [64]. The concept of a reduced number of resident macrophages predisposing to tumour development may be analogous to a reduced number or degree of maturation of blood monocytes as macrophage precursors. Depletion of Kupffer cells in chronic liver disease has been postulated [64] as a mechanism that reduces immunosurveillance, permitting neoplastic transformation of hepatocytes, which may help to explain the increased incidence of liver-cell carcinoma in this condition. Experimental rat evidence supports the association of progressive depletion of Kupffer cells with the tendency for chemical-induced hepatic nodules to develop into tumours [78]. In humans with liver fluke hepatic infestation, the periductular mononuclear cell infiltration is associated with Kupffer cell depletion and malignant transformation [79] not in the areas of the chronic inflammatory infiltrate but with hyperplastic and adenomatous biliary polyps [80]. The high incidence of metastatic cancer deposition in the liver would argue against the hypothesis, but the process of metastasis may not be a fair comparison with tumour development in situ [64], as the macrophage capacity is probably more limited in its ability to eliminate a tumor embolus than a single-cell neoplastic transformation. The analogy has been drawn to the reduced numbers of Paneth cells in coeliac disease [23] where there is an increased incidence of small-intestinal malignancy [81]. Paneth cells may function as immune surveillance cells, and their reduced numbers in coeliac disease are associated not only with an increased incidence of small-intestinal malignancy but also with other organ-unrelated autoimmune diseases. As well as functioning as immunosurveillance cells for local tumour development, these resident macrophages in the liver and small intestine may also act as filters for potential carcinogens of dietary or microbial origin; this may be a second mechanism whereby depletion of these cells predisposes to malignancy.

The number of macrophages infiltrating primary tumours and metastases has already been mentioned, and their study may be extremely important in helping us to understand the role of this heterogeneous cell line in malignant disease. However, the literature is confusing on this point and provides limited solid information, due mainly to the technical problems of accurately enumerating the macrophage content of a tumor. A prominent macrophage stromal tumour infiltrate has been interpreted as associated with a good prognosis [1,82]. Also, in some human tumours the macrophage content was inversely related to the tendency to metastasize [83], especially in human breast carcinoma [84]. In contrast to these reports, no correlation was found between the numbers of infiltrating macrophages and tumour behaviour in human colonic carcinoma [85], and in rodent tumours the macrophage content neither correlated with in vivo and in vitro growth rates nor with the metastatic potential of the tumours [86]. However, Gauci [87] has reported that a reduced macrophage content in the normally immunogenic rat sarcoma (HSBPA) is associated with a lack of immunogenicity, but thymectomy had little effect on the ease with which such tumours metastasized. Also, in 56 solid human tumours the macrophage content of metastasizing tumours was low (less than 10%) compared with primary or locally recurrent tumours (0 to 30%). Using macrophage-extraction techniques [70], it was shown that tumour-infiltrating macrophages were relatively reduced in colonic carcinoma, head and neck carcinomas, and benign breast disease, compared with ''normal'' numbers in breast carcinoma and increased numbers in lung cancer. Reports of the macrophage content of tumours must be interpreted cautiously because (1) different techniques have been employed that provide very differing sensitivities and (2) the mere enumeration of macrophages provides little information about their health or their functional capacity.

Macrophages and the induction of immune responses to tumours

The number of available normal functional monocytes/macrophages may be an important factor in the host's ability to respond to a tumour. However, the question of the functional significance of levels of peripheral blood monocytes, and of normal resident, exudate, and tumour-infiltrating macrophages, as raised earlier, is not resolved. The monocytosis observed in some patients with solid tumours [76] may be a proliferation of suppressor monocytes, which can actively depress the specific immune response and facilitate tumour development and spread. Little work has been done on the changes in macrophage function as inducer cells in the specific immune response, although indirect evidence suggests that this function is depressed in the tumour-bearing host [28].

Most of the work on the inducer function of macrophages in the malignant state has been done using indirect techniques. Monocytes/macrophages are as essential for the normal in vitro lymphocyte proliferative responses to mitogens such as PHA and allogeneic cells as they are for the in vivo induction of a specific immune response. Therefore the suppressor/stimulator status of monocytes from patients has been studied by adding their monocytes to mitogen-stimulated cultures of normal lymphocytes or by depleting or metabolically inhibiting monocytes in stimulated autologous cultures of patients' lymphocytes. In any of these systems a reduced lymphocyte proliferative response is considered to indicate monocyte suppressor activity.

Macrophage depletion techniques demonstrated adherent suppressor cells in lung and breast cancer patients [88]; the adherent cells could also suppress the mitogen response of lymphocytes from normal individuals. In a study of 78 patients with nonlymphoreticular tumours, Wood et al. [77] found that monocytosis in mononuclear cell preparations was associated with a suppressed T-cell response to mitogens; a depressed PHA response in the majority of 35 patients with untreated nonlymphoreticular tumours correlated with raised levels of monocytes in their mononuclear cell preparations [76]. In addition, patients with disseminated tumours had higher levels of blood monocytes and lower levels of mitogen-induced T-cell reactivity, compared with patients who had minimal local disease [76]. Schulof et al. [89] reported a suppressor cell for lymphocytes that was responsive to the mitogen concanavalin A (con-A) in patients with Hodgkin's disease, but were unable to prove whether the suppressor cell was a monocyte or a T-suppressor cell. They used a mixed-culture technique that involved the cocultivation of lymphocytes with artifactually high numbers of unfractionated putative suppressor cells, a process that makes interpretation of the data extremely difficult. However, adherent mononuclear cells were identified as suppressor cells of lymphoproliferation in a number of disseminated malignances [90].

The mixed lymphocyte reaction (MLR), coupled with adherent cell depletion/restoration techniques [91], was used to study immunoreactivity in 54 patients with carcinoma of the mouth, larynx, and pharynx; 67% had demonstrable deficient cell-mediated immunity of whom 56% had adherent monocyte suppressor cells. This work utilized the patient's peripheral mononuclear cells only as responder cells in the MLR; it would have been interesting to have used the patient's cells as stimulators in view of the important role of macrophages as inducers of an in vivo immune response to which the in vitro MLR has some counterparts. This approach was used in patients with Hodgkin's disease [92] and showed that adherent cells could act as suppressors in the stimulator MLR population, thus confirming the reduced MLR in this disease. Interestingly, the adherent suppressor cells could not alter the response of lymphocytes from unrelated individuals but could suppress the response in a histocompatible sibling, thus confirming the restriction of the major histocompatibility system on macrophage-lymphocyte interactions and suggesting that macrophage-mediated suppression may be a normal immunoregulatory mechanism that is altered in Hodgkin's disease. This concept was confirmed by the suppression of lymphoproliferation by high concentrations of normal human monocytes [93]. Increased suppressor monocytes in malignancy are best documented in relation to Hodgkin's disease [94–96]. However, other workers [97] did not detect monocyte abnormalities in active Hodgkin's and non-Hodgkin's lymphoma patients whose monocytes had normal helper and suppressor activity in homologous or heterologous lymphocyte responses to con-A. In addition, in lymphoma [98] monocyte enzyme activity did not correlate with lymphocyte function. However, in gastric cancer [99] although monocyte suppressor cells decreased after total tumour resection, in patients with advanced disease the occurrence of suppressor cells was associated with a significantly increased survival.

The functional capacity of monocytes/macrophages as inducer cells in cancer patients, and the possible existence of a separate suppressor population, has been studied in relation to prostaglandin (PG) synthesis by monocytes [30]. These studies are based on the suppressive effect of PGs on lymphocytes [31] and use assays outlined earlier. Evidence suggests an increase of prostaglandin-synthesizing monocytes/macrophages in cancer patients that are suppressive for T-lymphocytes. The well-documented depression of the lymphoproliferative response to mitogens in the majority of patients with Hodgkin's disease and non-Hodgkin's lymphoma could be abrogated by indomethacin [100]. However, the addition of indomethacin to the cultures did not eliminate the difference between the patients and controls. Indomethacin was usually incorporated for the full culture period, but prior exposure of putative suppressor cells in a few cases indicated a slight trend toward an increased lymphoproliferative response. In two small studies [95,101] in patients with Hodgkin's disease, indomethacin enhanced the in vitro lymphoproliferative response to PHA but no similar increase was observed in normal subjects; moreover, oral indomethacin treatment improved lymphocyte responsiveness to suboptimal concentrations of PHA in two patients [101].

A fourfold increase in PGE_2 synthesis after 48 hours of PHA-stimulated lymphocyte culture in Hodgkin's disease was detected compared with controls. Removal of adherent cells decreased the indomethacin enhancement, reduced PGE_2 production by more than 89%, and eliminated the differences in response to PHA between lymphocytes from Hodgkin's disease and controls [95]. Thus, there is evidence for excessive activity of PGE_2-synthesizing monocytes mediating the mitogen hyporesponsiveness of lymphocytes in patients with Hodgkin's disease. Similar techniques have been applied to demonstrate monocyte suppressor cells in patients with a variety of solid tumors [76] and melanoma [102]. In contrast, in a relatively large series of patients with lung carcinoma [103] the PHA response of purified T-lymphocytes was depressed in only 20% of 30 patients, but 87% of the patients had suppressor cells that appeared to be monocytes. However, cell characterisation was partly based upon the assumption that suppressor monocytes/macrophages are extremely radioresistant, but this criterion does not delineate a truly separate population and may merely indicate that the monocytes had been activated [104]. The use of carrageenan, which is toxic for monocytes/macrophages, provided evidence for active nonspecific suppressor monocytes in patients with colorectal, lung and head and neck carcinoma [105].

Multiple myeloma frequently presents as an immune paresis with considerably reduced synthesis of normal immunoglobulins. This was originally attributed to the homeostatic influence of the monoclonal immunoglobulin on the normal, unrelated, polyclonal immunoglobulins. However, in vitro culture of peripheral blood B-cells from 22 myeloma patients showed impaired synthesis of polyclonal immunoglobulins compared with healthy controls, and monocytes from some myeloma patients suppressed polyclonal immunoglobulin synthesis by normal cultured B-cells [106]. This finding was not observed in all patients but may be important in the induction of an immune paresis in multiple myeloma, where the relative paresis does not always correlate with levels or class of mono-clonal immunoglobulins.

Little work has been done on the immunoinduction activity of macrophages in tumour-bearing animals. Accumulation of peritoneal macrophages, delayed type hypersensitivity reactions to recall antigens [107], and reduced systemic and local resistance to microorganisms such as Listeria monocytogenes and Yersinia enterocolitica were depressed in tumour-bearing animals [108–110]. The clearance of inert particles of colloidal carbon was reduced in C57BL mice bearing the Lewis lung carcinoma [111], which emphasises the nonspecific depression of monocyte/macrophage function in tumour-bearing animals. In addition the clearance of colloidal carbon, peritoneal macrophage chemotaxis, and marrow-derived macrophage colony formation exhibited a triphasic response [111]—depressed ac-tivity was followed by normal or enhanced activity with a third phase featuring decline of all macrophage activity. The relative short duration of such animal experiments may be im-portant when relating the results to human cancers that may have been established for a considerable time before diagnosis.

A further interesting aspect of macrophage-inducer function in cancer is the influence of macrophages over natural killer (NK) cells. As described earlier, activated monocytes/macrophages may augment all lymphocyte reactivity, including NK and antibody-dependent cell-mediated cytotoxicity (ADCMC), probably by the synthesis of in-terleukin 1 (IL-1) and interferons [112]. Monocyte-depleted lymphocyte populations ex-hibited little NK activity [113], which could be restored by the addition of peripheral blood monocytes of low specific gravity. This monocyte subpopulation contained the lowest esterase, peroxidase, and ADCMC activity but induced T-cell proliferation in vitro and synthesized IL-1. Although denser monocytes produced IL-1, they not only failed to augment NK activity [114] but actually suppressed it, thus suggesting the operation of other factors. Interferon may be important, especially as macrophage IL-1 induces the syn-thesis of interferon [115], which enhances NK activity. These potential pathways by which monocytes/macrophages may modulate NK activity have been studied using normal murine peritoneal [116], human alveolar [117], and malignant plural effusion [118] macrophages, all of which suppressed in vitro NK activity. Possibly, mature cells of the macrophage series, especially if activated, can act as NK suppressors, in contrast to the enhancing effect observed in the low-density blood monocyte [114]. It is beyond the scope of this chapter to speculate on the importance of NK-cells and their modulation by macrophages in tumour immunity; undoubtedly, they are potentially important effector cells, although the high degree of specificity for in vitro tumour cell targets and variable macrophage effects implies that their role may be limited.

Most studies of monocytes/macrophages as inducer cells are indirect and few data relate directly to the role of these cells as inducers of tumour immunity or even of a normal specific immune response. Some of the studies reporting a monocytosis in cancer patients enumerated the monocytes in mononuclear cell preparations that may have been depleted or augmented of monocytes during the initial separation from whole blood; the results, therefore, must be interpreted cautiously. Separation techniques may not only alter the relative number of monocytes but may select for a functionally distinct population that might be a true subpopulation or a maturational variant that is increased or decreased in the cancer patient. Thus, variations in techniques may explain some of the conflicting data and effect the interpretations of much of the work in both experimental animals and cancer patients. However, the tumour state evidences a depression of the monocyte/macrophage ability to induce an immune response, which is generally explained by the predominance of a suppressor cell form rather than numerical lack or dysfunction of normal monocytes/ macrophages.

Macrophages as effector cells against tumours

This section covers the role of the macrophage in tumour killing in terms parallel to its normal function described earlier. Migration, attachment, phagocytosis, and killing will be considered separately; the interesting point of numbers and maturity of blood monocytes, resident macrophages, and tumour-infiltrating macrophages has already been covered.

Macrophage migration and tumours

Two aspects will be considered: first, the migration of monocytes/macrophages into tumours and their in vitro chemotaxis toward tumour cells or their extracts and, second, the migration of macrophages from patients and tumour-bearing animals toward nontumour chemotactins in vitro or spontaneously, in vivo, using skin window techniques.

Macrophages infiltrate a tumour in response to stimuli that may be principally of tumour origin, T-cell lymphokines such as LDCF, or complement activation. A reduced macrophage stromal infiltration could be accounted for by changes in any of these three mechanisms or by an antichemotactic effect of tumours depressing the normal chemotaxis. Tumour chemotactins have not been adequately characterized or assayed in vitro, and evidence supporting a generalized chemotactic defect of monocytes/macrophages in cancer is based upon the chemotactic response to nontumour stimuli. Peripheral blood monocytes from patients with various malignancies, including malignant melanoma, carcinoma, lymphoma, sarcoma, and multiple myeloma, all exhibited depressed responses in vitro to standard chemotactins [119–130]. This depression was generally related to the extent of the disease and was partially reversed following tumour removal [121,126] or immunotherapy [130,131]; uncharacterized chemotactic inhibiting factors for normal monocytes have been described in up to 90% of patients with lung and prostatic carcinoma [126]. However, local factors may be important, as the depressed chemotaxis of bronchopulmonary lavage monocytes from patients with primary lung carcinoma was greater in macrophages obtained from the vicinity of the tumour than in cells from the opposite, tumour-free lung [132].

Limited numbers of animal experiments support the general concept of depressed macrophage chemotaxis in the tumour-bearing host. Rats bearing subcutaneous transplants of chemically induced tumours [133] or with intramuscular transplants of syngeneic sarcomas [134] showed a decreased peritoneal macrophage response to inflammatory stimuli that was directly proportional to the degree of tumour growth and spread of disease [133]. Also, peritoneal macrophages in mice carrying the BP8 sarcoma subcutaneously showed decreased responses in vivo to PHA or proteose peptone and decreased in vitro chemotaxis [121]. Macrophage chemotaxis was also depressed in mice bearing the Lewis lung carcinoma [111], especially in animals bearing tumours for long periods.

In man, in vivo skin window studies of macrophage chemotaxis demonstrate a depression in Hodgkin's and non-Hodgkin's lymphoma patients [4] and also in solid tumours [135,136] irrespective of treatment. In untreated patients the depression of chemotaxis was more marked in advanced, widespread disease [135] and was partly reversed following immunotherapy or plasmapheresis. In contrast to disseminated disease, patients with localized carcinomas tended to exhibit increased macrophage chemotaxis that returned to normal after tumour resection [135,136].

Macrophages, phagocytosis, and tumours

Tumour cells may be phagocytosed [137] and killed by macrophages. However, most tumour cell killing may be an extracellular event but this requires adherence between the macrophage and tumour cell, which is probably of an identical nature to that preceding phagocytosis. Phagocytosis in the tumour-bearing state has usually been investigated indirectly using nontumour targets and in vitro techiques such as the uptake of microorganisms, erythrocytes, or latex particles; chemiluminescence; the reduction of nitroblue tetrazolium (NBT); and the expression of macrophage membrane lgG Fc receptors (γFcR). In vivo studies have been based upon the clearance of labeled albumin or lipid.

Studies of monocyte/macrophage phagocytic function in malignant states provide conflicting data ranging from reports of hypo- to hyperactivity [123,126,129,138–151]. Increased phagocytic activity was found in patients with untreated Hodgkin's disease [150] and with miscellaneous untreated carcinomas [129,138,139]. In contrast, decreased phagocytosis has been reported in Hodgkin's disease [140,141], especially in patients with more extensive disease. The increased NBT reduction by monocytes from patients with micrometastatic melanoma compared with disseminated melanoma was interpreted as indicating functionally reduced phagocytosis in advanced disease [142]. However, the quantitative NBT test is difficult to make reproducible, and NBT reduction may occur irrespective of phagocytosis and only indicates activation of the hexose monophosphate shunt pathway. Chemiluminescence is triggered by this pathway and was increased in phagocytosing monocytes from patients with various lymphomas but not with solid tumours [143]. The expression of monocyte γFcR was increased in patients with various untreated carcinomas [147], normal in cases of lung and prostatic carcinoma [126], and increased in patients with solid carcinomas following immunotherapy with *Corynebacterium parvum* [151]. In a group of untreated patients with solid tumours, enhanced monocyte phagocytosis of opsonized sheep erythrocytes was related to an increased rate of phagocytosis as well as cell numbers, although no association was found with the type or clinical staging of the tumour [139]. In contrast, monocyte phagocytosis of *Staphylococcus aureus* was normal in patients with lymphoma and lung carcinoma but depressed in patients receiving cytotoxic drugs [123].

In experimental mice bearing intrafootpad syngeneic fibrosarcomas, peritoneal macrophage phagocytosis of opsonized sheep erythrocytes was augmented considerably, especially during early tumour growth, compared with a marked depression of chemotactic responses [149], suggesting a dissociation of these two functions. The depression of macrophage chemotaxis contrasted with the four- to five-fold increase in phagocytosis, especially within one week of tumour transplantation, and was accounted for by an increased phagocytic rate and number of macrophages. However, the increased phagocytosis was transient, having returned to normal quite rapidly, and may be explained by an acute phase response to tumour implantation. In addition, peritoneal macrophages from mice bearing the 180-sarcoma showed enhanced phagocytosis of *Staphylococcus aureus* after tumour implantation but was followed by depressed function [152]. Increased binding of the ascites tumour line-10 hepatoma cells by peritoneal guinea pig macrophages was induced by activation with lymphocyte-derived factors such as macrophage-activating factor (MAF) or mitogen-induced lymphocyte factors [153]; the study suggested a specific macrophage-tumour cell binding mechanism that depended upon macrophage activation.

The results of studies of monocyte/macrophage phagocytosis in cancer patients and animals are conflicting, thus compounding the confusion concerning the role of this cell in tumour immunity. The study of opsonic factors in relation to the adherence of macrophages to tumour cells prior to extracellular killing is an interesting area, especially in relation to the role of fibronectin [57]. It must also be remembered that the balance between host and tumour is in constant flux and that tumour therapy and the intercurrent infections frequently suffered by cancer patients may further influence macrophage function [4].

Macrophages and tumour cell killing

The tumouricidal activity of macrophages must be regarded as their most important function, but it cannot be seen as a single entity because it depends upon other macrophage functions, variations in which may modulate tumouricidal activity. Most macrophage-mediated tumour cell killing is probably extracellular, although intracellular killing can occur [137,154] and the cytotoxic mechanisms are essentially similar. Macrophage tumour cell killing is essentially of a nonspecific "natural" nature, but this function can be enhanced by products of specific immunity such as lymphokines and opsonic antibody. The latter is the basis for the phenomenon of antibody-dependent cell-mediated cytotoxicity (ADCMC), which is slightly misleading because the cytotoxicity is innate and not truly dependent upon but is enhanced by specific antibody, although there may be differences in the predominant metabolic pathways activated. This section first covers basic tumouricidal macrophage mechanisms, then considers in vitro and in vivo macrophage activities in the tumour-bearing host, and finally includes the results of studies of intratumour macrophages.

MACROPHAGE TUMOURICIDAL MECHANISMS. Earlier, we considered that macrophages have two antitumour roles of true cytolysis and cytostasis, induced through an inhibition of DNA synthesis [155]. More likely, rather than two populations of effector macrophages, functional variants exist that depend upon the degree of macrophage activation. Some of the cytotoxic cytolytic/macrophage mechanisms exhibit a considerable increase following activation by a variety of agents such as lymphokines, complement cleavage and other products of inflammation, lipopolysaccharide (LPS), and whole microorganisms. Interestingly, whilst immune complexes may activate a macrophage through binding to γFcR, the cell might then be unable to bind to a tumour cell via cytophilic antibody. Binding of macrophages to tumour cells is probably prerequisite to extracellular killing and may be a major macrophage-activating mechanism [156]. An important aspect of binding in relation to cytolysis is that there are narrow clefts between activated macrophages and bound targets where diffusion of secreted cytotoxic agents might be limited and thus produce a concentration of these agents where they would be protected from any inhibitors in the extracellular fluid [157,158]. Macrophage-secreted cytotoxic agents have already been described; additionally, however, there are some mechanisms that may be peculiar to tumour targets.

Hydrogen peroxide is probably the major mediator in ADCMC [159–161]. The role of H_2O_2 in natural cytotoxicity may be more important than originally thought, as eosinophil peroxidases can convert it to very active halogen derivatives [162] and presumably other peroxidases can operate in the same way. In natural cytotoxicity, various macrophage-secreted antitumour proteins have been described. Murine macrophages contain an extremely potent tumouricidal serine protease of 40,000 molecular weight that can lyse a wide spectrum of tumour target cells [163]; one activated macrophage can secrete sufficient cytolytic protease (CP) to lyse between 10 and 20 tumour cells. CP has been partly characterized by demonstrating that low-molecular-weight inhibitors of serine protease inhibit macrophage natural cytotoxicity and that CP-deficient macrophages cannot become cytotoxic in response to activation with LPS. There is also synergistic action between CP and H_2O_2, which implies that H_2O_2 secretion may be important in natural cytotoxicity. In contrast, cytolytic proteases do not appear to be involved in ADCMC [156].

Other macrophage secretory products have been described that are capable of producing massive tumour cell necrosis (TNF) in vivo [164]. However, TNF remains uncharacterized and appears to be very heterogeneous. A better characterized potential antitumour macrophage-secreted product is arginase [165], which can deprive neoplastic cells of their high arginine requirement and thus be cytotoxic. However, in vivo studies [166] do not correlate well with the in vitro evidence for arginase as an important tumouricidal modulator [165,167]. Other secreted macrophage enzymes may be directly lytic; these are lysozyme, neutral proteases, and lysosomal hydrolases, of which β-glucuronidase and N-acetyl glucosaminidase are the best documented [168].

Although lysozyme is potentially an important tumouricidal enzyme, its secretion is not related to the degree of macrophage activation in vivo or in vitro, but complement enhancement of the lysozyme system is important, especially as most of the complement components are also synthesised by macrophages. Plasminogen activator, which converts plasminogen into plasmin, was the first macrophage secretory neutral protease to be identified. It is not actively secreted by resting macrophages but is secreted in considerable quantities by infiltrating and in vitro activated macrophages [168]. The lytic nature of plasmin would confer an important pathogenic role for excess secretion of plasminogen activator that could facilitate local tumour spread.

Acid hydrolases such as β-glucuronidase and N-acetyl glucosaminidase are secreted in small quantities by resting macrophages, but their secretion is greatly enhanced by phagocytosis or nonspecific activators [168]; such hydrolases could be effective if their pH optima could be maintained in the microclefts [157,158] between the macrophage and the tumour cell.

The study of the molecular tumouricidal mechanisms in malignant states has provided some indirect information about macrophage function in neoplasia, although the potential synergistic action of some of the cytotoxic systems makes interpretation difficult. Regrettably, owing to technical problems, direct evidence of effective macrophage tumouricidal function in human malignancies is sparse; only indirect evidence is available using either heterogeneous tumour or nontumour targets. Most work on macrophage tumouricidal mechanisms fails to stress the possible variation in susceptibilities of tumour cell targets and that successful neoplastic evolution may actually involve acquisition of properties that make tumour cells less susceptible to macrophage cytotoxic mechanisms. In addition, if tumour growth induces a state of anergy in the heterogeneous macrophage population, much of the tumouricidal potential of macrophages against tumour cells would be unavailable.

IN VIVO AND IN VITRO MACROPHAGE TUMOURICIDAL ACTIVITY IN EXPERIMENTAL TUMOURS AND IN HUMAN MALIGNANCIES. Macrophage tumouricidal activity may be studied in vitro against autologous or heterologous tumour cell targets, although the former target is usually unavailable in humans and thus necessitates the frequent use of nontumour targets. There is limited information about the role of macrophages in tumour cytotoxicity from in vivo experiments as regards the extrapolation to human malignancies because most studies of macrophage tumouricidal mechanisms in experimental animals have used peritoneal macrophages whereas most human studies have used blood monocytes. Technical problems also abound; the most careful separation techniques may still leave a few NK-cells in macrophage preparations, and the natural cytotoxicity of peritoneal macrophages may vary considerably compared with macrophages from other sites. In addition, the kinetics of spontaneous in vitro killing may be influenced by the nature of the macrophage-activating stimulus and the nature of the target.

It has been confirmed that macrophages must be activated in order to become tumouricidal. This applies to natural "spontaneous" cytotoxicity, lymphokine-directed cytotoxicity, and ADCMC, although the tumour recognition mechanisms are different; the altered topography of a tumour cell may account for how an activated macrophage can recognize it as different from a nontransformed cell and mediate natural cytotoxicity [169]. Direct tumour cell activation provides evidence for the separation of macrophage function into cytostasis and cytolysis by showing that macrophage-mediated arrest of the cell cycle of a replicating tumour cell is fully reversible within 16 to 24 hours, whereas the cytolytic process proceeds irreversibly after 8 to 12 hours of contact with activated macrophages [2,170,171]. However, this does not necessarily imply that there are subsets of effector macrophages because the effector capacity of a macrophage may be governed to an extent by the activating stimulus. A slow-acting form of spontaneous cytotoxicity by macrophages against a wide range of syngeneic, allogeneic, and xenogeneic tumour cells has been described [171–173] that is effective over 24 hours and requires particularly close effector/target contact. The mechanisms are not yet characterized but appear to be oxygen independent and are most likely to be mediated by the secretion of neutral or cytolytic proteases [158,163,174].

The most relevant macrophage activators in relation to cytotoxicity are probably lymphokines derived from antigen- or mitogen-stimulated lymphocytes. Human macrophages, derived from cultured monocytes, acquired enhanced cytotoxicity for human tumour cell targets following 24-hour preincubation with supernates from tumour-stimulated lymphocytes, but no change in activity was observed against nonmalignant target cells [175]. This lymphokinelike activation was effective after 8 hours of preincubation and persisted for at least 40 hours after removal of the lymphocyte-derived mediators. There is now strong evidence that immune interferon gamma (IFNγ) is the principal lymphokine that activates macrophage oxidative metabolism and antimicrobial activity [176] and induces γFcR expression [177]. However, IFNγ may not be the single identity of macrophage-activating factor (MAF), as nonimmune fibroblast interferon (IFNβ) can also activate macrophages [178], although IFNβ is also reported to reduce macrophage H_2O_2 production and bactericidal activity with an associated reduction in suppressive capacity [179]. It is probable [180] that the macrophage's own secreted lysozyme may potentiate monocyte tumour killing in addition to lipid changes in the macrophage membrane following tumour contact [181].

Monocytes from healthy humans exhibited natural cytotoxicity and ADCMC against the nonadherent tumour target cell lines K562 and CLA-4 [182]; the result was enhanced by stimulation with endotoxin-treated serum and was effective over a relatively long period of 24 to 72 hours. This cytotoxicity was not due to contaminating NK-cells and was abrogated by the addition of silica particles. In Hodgkin's disease, increased ADCMC was mediated by elutriation-purified blood monocytes [183], although the target was antibody-coated chicken erythrocytes and not a tumour cell. In contrast [184], monocyte cytotoxicity against *herpesvirus*-infected targets was reduced in a different group with Hodgkin's disease.

The considerable literature on macrophage tumouricidal activity in animal models has helped to confirm the similarity between basic bactericidal and tumouricidal mechanisms [185]. Evidence for lymphokine activation of macrophages comes from experiments that immunized mice intraperitoneally with an allogeneic lymphoma; subsequently the peritoneal macrophages were rapidly cytotoxic (8–12 hours) for the same lymphoma cells in vitro [186]. This targeting appeared to be lymphokine controlled because nonimmune macrophages could be made tumouricidal by prior culture with approximately equal numbers of appropriate alloimmune peritoneal lymphocytes [155,187–189]. This mechanism was confirmed in the mouse B16 melanoma model [190], where immune macrophages from tumour-bearing mice were cytotoxic for the B16 tumour in vitro and nonimmune macrophages were not. However, nonimmune macrophages became tumouricidal following preincubation with lymphocyte supernates from tumour-immunized syngeneic, allogeneic, or xenogeneic animals but not from corresponding unimmunized animals. Thus, genetic and species barriers did not apply to lymphokine macrophage activation in that model [190]. Similar lymphokine-modulated macrophage cytotoxicity has been demonstrated against mouse mastocytoma and EL-4 lymphoma tumour cells [191]. In animals, lymphokine activation of macrophage cytotoxicity may be effective only in the early stages of tumouricidal activity [169], but this study compared lymphokine activation with artificial stimuli such as LPS and amphotericin B. In addition, it was implied that tumouricidal activity was a late event in macrophage activation, which is in contrast to others [2]. Animal models of cancer facilitate the study of macrophage function and the evaluation of immunostimulants that are presumed to act on macrophages [171]. However, caution must be exercised in the extrapolation to man, especially in relation to the effect of a sudden, and often large, tumour burden imposed on an animal and the use of nontumour targets to assess macrophage cytotoxicity.

REDUCED MACROPHAGE CYTOTOXICITY IN VIVO AND IN VITRO IN EXPERIMENTAL TUMOURS AND IN HUMAN MALIGNANCY. In contrast to the generally effective tumouricidal activities of macrophages just reported, depressed cytotoxic function of macrophages has been widely reported in malignant states. This contrast is heightened by the differing reported cytotoxic capacity of macrophages not only in similar human malignant disease states but also in animal models that share a very similar design to each other. Reduced tumouricidal capacity could be due to enhanced tumour resistance or reduced cytotoxic capacity of macrophages; this latter possibility may be directly or indirectly related to tumour cells.

Information about depressed macrophage cytotoxicity has been derived directly and indirectly, the latter evidence being based upon the concept that tumouricidal mechanisms are also effective against bacteria and protozoa. Cultured human macrophages derived from monocytes of 66 patients with colonic, breast, and cervical carcinomas; leukaemias; and lymphomas were studied for their ability to kill the target cell lines SK-BR-3 and HT-29 derived from human adenocarcinomas of the breast and the colon, respectively [192]. Macrophage activation with LPS enhanced cytotoxicity in the colonic carcinoma and leukaemia/lymphoma group but not in the breast and cervical carcinoma group. A plasma factor that inhibited macrophage tumour cytotoxicity was found in a large proportion of the patients of all groups, although total abrogation of tumouricidal activity was uncommon. These cytotoxicity-inhibiting plasma factors have been partially purified and characterized as variously inhibiting lysozomal enzyme and protease activity [193]. In renal carcinoma adherent monocytes displayed reduced cytotoxicity against K-562 tumour target cells in studies designed to eliminate the influence of NK-cells [194]. The depressed cytotoxicity was partly restored two weeks after nephrectomy and appeared to be controlled in the cancer patients by the production of a monocyte-activating lymphokine that could reduce the cytotoxic ability of normal monocytes. In addition, the patients' monocytes showed an impaired response to lymphokine stimulation. Conflicting reports of monocyte cytotoxicity in Hodgkin's disease have been mentioned [183,184]; using the microbial targets *Candida albicans* and *Staphylococcus aureus*, cytotoxicity was depressed in a small series of treated Hodgkin's and non-Hodgkin's lymphoma patients [195], although therapies may have influenced monocyte function directly.

The potential side effect of tumour treatment upon monocyte function assays was clearly demonstrated, again using a bacterial target, in lymphoma and lung carcinoma patients [123] where bactericidal capacity was further reduced following chemotherapy over the already depressed function in the malignant state. In contrast, using human erythrocyte targets no depression of monocyte ADCMC and spontaneous cytotoxicity was observed in 90 patients with breast, colonic, head and neck, and lung carcinomas and melanoma [70]. In fact, increased ADCMC and spontaneous cytotoxicity were observed in the 32 cases of colonic carcinoma, but the gross difference in the nature of the targets for the cytotoxicity assays renders comparison to other studies extremely tenuous—although using similar techniques depressed monocyte spontaneous cytotoxicity was confirmed in a variety of malignancies [145]. Recently, attention has focused upon the role of macrophages in the activation of NK-cells [114,196] because, as previously described, they may activate NK-cells via interleukin 1 and interferon. However, activated monocytes may be unable to induce NK activity, as was the case following activation using diterpene esters [196].

Peritoneal macrophages from mice bearing a chemically induced fibrosarcoma, a radiation-induced lymphoma, and a spontaneous melanoma all enhanced tumour growth in vivo and abolished the effect of tumour-inhibitory lymphocytes [197]. Macrophage activation by *Corynebacterium parvum* reversed this pattern and markedly inhibited tumour growth. It has also been shown [185] that macrophages from tumour-bearing animals have an impaired ability to kill protozoa. Interesting differences in systemic and local macrophage antimicrobial activity were observed [198] in tumour-bearing mice. There was an increase in macrophage capacity to inactivate bacteria systemically but a defect in macrophage ability to eliminate bacteria within a solid or ascitic tumour.

Serum lysozyme levels have been interpreted as reflecting macrophage activity. The level is frequently raised in neoplastic disease [199], which may correlate with the previously described monocytosis observed in many malignant states. However, reduced serum lysozyme levels were found in patients with chronic lymphocytic leukaemia [200], and in a large series of untreated patients with malignant melanoma, hypernephroma, and breast carcinoma raised levels were found only where the disease was localized [199]. This suggests that reduced serum lysozyme could result from ineffective activation of macrophages in the neoplastic state or by the reduced tumour infiltration of macrophages, as confirmed in a rat fibrosarcoma model where the elevation of the serum lysozyme level reflected the increased macrophage content of the tumour [201].

THE FUNCTION OF MACROPHAGES WITHIN TUMOURS. The study of intratumour macrophages may provide information about the role of macrophages in tumour immunity. However, apart from the enumeration and morphological examination of macrophages within tumours, technical problems have presented major difficulties in the study of their functional capacity. The immunohistochemical examination of functionally related membrane and cytoplasmic markers has provided useful data, but this type of investigation is always limited by the small sample size imposed by histological techniques. Moreover, in relation to an individual cell, information is usually only qualitative and lacks the potentially important quantitative component. Functional assays involve enzymatic and mechanical extraction procedures that may actually damage the functional capacity of the cells. In addition, such extraction may select for macrophages of a specific degree of maturation or activation so that the extracted cells are not a representative sample of the intratumour macrophage population. However, studies have been performed that generally indicate a depressed function of macrophages within tumours.

The intratumour macrophages in experimental murine carcinomas and sarcomas expressed γFcR [202], and in hamsters bearing transplantable lymphomas there was microscopic evidence that intratumour macrophages were more phagocytic in nonmetastasizing than in metastasizing tumours [203]. Immature, potentially proliferative macrophages were reported [204] in rat sarcomas where macrophage proliferation was apparently inhibited by the tumour, as division occurred in vitro in the absence of the tumour. Studies of the intratumour macrophages obtained from the antigenic SL2 lymphoma in DBA/2 mice and the antigenic 488 rat hepatoma showed that they were cytotoxic for the autologous tumour in vitro [205]. However, macrophages derived from the nonimmunogenic C57 BL mouse TLX9 lymphoma were not cytotoxic for the autologous tumour. This emphasises that in vitro effective cytotoxic macrophages may not be adequately cytotoxic in vivo; an important point is that many in vitro cytotoxicity assays use extremely high ratios of macrophages to target cells, which may be grossly different from their relative numbers in the tumour.

In mice, macrophages isolated from progressive Moloney sarcomas were less cytotoxic for target cells than were those isolated from nonprogressive tumours [206], and intra-tumour macrophages could not be activated to become cytotoxic compared with normal peritoneal macrophages [207]. Intratumour macrophages from mice bearing footpad tumours were incapable of eliminating *Listeria monocytogenes* from the tumour, although the organism was rapidly eliminated from other sites in the animals [110]. Further evidence that intratumour macrophage function is depressed comes from a study [208] where murine sarcomas containing macrophages with the lowest phagocytic activity spread more rapidly than tumours containing macrophages of higher phagocytic activity. In this area parallels with human tumours are infrequent and often tenuous, but the intralesional inoculation into the lesions of melanoma and breast carcinoma of glucan as a macrophage activator resulted in a regression of some tumours that was associated with the presence of large foamy macrophages [209]. Lysozyme has been used as a marker of macrophage activity within tumours using immunohistochemical techniques. However, it is difficult to quantify lysozyme at the level of a single cell and reports are usually based on the total number of re-active cells and staining intensity. Enhanced lysozyme levels in intratumour macrophages were associated with a good prognosis in Hodgkin's disease [210]. However, a complication in this area is that the Reed-Sternberg cell itself contains and may synthesize lysozyme [211].

The general picture emerging is that macrophages that infiltrate tumours may become reduced in their capacity to kill tumour cells, some of which may be relatively resistant to killing. The other aspect is that some tumours may reduce the ability of macrophages to in-filtrate. This leads into an important discussion, one that reports studies of how tumours may have a direct effect on macrophage function and, thus in a variety of ways, depress an-titumour macrophage activities.

THE DIRECT EFFECTS OF TUMOURS UPON MACROPHAGE FUNCTION

This section covers in vitro evidence that tumour cells, their extracts, and their products can modify monocyte/macrophage function. A number of studies describe the effects of serum or plasma from the tumour-bearing host upon macrophage function and assume that these "serum factors" are due to the tumour, yet, strictly, such evidence is indirect. Some of the work cited has already been mentioned earlier, but it is appropriate to correlate in vitro findings to related in vivo studies in order to gain knowledge about the relevance of the in vitro effects of tumours upon macrophages.

In patients with breast cancer a serum factor inhibited macrophage maturation, particu-larly in cases with metastatic spread [72]. Although depression of macrophage maturation in malignancies has been attributed to a cellular defect by some workers [69], it is possible that tumour factors may influence the reported immature forms in neoplasia.

Chemotaxis is the best documented macrophage function reported to be perturbed by tumours, and their metabolism and could account for the reduced accumulation of macro-phages within certain tumours. Factors that inhibit macrophage chemotaxis occur naturally and may play an important role in the regulation of chronic inflammation. Possibly, tumour growth in the malignant state may induce increased host synthesis of chemotactic inhibitory factors, but there is also evidence that specific antichemotactic factors may be synthesized by some tumours. Monocyte chemotaxis was depressed in patients with untreated bronchogenic carcinoma [129], most profoundly in cases where the tumour was poorly differentiated and the patient's plasma depressed chemotaxis of normal monocytes. However, patients' monocytes could not be restored to normal function by washing and the assay for plasma-induced chemotaxis inhibition was rather indirect, as it involved prior incubation with the chemotactin casein and then studying changes in the potency of the treated casein. Defective monocyte chemotaxis in Hodgkin's disease was explained by abnormally high levels of a normal chemotactic inhibitor, which could account for the reduced delayed hypersensitivity reactions frequently encountered in this and in other malignancies [212]. Similar tumour-associated plasma factors have been described, but frequently merely postulated, in relation to a variety of human neoplasmas [130,213,214], including breast cancer [127], melanoma [125], and mycosis fungoids [215]; in the latter study the underlying effect of the tumour may have been on helper T-cells. Monocyte chemotaxis-inhibiting factors correlated with a poor prognosis and an increased incidence of metastasis [125,127]. These monocyte chemotaxis inhibitors are poorly characterized in man, with reported molecular weights ranging from 6,000 to 600,000, although chemotactic inhibitors have been identified in malignant pleural effusions and roughly characterized as of low molecular weight [130].

Animal studies confirm the existence of antichemotactic tumour factors and plasma factors in the tumour-bearing host. A low-molecular-weight (6,000 to 10,000), heat-stable factor was present in the supernatant of cultured murine tumours, which inhibited macrophage chemotaxis and actually enhanced the growth of transplantable tumours [216]. In mice an attenuated lymphoma that was associated with little macrophage chemotactic-inhibitory factor behaved in a more malignant fashion when chemotactic-inhibitory factor was injected concurrently [217]. A triphasic effect of the tumour upon in vivo and in vitro macrophage function including chemotaxis was observed [111] in the mouse Lewis lung carcinoma model. Tumour cell extracts and sera from tumour-bearing mice depressed normal peritoneal macrophage chemotaxis initially after tumour implantation, which was followed by a period of normal or even enhanced function and always by a chemotaxis depressive effect in the longer tumour-bearing term. Lewis lung carcinoma culture supernates inhibited macrophage spreading [218], probably by inhibiting the fixation and thus the natural spreading enhancement property of bradykinin.

Normann et al. [219], using a subcutaneous implanted filter technique, confirmed the depressed macrophage chemotaxis in rats bearing a dimethylbenzanthracene- (DMBA) induced tumour and showed that the depression was abrogated by tumour resection. However, the defect occurred late in tumour growth and required a high threshold of tumour cells, often exceeding 1×10^8 cells. Thus, it could be concluded that the defect in monocyte chemotaxis arises as a result of tumour growth and is not a factor that restricts immunosurveillance thus potentiating the emergence of nascent neoplastic cells [219–221]. This finding conflicts with those reported using the Lewis lung carcinoma model [111], but, in animal models, the sudden introduction of large numbers of malignant cells into an animal may not be as good a model of human cancer as the slower development of a chemical carcinogen-induced tumour, which probably arises from relatively few transformed cells. Supernatants from well-characterized tumour-derived cell lines have been shown to be inhibitory in standard macrophage spreading [222] and chemotaxis [223] assays. A "tumour facilitating factor" (TFF) was derived from the supernatants of B16 melanoma cell line cultures, which reduced macrophage spreading [222]. The TFF enhanced the in vivo growth of small inocula of the B16 melanoma and was not toxic for macrophages. Culture supernatants from a variety of neoplastic and other rapidly proliferating cell lines including polyomavirus-induced, DMBA-induced, SV-4O virus-transformed tumours, and Chinese hamster fibroblasts all exhibited macrophage chemotaxis inhibition activity [223]. The inhibiting factor bound to be macrophage plasma membrane and was actually weakly chemotactic for polymorphs, which may help to explain the mechanisms whereby the tumour-bearing state produces a cell-specific defect in chronic but not in acute inflammation. In contrast to the results of these studies, culture supernatants from a variety of solid and non-solid mouse and human tumours had appreciable chemotactic activity for mouse macrophages and human monocytes [224,225]. The effect was not species specific and was mediated by a low-molecular-weight (12,000), heat-stable protein that may help to regulate the accumulation of macrophages in tumours.

The direct effects of tumours upon the phagocytic and cytotoxic function of macrophages are poorly documented. Depressed peritoneal macrophage phagocytosis of bacterial targets was observed in sarcoma-bearing mice [152]. Phagocytosis-inhibiting factors have been identified in the culture supernatants of human colonic carcinoma cells [226] and mouse sarcoma cells [227], the latter being of approximately 12,000 molecular weight and heat stable. Studies on the monocyte γFcR expression in humans indicate alterations in malignant states that may be modulated by the tumour. Inhibition of γFcR expression by normal monocytes was induced by supernatants of human carcinoma explant cultures [148], although a low-molecular-weight, heat-stable factor in normal human serum was also inhibitory. In contrast, enhanced γFcR expression was induced by serum from patients with various untreated solid tumours [228]. Immune complexes may bind to macrophage γFc receptors and thus reduce phagocytic capacity [229] and also block ADCMC. Some tumour cells shed copious quantities of antigens [230], which may form part of an immune complex, but the significance in relation to cancer is difficult to evaluate because if immune complexes are effectively blocking receptors, they are bound to the cells, which would render them undetectable in serum using conventional techniques. However, there is limited evidence [231] that plasmapheresis may be beneficial in some cancer patients, although the results of the procedure are complicated and interpretation is difficult. Monocyte-mediated cytotoxicity was depressed in vitro by factors in the serum of patients with multiple myeloma and malignant lymphoma [232]. Tumour-bearing mice produced a low-molecular-weight, heat-stable serum factor that induced a severe impairment of macrophage microbial cytotoxicity [108,109], suggesting that similar impairment existed toward tumour cells.

The study of the direct effect of tumours and their products upon the macrophage warrants further investigation. In particular, much more precise characterization is required of macrophage depressive factors either in cultured tumours or derived from a tumour-bearing host. There is also considerable scope for parallel in vivo and in vitro studies in order to evaluate better the significance of some of the phenomena described in this section.

INDIRECT EFFECTS OF MACROPHAGE ACTIVATION IN THE TUMOUR-BEARING HOST

The establishment and growth of metastatic tumour deposits in bone must be facilitated by local osteoclast activity. This would also apply to the local spread of some tumours that are sited close to bone. Osteoclasts may become activated by the poorly characterized osteo-clast-activating factor (OAF), which is produced by activated T-cells. This raises an inter-esting contrast to previous descriptions of the direct effect of a lack of macrophage activity facilitating tumour growth. Therefore, it is possible that some tumours may depress osteo-clast activity in a fashion comparable with monocyte/macrophage depression and thus reduce the tumour's metastatic potential. However, the osteoclast is a highly specialized macrophage, and OAF synthesis by infiltrating T-cells may be a dominant mechanism in the control of osteoclast activation. Extensive tumour deposits in bone may result in hyper-calcaemia, which is thought to be due to excessive osteoclast activity. This indirect effect of activation of osteoclastas is commonly encountered in multiple myeloma and is an extreme-ly important consideration in the management of this condition.

THE RELEVANCE OF IN VIVO AND IN VITRO STUDIES OF MACROPHAGES AS PROGNOSTIC INDICATORS IN CANCER

It is unlikely that monocyte/macrophage studies will ever play an important role in the diagnosis of cancer, but they may have a future role as prognostic indicators and contribute to the evaluation of therapy by monitoring macrophage function during treatment. The central role of the macrophage in immune responses means that the results of any in vivo or in vitro test of immune function in cancer may be influenced by macrophages. However, this section will cover only direct studies of macrophages.

The most frequently recorded depressed monocyte function in cancer is chemotaxis, which correlated with clinical staging in malignant melanoma [122] and led to the suggestion that monitoring of melanoma patients' macrophage chemotactic responsiveness might provide a useful indication of prognosis and therapy. The only established in vitro test of mono-cyte/macrophage function as a prognostic indicator in cancer is the leucocyte adherence in-hibition (LAI) assay. However, the LAI test has been widely criticized as being unreliable and too susceptable to minor technical variations. The test as originally described by Halliday et al. [233,234] was based upon the fact that cancer patients' leucocytes exhibited reduced adherence to glass surfaces in the presence of tumour extracts. This adherence inhibition effect could be blocked by the serum of cancer patients, which, without any direct evidence, was at-tributed to immune complexes. The technique was modified slightly and applied to cases of breast cancer [235], where leucocytes from 40 of 47 patients exhibited adherence inhibition compared with 2 of 32 control subjects. However, these techniques used a buffy coat prepara-tion of whole blood leucocytes, and most studies made no attempt to verify their assumption that the monocyte was the predominant cell to lose adhesive qualities in the presence of tumour extracts. Claims were made not only for the sensitivity but also the specificity of the test in terms of the nature of the inhibiting tumour cell extract in relation to that of the pa-tients neoplasm [234]. However, these claims have not been substantiated by other studies, where in cases of breast cancer a high proportion of healthy controls exhibited LAI activity [236] and LAI positivity was also induced by extracts of normal breast tissue [237].

Animal models of the LAI phenomena [238] indicate that the LAI test may have a scien-tific basis but that approaches in humans have been naive and existing techniques inade-quately sophisticated. In a mouse virus-induced sarcoma model, macrophage adherence could be promoted or inhibited by subpopulations of mouse T-cells whose effect was, in turn, modulated by macrophages. The phenomenon of macrophage adherence in the tumour-bearing state is complex, and the implication is that the adherence of unfractionated and usually uncharacterized human leucocytes is varied. The human LAI test may have a future role as a prognostic indicator and as a monitor of cancer therapy. However, considerable development is required, particularly in the purification and characterization of indicator cells and of potential modulating cells, in order to understand what the test means before it can rationally be applied as a guide to the prognosis of cancer and monitoring of therapy.

SUMMARY

There is now considerable evidence that macrophages can play a major role in the body's defense against neoplasia. They can destroy tumour cells in vitro and can be effective in vivo against experimental tumours. The puzzle is why a neoplastic process starts when macrophages should be capable of dealing with it and why tumours grow when their stroma frequently contain many macrophages. It is difficult to accept that all the reports of effective macrophage antitumour activity are experimental artifacts; it is more likely that macrophages usually do deal effectively with neoplastic cell transformations.

The failure of macrophages to control an established tumour may relate to a tumour-mediated depression of macrophage function. Some of the experimental work cited in this chapter provides evidence for a progressive localized and then a systemic depression of macrophage function during tumour growth and spread. The best documented macrophage functions that appear to be disturbed in cancer are chemotaxis and, to a lesser extent, cytotoxicity and immunoregulation. However, this may give an erroneous impression of the relationship of the macrophage to cancer because much work has been designed to investigate specific functions without attempting to compare other macrophage functions in the same tumour-bearing state. In addition, much in vitro work is based upon the use of nontumour cell targets and frequently uses crude peripheral mononuclear cell preparations where monocytes would be a relatively small population. Despite reservations about some studies there is the general impression of a depression of monocyte/macrophage function in many malignancies. This is substantiated by reports of increased numbers of suppressor monocytes in malignancy, which may account for the unexplained and apparently ineffective monocytosis that is frequently observed in cancer patients.

The role of the macrophage in cancer requires further investigation. In vitro studies require the use of more appropriate cytotoxicity target cells, more closely defined effector cell populations, and better characterization of described antimacrophage tumour products and serum factors. In vivo studies require the development of better animal models, especially to achieve kinetics of tumour growth and tumour immunogenicity that closely resemble human cancer. In addition, technical developments in functional studies of intratumour macrophages would provide valuable information about why a macrophage-laden tumour grows. The macrophage is an obvious target cell for the use of immunostimulatory compounds in malignancy, and increased interest will undoubtedly be focused upon this potentially important aspect of cancer immunotherapy. Macrophage studies will become valid as prognostic indicators in malignancy only when considerably more is understood about the role of this fascinating cell line in neoplastic disease.

REFERENCES

1. Alexander, P. The functions of the macrophage in malignant disease. Annu Rev Med 27: 207–224, 1976.
2. Keller R. Characteristics of cytotoxic macrophages as natural effectors of resistance to cancer. Clinics Immunol Allergy 3: 523–537, 1983.
3. Rhodes J. Resistance of tumour cells to macrophages: A short review. Cancer Immunol Immunother 7: 211–215, 1980.
4. Sokol RJ, Hudson G. Disordered function of mononuclear phagocytes in malignant disease. J. Clin Pathol 36: 316–323, 1983.
5. Levy MH, Wheelock EF. The role of macrophages in defense against neoplastic disease. Adv Cancer Res 20: 131–163, 1974.
6. Nelson DS (ed.). Immunobiology of the macrophage. New York: Academic Press, 1976.
7. Bellanti JA, Dayton DH (eds.). The phagocytic cell in hose resistance. New York: Raven Press, 1975.
8. Fink MA (ed.). The macrophage in neoplasia. New York: Academic Press, 1976.
9. van Furth R (ed.). Mononuclear phagocytes in immunity, infection and pathology. Oxford: Blackwell Scientific Publications, 1975.
10. van Furth R (ed.). Mononuclear phagocytes—Functional aspects. The Hague: Martinus Nijhoff, 1980.
11. James K, McBride B, Stuart A (eds.). The macrophage and cancer. Edinburgh: University of Edinburgh Medical School, 1977.
12. Braunsteiner H, Schmalzl F. Cytochemistry of monocytes and macrophages. In van Fruth R (ed.), Mononuclear phagocytes. Oxford: Blackwell, 1970, pp. 62–81.
13. Klockars M, Osserman EF. Localisation of lysozyme in normal rat tissues by an immunoperoxidase method. J Histochem Cytochem 22: 139–146, 1974.
14. McClelland DBL, van Furth R. In vitro synthesis of lysozyme by human and mouse tissues and leukocytes. Immunology 28: 1099–1114, 1975.
15. Bainton DF. Changes in peroxidase distribution within organelles of blood monocytes and peritoneal macrophages after surface adherence in vitro and in vivo. In van Furth R (ed.), Mononuclear phagocytes, functional aspects. The Hague: Martinus Nijhoff, 1980, pp. 61–86.
16. van Furth R. Cells of the mononuclear phagocyte system—Nomenclature in terms of sites and conditions. In van Furth R (ed.), Mononuclear phagocytes, functional aspects. The Hague: Martinus Nijhoff, 1980, pp. 1–40.
17. Unanue ER. The regulatory role of macrophages in antigen stimulation. Adv Immunol 15: 95–165, 1972.
18. Pierce CW, Kapp JA. The role of macrophages in antibody responses in vitro. In Nelson DS (ed.), Immunobiology of the macrophage. New York: Academic Press, 1976, pp. 1–33.
19. Daems WTh, Wisse E, Brederoo P. Emeis JJ. Peroxidatic activity in monocytes and macrophages. In van Furth R (ed.), Mononuclear phagocytes in immunity, infection and pathology. Oxford: Blackwell Scientific Publications, 1975, pp. 57–77.
20. Unanue ER. The regulation of lymphocyte function by macrophages. Immunol Rev 40: 227–255, 1978.
21. Erb P, Feldmann M, Gisler R, Meier B, Stern A, Vogt P. Role of macrophages in the in vitro induction and regulation of antibody responses. In van Furth R (ed.), Mononuclear phagocytes, functional aspects. The Hague: Martinus Nijhoff, 1980, pp. 1857–1885.
22. Crofton RW, Diesselhoff-den Dulk MMC, van Furth R. The origin, kinetics and characteristics of the Kupffer cells in the normal steady state. J Exp Med 148: 1–17, 1978.
23. Ward M, Ferguson A, Eastwood MA. Jejunal lysozyme activity and the Paneth cell in coeliac disease. Gut 20: 55–58, 1979.
24. Katz SI, Tamaki K, Sachs DH. Epidermal Langerhans cells are derived from cells originating in bone marrow. Nature (Lond.) 282: 324–326, 1979.
25. Gassmann AE, van Furth R. The effect of azathioprine (Imuran) on the kinetics of monocytes and macrophages during normal steady state and the acute inflammatory reaction. Blood 46: 51–64, 1975.
26. Nichols BA, Bainton DF. Ultrastructure and cyto-chemistry of mononuclear phagocytes. In van Furth R (ed.), Mononuclear phagocytes in immunity, infection and pathology. Oxford: Blackwell Scientific Publications, 1975, pp. 17–55.
27. Stingl G. Role of epidermal Langerhans cells in the immune response. Recent Adv Immunol 3: 1–7, 1983.
28. Kirchner H. Suppressor cells of immune reactivity in malignancy. Europ J Cancer 14: 453–459, 1978.
29. Rice L, Laughter AH, Twomey JJ. Three suppressor systems in human blood that modulate lymphoproliferation. J Immunol 122: 991–996, 1979.
30. Goodwin JS, Messner RP, Peake GT. Prostaglandin suppression of mitogen-stimulated lymphocytes in vitro. J Clin Invest 62: 753–760, 1978.

31. Goodwin JS, Bankhurst AD, Messner RP. Suppression of human T-cell mitogenesis by prostaglandin. J Exp Med 146: 1719–1734, 1977.
32. Bandeira A, Pobor S, Pettersson S, Coutinhos A. Differential macrophage requirements for T helper cell and T helper-cell induced B lymphocyte proliferation. J Exp Med 157: 312–323, 1983.
33. Wilkinson PC. Cell-membrane activation of macrophage function. Recent Results in Cancer Res 56: 41–48, 1976.
34. Silverstein SC, Loike JD. Phagocytosis. In van Furth R (ed.), Mononuclear phagocytes, functional aspects. The Hague: Martinus Nijhoff, 1980, pp. 895–917.
35. Kohler PF. Human complement system. In Samter M (ed.), Immunological diseases, 3rd edn. Boston: Little Brown, 1978, pp. 224–280.
36. Brade V, Bentley C. Synthesis and release of complement components by macrophages. In van Furth R (ed.), Mononuclear phagocytes—Functional aspects. The Hague: Martinus Nijhoff, 1980, pp. 1385–1417.
37. Temple TR, Synderman R, Jordan HV, Mergenhagen SE. Factors from saliva and oral bacteria, chemotactic for polymorphonuclear leukocytes: Their possible role in gingival inflammation. J Periodont 41: 71–80, 1970.
38. Schiffmann E, Corcoran BA, Wahl SM. N-formylmethionyl peptides as chemoattractants for leucocytes. Proc Natl Acad Sci 72: 1059–1062, 1975.
39. Ward PA, Hill JH. C5 chemotactic fragments produced by an enzyme in lysosomal granules of neutrophils. J Immunol 104: 535–543, 1970.
40. Altman LC, Synderman R, Oppenheim JJ, Mergenhagen SE. A human mononuclear leukocyte chemotactic factor: Characterization, specificity and kinetics of production by homologous leukocytes. J Immunol 110: 801–810, 1973.
41. Mackler BF, Altman LC, Rosenstreich DL, Oppenheim JJ. Induction of lymphokine production by EAC and of blastogenesis by soluble mitogens during human B-cell activation. Nature (Lond.) 249: 834–837, 1974.
42. Wahl SM, Altman LC, Oppenheim JJ, Morgenhagen SE. In vitro studies of a chemotactic lymphokine in the guinea pig. Inter Arch Allergy Appl Immunol 46: 768–784, 1974.
43. Wahl SM, Iverson GM, Oppenheim JJ. Induction of guinea pig B-cell lymphokine synthesis by mitogenic and nonmitogenic signals to Fc, Ig and C3 receptors. J Exp Med 140: 1631–1645, 1974.
44. Wahl SM, Wilton JM, Rosenstreich DL, Oppenheim JJ. The role of macrophages in the production of lymphokines by T and B lymphocytes. J Immunol 114: 1296–1301, 1975.
45. Steinman RM, Brodier SE, Cohn ZA. Membrane flow during pinocytosis. A stereologic analysis. J Cell Biol 68: 665–687, 1976.
46. Machoney EM, Hamill AL, Scott WA, Cohn ZA. Response of endocytosis to altered fatty acyl compositions of macrophage phospholipids. Proc Natl Acad Sci 74: 4895–4899, 1977.
47. Unkeless JC, Eisen HN. Binding of monomeric immunoglobulins to Fc receptors of mouse macrophages. J Exp Med 142: 1520–1533, 1975.
48. Unkeless JC. The presence of two Fc receptors on mouse macrophages. Evidence from a variant cell line and differential trypsin sensitivity. J Exp Med 145: 931–947, 1977.
49. Heusser CH, Anderson CL, Grey HM. Receptors for IgG: Subclass specificity of receptors on different mouse cell types and the definition of two distinct receptors on a macrophage cell line. J Exp Med 145: 1316–1327, 1977.
50. Coupland K, Leslie RGQ. The expression of Fc receptors on guinea-pig peritoneal macrophages and neutrophils. Immunol 48: 647–656, 1983.
51. Michl J, Unkeless JC, Silverstein SC. Modulation of macrophage plasma membrane receptors for IgG and complement. In van Furth R (ed.), Mononuclear phagocytes—Functional aspects. The Hague: Martinus Nijhoff, 1980, pp. 921–937.
52. Griffin FM Jr, Bianco C, Silverstein SC. Characterization of the macrophage receptor for complement and demonstration of its functional independence from the receptor for the Fc portion of immunoglobulin G. J Exp Med 141: 1269–1277, 1975.
53. Griffin FM Jr, Silverstein SC. Segmental response of the macrophage plasma membrane to a phagocytic stimulus. J Exp Med 139: 323–336, 1974.
54. Griffin FM Jr, Griffin JA, Leider JE, Silverstein SC. Studies on the mechanisms of phagocytosis. I. Requirements for circumferential attachment of particle bound ligands to specific receptors on the macrophage plasma membrane. J Exp Med 142: 1263–1282, 1975.
55. Griffin FM Jr, Griffin JA, Silverstein SC. Studies on the mechanism of phagocytosis. II. The interaction of macrophages with anti-immunoglobulin IgG-coated bone marrow-derived lymphocytes. J Exp Med 144: 788–809, 1976.
56. Hartwig JH, Davies WA, Stossel TP. Evidence for contractile protein translocation in macrophage spreading, phagocytosis and phagolysozome formation. J Cell Biol 75: 956–967, 1977.

57. Choate JJ, Mosher DF. Fibronectin concentration in plasma of patients with breast cancer, colon cancer and acute leukaemia. Cancer 51: 1142–1147, 1983.

58. Klebanoff SJ. Oxygen intermediates and the microbicidal event. In van Furth R (ed.), Mononuclear phagocytes—Functional aspects. The Hague: Martinus Nijhoff, 1980, pp. 1105–1137.

59. Johnston RB Jr, Chadwick DA, Pabst MJ. Release of superoxide anion by macrophages: Effect of in vivo or in vitro priming. In van Furth R. (ed.), Mononuclear phagocytes, functional aspects. The Hague: Martinus Nijhoff, 1980, pp. 1143–1158.

60. Daems WTh, Poelmann RE, Brederoo P. Peroxidatic activity in resident peritoneal macrophages and exudate monocytes of the guinea pig after ingestion of latex particles. J Histochem Cytochem 21: 93–95, 1973.

61. Gordon S, Todd J, Cohn ZA. In vitro synthesis and secretion of lysozyme by mononuclear phagocytes. J Exp Med 139: 1228–1248, 1974.

62. Zeya HI, Spitznagel JK. Arginine-rich proteins of polymorphonuclear leukocyte lysosomes. Antimicrobial specificity and biochemical heterogeneity. J Exp Med 127: 927–941, 1968.

63. Rees RC, Underwood JCE. Tumour immunology. In Hancock BW (ed.), Assessment of tumour response. The Hague: Martinus Nijhoff, 1982, pp. 181–210.

64. Manifold IH, Triger DR, Underwood JCE. Kupffer-cell depletion in chronic liver disease: Implications for hepatic carcinogenesis. Lancet 2: 431–433, 1983.

65. Rebuck JW, Monto RW, Monaghan EA, Riddle JM. Potentialities of the lymphocyte, with an additional reference to its dysfunction in Hodgkin's disease. Ann N Y Acad Sci 73: 8–38, 1958.

66. Sokol RJ, Durrant TE, Lambourne CA, Hudson G. Scanning electron microscopy of exudate macrophages in malignant lymphoma. Scand J Haematol 22: 129–140, 1979.

67. Dent RG, Cole P. "In vitro" monocyte maturation in squamous carcinoma of the lung. Br J Cancer 43: 486–495, 1981.

68. Currie GA, Hedley DW. Monocytes and macrophages in malignant melanoma. I. Peripheral blood macrophage precursors. Br J Cancer 36: 1–6. 1977.

69. Krishnan EC, Menon CD, Krishnan L, Jewell WR. Deficiency in maturation process of macrophages in human cancer. J Natl Cancer Inst 65: 273–276, 1980.

70. Unger SW, Bernhard MI, Pace RC, Wanebo HJ. Monocyte dysfunction in human cancer. Cancer 51: 669–674, 1983.

71. Krishnan EC, Mebust WK, Weigel JW, Jewell WR. Maturation of monocytes in patients with renal cell carcinoma. Invest Urol 19: 4–7, 1981.

72. Palmer BV, Currie G. Monocyte maturation and breast cancer. Clin Oncol 6: 377, 1980.

73. Hedley DW, Nylholm RE, Currie GA. Monocytes and macrophages in malignant melanoma. IV. Effects of C.parvum on monocyte function. Br J Cancer 39: 558–565, 1979.

74. Taylor SA, Currie GA. Monocyte maturation and prognosis in primary breast cancer. Br Med J i: 1050–1051, 1979.

75. Dent RG, Cole P. In vitro monocyte maturation as a prediction of survival in squamous cell carcinoma of the lung. Thorax 36: 446–451, 1981.

76. Braun DP, Harris JE. Relationship of leukocyte numbers, immunoregulatory cell function, and phytohaemagglutinin responsiveness in cancer patients. J Natl Cancer Inst 67: 809–814, 1981.

77. Wood GW, Neff JE, Stephens R. Relationship between monocytosis and T-lymphocyte function in human cancer. J Natl Cancer Inst 63: 587–592, 1979.

78. Popper H, Sternberg SS, Osler BL, Osler M. The carcinogenic effect of Aramite in rats. A study of hepatic nodules. Cancer 13: 1035–1046, 1960.

79. Flavell DJ. Liver-fluke infection as an aetiological factor in bile-duct carcinoma of man. Trans R Soc Trop Med Hyg 75: 814–824, 1981.

80. Hou PC. The relationship between primary carcinoma of the liver and infestation with Clonorchis sinensis. J Path Bacteriol 72: 239–246, 1956.

81. Swinson CM, Slavin G, Coles EC, Booth CC. Coeliac disease and malignancy. Lancet i: 111–115, 1983.

82. Underwood JCE. Lymphoreticular infiltration in human tumours: Prognostic and biological implications: A review. Br J Cancer 30: 538–548, 1974.

83. Alexander P, Eccles SA, Ganci CL. The significance of macrophages in human and experimental tumors. Ann N Y Acad Sci 276: 124–133, 1976.

84. Lauder I, Aherne W, Stewart J, Sainsbury R. Macrophage infiltration of breast tumors: A prospective study. J Clin Pathol 30: 563–568, 1977.

85. Skinner JM, Jarvis LR, Whitehead R. The cellular response to human colonic neoplasms: Macrophage numbers. J Pathol 139: 97–103, 1983.

86. Talmadge JE, Key M, Fidler IJ. Macrophage content of metastatic and nonmetastatic rodent neoplasms. J Immunol 126: 2245–2248, 1981.

87. Gauci CL. The significance of the macrophage content of human tumours. Recent Results Cancer Res 56: 122–130, 1976.
88. Jerrells TR, Dean JH, Richardson GL, McCoy JL, Herberman RB. Role of suppressor cell in depression of in vitro lymphoproliferative responses of lung cancer and breast cancer patients. J Natl Cancer Inst 61: 1001–1009, 1978.
89. Schulof RS, Lee BJ, Lacher MJ, Straus DJ, Clarkson BD, Good RA, Gupta S. Concanavalin A-induced suppressor cell activity in Hodgkin's disease. Clin Immunol Immunopathol 16: 454–462, 1980.
90. Zembala M, Mytar B, Popiela T, Asherson G. Depressed in vitro peripheral blood lymphocyte response to mitogens in cancer patients: The role of suppressor cells. Int J Cancer 19: 605–613, 1977.
91. Berlinger NT, Hilal EY, Oettgen HF, Good RA. Deficient cell-mediated immunity in head and neck cancer patients secondary to autologous suppressive immune cells. Laryngoscope 88: 470–483, 1978.
92. Hillinger SM, Herzig GP. Impaired cell-mediated immunity in Hodgkin's disease mediated by suppressor lymphocytes and monocytes. J Clin Invest 61: 1620–1627, 1978.
93. Laughter AH, Twomey JJ. Suppression of lympho-proliferation by high concentrations of normal human mononuclear leukocytes. J Immunol 119: 173–179, 1977.
94. Twomey JJ, Laughter AH, Farrow S, Douglas CD. Hodgkin's disease. An immunodepleting and immuno-suppressive disorder. J Clin Invest 56: 467–475, 1975.
95. Goodwin JS, Messner RP, Bankhurst AD, Peake GT, Saiki JH, Williams RC Jr. Prostaglandin-producing suppressor cells in Hodgkin's disease. New Eng J Med 297: 963–968, 1977.
96. Broder S, Muul L, Waldmann TA. Suppressor cells in neoplastic disease. J Natl Cancer Inst 61: 5–11, 1978.
97. Holm G, Bjorkholm M, Johansson B, Mellstedt H, Lindemalm C. Monocyte function in Hodgkin's disease. Clin Exp Immunol 47: 162–168, 1982.
98. Sagone AL Jr, Kamps S, Campbell R, King GW. Lack of correlation of activated monocytes with lymphocyte function in patients with lymphoma. J Reticuloendothelial Soc 21: 377–383, 1977.
99. Zembala M, Mytar B, Ruggiero I, Uracz W, Popiela T, Czupryna A: Suppressor cells and survival of patients with gastric cancer. J Natl Cancer Inst 70: 222–228, 1983.
100. Han T, Winnicki MS. Indomethacin-mediated enhancement of lymphocyte response to mitogens. N Y State J Med 80: 1070–1075, 1980.
101. De Shazo RD. Indomethacin-responsive mononuclear cell dysfunction in Hodgkin's disease. Clin Immunol Immunopathol 17: 66–75, 1980.
102. Tilden AB, Balch CM. Indomethacin enhancement of immunocompetence in melanoma patients. Surgery 90: 77–84, 1981.
103. Han MD, Takita H. Depression of T-lymphocyte response by non-T suppressor cells in lung cancer patients. Cancer 44: 2090–2098, 1979.
104. Den Otter W, Evans R, Alexander P. Differentiation of immunologically specific cytotoxic macrophages into two types on the basis of radiosensitivity. Transplant 18: 421–428, 1974.
105. Quan PC, Burtin P. Demonstration of nonspecific suppressor cells in the peripheral lymphocytes of cancer patients. Cancer Res 38: 288–296, 1978.
106. Broder S, Humphrey R, Durm M, Blackman M, Mead B, Goldman C, Strober W, Waldman T. Impaired synthesis of polyclonal (non-paraprotein) immunoglobulins by circulating lymphocytes from patients with multiple myeloma. New Engl J Med 293: 887–892, 1975.
107. Eccles SA, Alexander P. Macrophage content of tumours in relation to metastatic spread and host immune reaction. Nature 250: 667–669, 1974.
108. North RJ, Kirstein DP, Tuttle RL. Subversion of host defense mechanisms by murine tumours. I. A circulating factor that suppresses macrophage-mediated resistance to infection. J Exp Med 143: 559–573, 1976.
109. North RJ, Kirstein DP, Tuttle RL. Subversion of host defense mechanisms by murine tumours. II. Counter-influence of concomitant antitumour immunity. J Exp Med 143: 574–584, 1976.
110. Spitalny GL, North RJ. Subversion of host defense mechanisms by malignant tumours: An established tumour as a privileged site for bacterial growth. J Exp Med 145: 1264–1277, 1977.
111. Otu AA, Russell RJ, Wilkinson PC, White RG. Alterations of mononuclear phagocyte function induced by Lewis lung carcinoma in C57BL mice. Br J Cancer 36: 330–340, 1977.
112. Stutman O, Lattime EC. Natural cytotoxic cells against tumours in mice. Clinics Immunol Allergy 3: 507–521, 1983.
113. de Vries JE, Mendelsohn J, Bont WS. Requirement for monocytes in the spontaneous cytotoxic effects of human lymphocytes against non-lymphoid target cells. Nature 283: 574–576, 1980.
114. de Vries JE, Figdor CG, Spits H. Regulation of human NK activity against adherent tumour target cells by monocyte subpopulations, interleukin 1 and interferons. In Herberman RB (ed.), NK cells and other natural effector cells. New York: Academic Press, 1982, pp. 657–668.

115. Farrar WL, Johnson HM, Farrar JJ. Regulation of the production of immune interferon and cytotoxic T lymphocytes by interleukin 2. J Immunol 126: 1120–1125, 1981.
116. Brunda MJ, Taramelli D, Holden HT, Varesio L. Suppression of murine natural killer cell activity by normal peritoneal macrophages. In Herberman RB (ed.), NK cell and other natural effector cells. New York: Academic Press, 1982, pp. 535–546.
117. Bordignon C, Allavena P, Introna M, Biondi A, Bottazzi, B, Mantovani A. Modulation of NK activity by human mononuclear phagocytes: Suppressive activity of broncho-alveolar macrophages. In Herberman RB (ed.), NK cells and other natural effector cells. New York: Academic Press, 1982, pp. 581–588.
118. Uchida A, Micksche M. Suppression of NK cell activity by adherent cells from malignant pleural effusions of cancer patients. In Herberman RB (ed.), NK cells and other natural effector cells. New York: Academic Press, 1982, pp. 589–594.
119. Boetcher DA, Leonard EJ. Abnormal monocyte chemotactic response in cancer patients. J Natl Cancer Inst 52: 1091–1099, 1974.
120. Hausman MS, Brosman S, Synderman R, Mickey MJ, Fahey J. Defective monocyte function in patients with genito-urinary carcinoma. J Natl Cancer Inst 55: 1047–1054, 1975.
121. Snyderman R, Pike MC, Meadows L, Hemstreet G, Wells S. Depression of monocyte chemotaxis by neoplasms. Clin Res 23: 297, 1975.
122. Rubin RH, Cosimi AB, Goetzl EJ. Defective human mononuclear leukocyte chemotaxis as an index of host resistance to malignant melanoma. Clin Immunol Immunopathol 6: 376–388, 1976.
123. McVie JG, Logan EGM, Kay AB. Monocyte function in cancer patients. Eur J Cancer 13: 351–353, 1977.
124. Seitz LE, Golitz LE, Weston WL, Aeling JE, Dustin RD. Defective monocyte chemotaxis in mycosis fungoides. Arch Dermatol 113: 1055–1057, 1977.
125. Snyderman R, Seigler HF, Meadows L. Abnormalities of monocyte chemotaxis in patients with melanoma: Effects of immunotherapy and tumor removal. J Natl Cancer Inst 58: 37–41, 1977.
126. Kjeldesberg CR, Pay GD. A qualitative and quantitative study of monocytes in patients with malignant solid tumours. Cancer 41: 2236–2241, 1978.
127. Snyderman R, Meadows L, Holder W, Wells S. Abnormal monocyte chemotaxis in patients with breast cancer: Evidence for a tumour-mediated effect. J Natl Cancer Inst 60: 737–740, 1978.
128. Dammacco F, Miglietta A, Ventura MT, Bonomo L. Defective monocyte chemotactic responsiveness in patients with multiple myeloma and benign monoclonal gammapathy. Clin Exp Immunol 47: 481–486, 1982.
129. Nielsen H, Bennedsen J, Larsen SO, Dombernowsky P, Viskum K. A quantitative and qualitative study of blood monocytes in patients with bronchogenic carcinoma. Cancer Immunol Immunother 13: 93–97, 1982.
130. Snyderman R, Pike MC. Quantification of monocyte function in patients with cancer: Evidence for tumour-mediated dysfunction. In Hersh EM, Chirigos MA, Mastrangelo MJ (eds.), Augmenting agents in cancer therapy. New York: Raven Press, 1981. pp. 285–293.
131. Nielsen H, Bennedsen J, Dombernowsky P. Normalization of defective monocyte chemotaxis during chemotherapy in patients with small cell anaplastic carcinoma of the lung. Cancer Immunol Immunother 14: 13–15, 1982.
132. Renoux G, Lemarie G, Legrand MF, Renoux M, Lavandier M. Pulmonary alveolar macrophage chemotaxis in malignant tumours of the lung. In Norman SJ, Sorkin E (eds.), Macrophages and natural killer cells: Regulation and function. New York: Plenum Press, 1982, pp. 361–367.
133. Normann SJ, Sorkin E. Cell specific defect in monocyte function during tumor growth. J Natl Cancer Inst 57: 135–140, 1976.
134. Alexander P. Entry of inflammatory cells into tumours and the suppression of chronic inflammation by tumors. In Weissermann G, Samuelsson B, Paoletti R (eds.), Advances in inflammation research. New York: Raven Press, 1979, pp. 197–204.
135. Samak P, Israel L, Edelstein R. Influence of tumour burden, tumour removal, immune stimulation, plasmapheresis on monocyte mobilisation in cancer patients. In Escobar MR, Friedman H (eds.), Advances in experimental medicine and biology: Macrophages and lymphocytes. New York: Plenum Press, 1980, pp. 411–423.
136. Israel L, Samak R. A modified skin window technique as a staging tool in solid tumours. Correlation between nonspecific monocyte mobilization "in vivo" and spread of disease. Am Assoc Cancer Res Proc 20: 49, 1979.
137. Bennett B, Old LJ, Boyse EA. The phagocytosis of tumour cells in vitro. Transplant 2: 183–202, 1964.
138. Kuntz BME, Kuntz RM, Albert ED. Phagocytosis of monocytes in cancer patients. Zeit Krebsforchung Klin Onk 91: 11–17, 1978.
139. Ruco LP, Procopio A, Uccini S, Baroni CD. Increased monocyte phagocytosis in cancer patients. Eur J Cancer 16: 1315–1320, 1980.
140. Urbanitz D, Fechner I. Gross R. Reduced monocyte phagocytosis in patients with advanced Hodgkin's disease and lymphosarcoma. Klin Wochenschr 53: 437–440, 1975.

141. Estevez ME, Sen L, Bachmann AE, Paulovsky A. Defective function of peripheral blood monocytes in patients with Hodgkin's disease and non-Hodgkin's lymphomas. Cancer 46: 299–302, 1980.
142. Hedley DW, Currie GA. Monocytes and macrophages in malignant melanoma. III. Reduction of nitroblue tetrazolium by peripheral blood monocytes. Br J Cancer 37: 747–752, 1978.
143. Kitahara M, Eyre H, Hill HR. Monocyte functional and metabolic activity in malignant and inflammatory diseases. J Lab Clin Med 93: 472–479, 1979.
144. Gill PG, Waller CA. Quantitative aspects of human monocyte function and its measurement in cancer patients. In James K, McBride B, Stuart A (eds.), The macrophage and cancer. Edinburgh: University of Edinburgh Medical School, 1977, pp. 375–385.
145. Kleinerman ES, Howser D, Young RC et al. Defective monocyte killing in patients with malignancies and restoration of function during chemotherapy. Lancet ii: 1102–1105, 1980.
146. Cline MJ. Defective mononuclear phagocyte function in patients with myelomonocytic leukaemia and in some patients with lymphoma. J Clin Invest 52, 2185–2190, 1973.
147. Rhodes J. Altered expression of human monocyte Fc receptors in malignant disease. Nature 265: 253–255, 1977.
148. Rhodes J, Plowman P, Bishop M, Lipscomb D. Human macrophage function in cancer: Systemic and local changes detected by an assay for Fc receptor expression. J Natl Cancer Inst 66: 423–429, 1981.
149. Meltzer MS, Stevenson MM. Macrophage function in tumour bearing mice: Dissociation of phagocytic and chemotactic responsiveness. Cellular Immunol 35: 99–111, 1978.
150. Steigbigel RT, Lambert LH, Remington JS. Polymorphonuclear leukocyte, monocyte and macrophage bactericidal function in patients with Hodgkin's disease. J Lab Clin Med 88: 54–62, 1976.
151. Scheinberg MA, Masuda A, Maluf JA, Mendes NF. Monocyte function in patients with solid neoplasms during immunotherapy with Corynebacterium parvum. Cancer 41: 1761–1764, 1978.
152. Saito H, Tomioka H. Suppressive factor of tumour origin against macrophage phagocytosis of Staphylococcus aureus. Br J Cancer 41: 259–267, 1980.
153. Piessens WF. Increased binding of tumour cells by macrophages activated in vitro with lymphocyte mediators. Cell Immunol 35: 303–317, 1978.
154. Chambers VC, Weiser RS. The ultrastructure of target cells and immune macrophages during their interaction in vitro. Cancer Res 29: 301–317, 1969.
155. Evans R. Macrophage cytotoxicity. In van Furth R. (ed.), Mononuclear phagocytes in immunity, infection and pathology. Oxford: Blackwell, 1975, pp. 827–843.
156. Adams DO, Nathan CF. Molecular mechanisms in tumour-cell killing by activated macrophages. Immunol Today 4: 166–170, 1983.
157. Nathan CF, Cohn ZA. Role of oxygen-dependent mechanisms in antibody induced lysis of tumour cells by activated macrophages. J Exp Med 152: 198–208, 1980.
158. Adams DO. Effector mechanisms of cytolytically activated macrophages. I. Secretion of neutral proteases and effect of protease inhibitors. J Immunol 124: 286–292, 1980.
159. Nathan CF, Brukner LH, Silverstein SC, Cohn ZA. Extracellular cytolysis by activated macrophages and granulocytes. I. Pharmacologic triggering of effector cells and the release of hydrogen peroxide. J Exp Med 149: 84–99, 1979.
160. Cohen MS, Taffet SM, Adams DO. The relationship between competence for secretion of H_2O_2 and completion of tumour cytotoxicity by BCG-elicited murine macrophages. J Immunol 128: 1781–1785, 1982.
161. Nathan CF, Arrick BA, Murray HW, DeSantis NM, Cohn ZA. Tumour cell anti-oxidant defenses. Inhibition of glutathione redox cycle enhances macrophage-mediated cytolysis. J Exp Med 153: 766–782, 1981.
162. Nathan CF, Klebanoff SJ. Augmentation of spontaneous macrophage-mediated cytotoxicity by eosinophil peroxidase. J Exp Med 155: 1291–1308, 1982.
163. Adams DO, Kao K-J, Farb R, Pizzo SV. Effector mechanisms of cytolytically activated macrophages. II. Secretion of cytolytic factor by activated macrophages and its relationship to secreted neutral proteases. J Immunol 124: 293–300, 1980.
164. Ruff MR, Gifford GE. Purification and physicochemical characterization of rabbit tumour necrosis factor. J Immunol 125: 1671–1677, 1980.
165. Currie GA. Activated macrophages kill tumour cells by releasing arginase. Nature (Lond.) 273: 758–759, 1978.
166. Fishman M. Functional heterogeneity among peritoneal macrophages. III. No evidence for the role of arginase in the inhibition of tumor cell growth by supernatants from macrophages or macrophage subpopulation culture. Cell Immunol 55: 174–184, 1980.
167. Farram E, Nelson DS. Mechanism of action of mouse macrophages as antitumour effector cells: Role of arginase. Cell Immunol 55: 283–293, 1980.
168. Baggiolini M, Schnyder J. Synthesis and release of lytic enzymes by macrophages in chronic inflammation. Adv Exp Med Biol 155: 305–312, 1982.

169. Hibbs JB Jr, Chapman HA Jr, Weinberg JB. Regulation of macrophage non-specific tumouricidal capability. In van Furth R (ed.), Mononuclear phagocytes, functional aspects. The Hague: Martinus Nijhoff, 1980, pp. 1681–1724.

170. Keller R. Cytostatic killing of syngeneic tumour cells by activated non-immune macrophages. In van Furth R (ed.), Mononuclear phagocytes in immunity, infection and pathology. Oxford: Blackwell, 1975, pp. 857–868.

171. Keller R. Distinctive characteristics of host tumor resistance in a rat fibrosarcoma model system. In van Furth R (ed.), Mononuclear phagocytes: Functional aspects. The Hague: Martinus Nijhoff, 1980, pp. 1725–1740.

172. Keller R. Regulatory capacities of mononuclear phagocytes with particular reference to natural immunity against tumours. In Herberman RB (ed.), Natural cell-mediated immunity against tumours. New York: Academic Press, 1980, pp. 1219–1269.

173. Somers SD, Adams DO. Augmented binding of tumour cells by activated murine macrophages and its relevance to tumour cytotoxicity. In Herberman RB (ed.), NK cells and other natural effector cells. New York: Academic Press, 1982, pp. 1003–1009.

174. Johnson WJ, Weiel JE, Adams DO. The relationship between secretion of a novel cytolytic protease and macrophage-mediated tumour cytotoxicity. In Herberman RB (ed.), NK cells and other natural effector cells. New York: Academic Press: 1982, pp. 949–954.

175. Cameron DJ, Churchill WH. Cytotoxicity of human macrophages for tumour cells—Enhancement by human lymphocyte mediators. J Clin Invest 63: 977–984, 1979.

176. Nathan CF, Murray HW, Wiebe E, Rubin BY. Identification of interferon – γ as the lymphokine that activates human macrophage oxidative metabolism and antimicrobial activity. J Exp Med 158: 670–689, 1983.

177. Perussia B, Dayton ET, Lazarus R, Fanning V, Trinchieri G. Immune interferon induces the receptor for monomeric IgG 1 on human monocytic and myeloid cells. J Exp Med 158: 1092–1113, 1983.

178. Schultz RM, Chirigos MA, Heine UI. Functional and morphologic characteristics of interferon-treated macrophages. Cell Immunol 35: 84–91, 1978.

179. Boraschi D, Ghezzi P, Pasqualetto E, Salmona M, Nencioni L, Soldateschi D, Villa L, Tagliabue A. Interferon decreases production of hydrogen peroxide by macrophages; correlation with reduction of suppressive capacity and of antimicrobial activity. Immunology 50: 359–368, 1983.

180. Le Marbre P, Rinehart JJ, Kay NE, Vasella R, Jacob HS. Lysozyme enhances monocyte-mediated tumoricidal activity: A potential amplifying mechanism of tumour killing. Blood 58: 994–999, 1981.

181. Schlager SI, Meltzer MS. Role of macrophage lipids in regulating tumoricidal activity. II. Internal genetic and external physiologic regulatory factors controlling macrophage tumor cytotoxicity also control characteristic lipid changes associated with tumoricidal cells. Cell Immunol 80: 10–19, 1983.

182. Horwitz DA, Kight N, Temple A, Allison AC. Spontaneous and induced cytotoxic properties of human adherent mononuclear cells: Killing of non-sensitized and antibody-coated non-erythroid cells. Immunol 36: 221–228, 1979.

183. De Mulder PHM, De Pauw BE, Pennings A, Wagener DJTh, Haanen C: Increased antibody-dependent cytotoxicity mediated by purified monocytes in Hodgkin's disease. Clin Immunol Immunopathol 26: 406–414, 1983.

184. Kohl S. Pickering LK, Sullivan MP, Walters DL. Impaired monocyte-macrophage cytotoxicity in patients with Hodgkin's disease. Clin Immunol Immunopathol 15: 577–585, 1980.

185. Remington JS, Krahenbuhl JJ, Hibb JB Jr: A role for the macrophage in resistance to tumour development and tumour destruction. In van Furth R (ed.), Mononuclear phagocytes in immunity, infection and pathology. Oxford: Blackwell, 1975, pp. 869–891.

186. Den Otter W, Evans R, Alexander P. Cytotoxicity of murine peritoneal macrophages in tumour allograft immunity. Transplant 14: 220–226, 1972.

187. Evans R, Alexander P. Co-operation of immune lymphoid cells with macrophages in tumour immunity. Nature 228: 620–622, 1970.

188. Evans R, Alexander P. Role of macrophages in tumour immunity. I. Co-operation between macrophages and lymphoid cells in syngeneic tumour immunity. Immunol 23: 615–626, 1972.

189. Evans R, Alexander P. Rendering macrophages specifically cytotoxic by a factor released from immune lymphoid cells. Transplant 12: 227–229, 1971.

190. Fidler IJ. Activation of mouse macrophages by syngeneic, allogeneic, or xenogeneic lymphocyte supernatants. J Natl Cancer Inst 55: 1159–1163, 1975.

191. Lohmann-Matthes M-L, Fischer H. Macrophage-mediated cytotoxic induction by a specific T-cell factor. In van Furth R. (ed.), Mononuclear phagocytes in immunity, infection and pathology. Oxford: Blackwell, 1975, pp. 845–854.

192 Cameron DJ, O'Brien P. Cytotoxicity of cancer patients' macrophages for tumour cells. Cancer 50: 498–502. 1982.

193. Cameron DJ, Collawn SS. Cytotoxicity of cancer patients' macrophages for tumour cells: Purification and characterization of plasma inhibitory factors obtained from colon cancer patients. Intern J Immunopharmacol 5: 55–66, 1983.

194. Unsgaard G, Eggen BM, Lamvik J. Depression of monocyte mediated cytotoxicity by renal carcinoma and restoration through therapy. J Surg Oncol 22: 51–55, 1983.

195. King GW, Yanes B, Hurtubise PE, Balcerzak SP, Lobuglio AF. Immune function of successfully treated lymphoma patients. J Clin Invest 57: 1451–1460, 1976.

196. Keller R: Tumor-promoting diterpene esters induce macrophage activation, but prevent activation for tumoricidal activity of macrophage and NK cells. In Herberman RB (ed.), NK cells and other natural effector cells. New York: Academic Press, 1982, pp. 601–606.

197. Gabizon A, Lelbovich SJ, Goldman R. Contrasting effects of activated and non-activated macrophages and macrophages from tumor-bearing mice on tumor growth in vivo. J Natl Cancer Inst 65: 913–920, 1980.

198. North RJ, Spitalny GL, Berendt MJ. Significance of systemic macrophage activation in response to tumour growth. In van Furth (ed.), Mononuclear phagocytes: Functional aspects. The Hague: Martinus Mijhoff, 1980, pp. 1655–1676.

199. Currie GA. Serum lysozyme as a marker of host resistance. II. Patients with malignant melanoma, hypernephroma or breast carcinoma. Br J Cancer 33: 593–599, 1976.

200. Zeya HI, Keku E, Richards F, Spurr CL. Monocyte and granulocyte defect in chronic lymphocytic leukaemia. Am J Pathol 95: 43–54, 1979.

201. Currie GA, Eccles SA. Serum lysozyme as a marker of host resistance. I. Production by macrophages in rat sarcomata. Br J Cancer 33: 51–59, 1976.

202. Kerbel RS, Pross HF, Elliott EV. Origin and partial characterization of Fc receptor-bearing cells found within experimental carcinomas and sarcomas. Int J Cancer 15: 918–932, 1975.

203. Birbeck MSC, Carter RL. Observations on the ultrastructure of two hamster lymphomas with particular reference to infiltrating macrophages. Int J Cancer 9: 249–257, 1972.

204. Haskill JS, Proctor JW, Yamamura A. Host responses within solid tumours. I. Monocytic effector cells within rat sarcomas. J Natl Cancer Inst 54: 387–393, 1975.

205. Van Loveren H, Den Otter W. Macrophages in solid tumours. I. Immunlogically specific effector cells. J Natl Cancer Inst 53: 1057–1060, 1974.

206. Russell SW, McIntosh AT. Macrophages isolated from regressing Moloney sarcomas are more cytotoxic than those recovered from progressing sarcomas. Nature (Lond.) 268: 69–71, 1977.

207. Mantovani A. In vitro effects on tumour cells of macrophages isolated from an early-passage chemically-induced murine sarcoma and from its spontaneous metastases. Int J Cancer 27: 221–228, 1981.

208. Pross HF, Kerbel RS. An assessment of intratumor phagocytic and surface marker-bearing cells in a series of autochthonous and early passaged chemically induced murine sarcomas. J Natl Cancer Inst 57: 1157–1167, 1976.

209. Mansell PWA, Di Luzio NR. The in vivo destruction of human tumor by glucan activated macrophages. In Fink MA (ed.), The macrophage in neoplasia. New York: Academic Press, 1976, pp. 227–243.

210. Ree HJ, Crowley JP, Leone LA. Macrophage-histiocyte lysozyme activity in relation to the clinical presentation of Hodgkin's disease: An immunohistochemical study. Cancer 47: 1988–1993, 1981.

211. Hansen NE, Clausen PP, Karle H, Christoffersen P. Tissue and plasma lysozyme in Hodgkin's disease. Scand J Haematol 27: 186–192, 1981.

212. Ward PA, Berenberg JL. Defective regulation of inflammatory mediators in Hodgkin's disease. Super normal levels of chemotactic-factor inactivator. New Engl J Med 290: 76–80, 1974.

213. Pike MC, Snyderman R. Depression of macrophage function by a factor produced by neoplasmas: A mechanism for abrogation of immune surveillance. J Immunol 117: 1243–1249, 1976.

214. Bice DE, Gruwell D, Salvaggio J. Inhibition of macrophage migration by plasma factor(s) from patients with neoplasms and normal individuals. J Reticuloendothel Soc 19: 281–289, 1976.

215. Norris DA, Perez RE, Golitz LE, Seitz LE, Weston WL. Defective monocyte chemotaxis in mycosis fungoides: Lack of essential helper lymphocytes. Cancer 44: 124–130, 1979.

216. Snyderman R, Pike MC. Biological activities of a macrophage chemotaxis inhibitor (MCI) produced by neoplasms. In Quastel MR (ed.), Cell biology and immunology of leukocyte function. New York: Academic Press, 1979, pp. 535–546.

217. Pasternack GR, Snyderman R, Pike MC, Johnson RJ, Shin HS. Resistance of neoplasms to immunological destruction: Role of a macrophage chemotaxis inhibitor. J Exp Med 148: 92–102, 1978.

218. Fauve RM, Hevin M-B. Toxic effects of tumour cells on macrophages. In James K. McBride B, Stuart A. (eds.), The macrophage and cancer. Edinburgh: University of Edinburgh Medical School, 1977, pp. 264–270.

219. Normann SJ, Schardt M, Sorkin E. Do tumours escape surveillance by depression of macrophage inflammation? In James K, McBride B, Stuart A (eds.), The Macrophage and cancer. Edinburgh: University of Edinburgh Medical School, 1977, pp 247–257.

220. Normann SJ. Tumour cell threshold required for suppression of macrophage inflammation. J Natl Cancer Inst 60: 1091–1096, 1978.

221. Normann SJ, Schardt M, Sorkin E. Cancer progression and monocyte inflammatory dysfunction: Relationship to tumour excision and metastasis. Int J Cancer 23: 110–113, 1979.

222. Kalish R, Brody NI. The effects of a tumour facilitating factor of B16 melanoma on the macrophage. J Invest Dermatol 80: 162–167, 1983.

223. Normann SJ, Sorkin E. Inhibition of macrophage chemotaxis by neoplastic and other rapidly proliferating cells "in vitro." Cancer Res 37: 705–711, 1977.

224. Bottazzi B, Polentarutti N, Acero R, Balsari A, Boraschi D, Ghezzi P, Salmona M, Mantovani A. Regulation of macrophage content of neoplasms by chemoattractants. Science 220: 210–212, 1983.

225. Bottazzi B, Polentarutti N, Balsari A, Boraschi D, Ghezzi P, Salmona M, Mantovani A. Chemotactic activity for mononuclear phagocytes of culture supernatants from murine and human tumor cells: Evidence for a role in the regulation of the macrophage content of neoplastic tissues. Int J Cancer 31: 55–63, 1983.

226. Ramaroo GVSV, Tompkins WAF. Inhibition of macrophage phagocytosis by a human colon tumour cell factor. J Reticuloendothel Soc 23: 373–382, 1978.

227. Saito H, Tomioka H. Suppressive factor against macrophage phagocytosis produced by cultured sarcoma-180 cells. Gann 70: 671–675, 1979.

228. Rhodes J, Bishop M, Benfield J. Tumour surveillance: How tumours may resist macrophage-mediated host defense. Science 203: 179–182, 1979.

229. Griffin FM. Effects of soluble immune complexes on Fc receptor and C3b receptor mediated phagocytosis by macrophages. J Exp Med 152: 905–919, 1980.

230. Currie GA, Alexander P. Spontaneous shedding of TSTA by viable sarcoma cells: Its possible role in facilitating metastatic spread. Br J Cancer 29: 72–75, 1974.

231. Israel L, Edelstein R. "In vivo" and "in vitro" studies on non-specific blocking factors of host origin in cancer patients. Role of plasma exchange as an immunotherapeutic modality. Isr J Med Sci 14: 105–130, 1977.

232. Eggen BM, Lamvik J, Ungsgaard G. Inhibitory effect on monocyte-mediated cytotoxicity of sera from patients with multiple myeloma and malignant lymphoma. Scand J Haematol 29: 381–388, 1982.

233. Halliday WJ, Miller S. Leukocyte adherence inhibition: A simple test for cell-mediated immunity and serum blocking factors. Int J Cancer 9: 477–483, 1972.

234. Halliday WJ, Maluish A, Isbister WH. Detection of anti-tumour cell-mediated immunity and serum blocking factors in cancer patients by the leucocyte adherence inhibition test. Br J Cancer 29: 31–35, 1974.

235. Grosser N, Thomson DMP. Cell-mediated anti-tumour immunity in breast cancer patients evaluated by antigen-induced leukocyte adherence inhibition in test tubes. Cancer Res 35: 2571–2579, 1975.

236. Vose BM, Hughes R, Bazill GW. Failure of leucocyte-adherence inhibition assays to discriminate between benign and malignant breast diseases. Br J Cancer 40: 954–956, 1979.

237. Fritze D, Fedra G, Kaufmann M. Prospective evaluation of the leukocyte adherence inhibition (LAI) test in breast cancer using a panel of extracts from known and unknown primary tumours. Int J Cancer 29: 261–264, 1982.

238. Sarlo KT, Mortensen RF. Leukocyte adherence inhibition response to murine sarcoma-virus-induced tumours. II. Requirement of T-cell subpopulations and macrophages. Cell Immunol 79:'211–219, 1983.

4. TUMOUR MARKERS

A. MILFORD WARD

INTRODUCTION

Tumour markers may be defined as serum or body fluid constituents found in inappropriate concentrations in tumour-bearing patients. As such they encompass not only those products of tumour cells that may correctly be termed tumour antigens but also normal body constituents that are produced in excessive amounts in response to the tumour load. Tumour antigens are "synthetic" markers, which may be tumour specific like the oncofetal antigens or nonspecific like the various enzymes and hormones that may demonstrate inappropriate secretion. Those substances produced by host tissues as a response to the presence of tumour are "reactive" markers and include such substances as the acute phase reactive proteins and many enzymes. These reactive markers can never be considered as specific for the tumour-bearing state, and their interpretation should always be approached with caution. Table 4–1 lists the synthetic and reactive tumour markers.

With few notable exceptions, the specificity of tumour markers for any particular malignancy is poor. Indeed, many of the synthetic markers may, on occasions, be considered as acute phase reactive substances, found as they are in increased concentrations in some inflammatory diseases. These synthetic markers with acute phase properties are, for the most part, cell surface antigens that are liberated during situations of increased cell turnover, which may occur in regenerative states as well as in malignancy.

The advent of the hybridoma has increased the impetus for research into antibodies reacting with cell surface antigens of malignant cells. This research has produced a plethora of "new" tumour markers, some of which show considerable promise both for diagnosis and for monitoring of the tumour-bearing patient and his or her treatment. The monoclonal

B.W. Hancock and A.M. Ward (eds.), Immunological Aspects of Cancer. Copyright © 1985, Martinus Nijhoff Publishing, Boston/Dordrecht/Lancaster.

Table 4–1. Tumour markers

Type	Specific/nonspecific	Substances produced
Synthetic	Specific	Oncofetal antigens/proteins Proteins
	Nonspecific	Proteins Hormones Enzymes Nucleosides
Reactive	Nonspecific	Acute phase proteins Enzymes

antibodies are not without their problems, however, and their extreme specificity may even be a disadvantage when considering the more heterogeneous markers such as carcinoembryonic antigen.

Tumour markers are conventionally thought of as recent innovations dependent on modern technology for their characterisation and measurement. It is salutary, therefore, to remember that the most specific and sensitive marker in the armamentarium of the laboratory was first described in 1847. Bence Jones [1] characterised the protein by which he is eponymously remembered but which had been previously isolated by MacIntyre [2] from the patient described by Dalrymple [3]. Bence Jones protein (or, more correctly, monoclonal free immunoglobulin light chains) in the urine is specific for plasma cell malignancy and is virtually never seen in any other situation. Such specificity cannot be claimed for any other tumour marker in general use today.

Despite the veritable plethora of tumour markers described in the last two decades, relatively few have stood the test of time and been shown to be of clinical value. The major question that must be asked of all putative markers is, Does the marker level allow the clinician to plan patient management? The answer to this question is, at best, a qualified yes in a small group of marker substances and then only in the light of the established clinical status.

Alphafetoprotein (AFP)

First described by Bergstrand and Czar [4], alphafetoprotein (AFP) is a normal serum protein of the fetus. A glycoprotein of 65,000 daltons, it has a biological half-life of 3.5 to 4.0 days. It is synthesised in the fetal liver, foregut, and yolk sac from the tenth gestational week [5]. Molecular heterogeneity based on the structure of the carbohydrate moiety has been described [6] and allows distinction to be made between AFP of hepatic and yolk sac origin.

The role of AFP as a tumour marker was first claimed by Abelev et al. [7] in their description of elevated levels in the serum of mice with transplantable hepatocellular carcinomas. This was closely followed by Tatarinov's description of elevated levels in human hepatocellular carcinoma [8] and somewhat later by the description of similar elevations in certain germ cell tumours [9]. The origin of the gonadal tumour AFP in yolk sac elements [10] of the teratomatous tumours successfully linked the physiological state described by Gitlin with the pathological morphology of Teilum [11].

Human chorionic gonadotrophin (HCG)

Human chorionic gonadotrophin (HCG) is a placental glycoprotein hormone of 38,000 daltons with a biological half-life of rather less than 24 hours. It is synthesised by the syncytial trophoblast and by nongestational trophoblast elements in both gonadal and extragonadal tumours. HCG is composed of two dissimilar polypeptide chains. The α chain is identical to the α chains of human luteinising hormone (LH) and follicle-stimulating hormone (FSH). The β chain, whilst being distinct from that of FSH, shares 86 identical residues with the β chain of LH and differs only in the extra C terminal domain of 26 residues. Whereas total HCG is used as a marker for intrauterine choriocarcinoma, tumour specificity for extrauterine malignancy is achieved by assay of the β subunit. In addition to its secretion by trophoblastic elements in germ cell tumours, inappropriate secretion has been described in a wide variety of malignancies [12].

The lack of total specificity of most antisera for the β subunit of HCG leads to varying degrees of cross-reactivity with endogenous LH with spurious elevations of the marker, particularly in female patients. LH is also known to rise after orchidectomy. This, together with the rise associated with chemotherapy-induced hypogonadism, will explain some of the spurious elevations noted in males undergoing regular βHCG monitoring of gonadal tumour therapy. Reassay after administration of testosterone may resolve any diagnostic problems that arise [13].

Carcinoembryonic antigen (CEA)

Carcinoembryonic antigen (CEA) is a family of acid glycoproteins of about 200,000 daltons that demonstrate considerable intermolecular and intramolecular heterogeneity. Originally, it was described as carcinoembryonic antigen (CEA) of the human digestive system to denote its site of isolation and preparation. It is expressed in considerable amounts by the fetal intestinal epithelium, where it can be found in the glycocalyx surrounding the cell membrane and from whence it can be shed into the circulation [14]. CEA can be detected as a normal serum protein in the adult in concentrations of less than $2.5\mu g/l$. Modest elevations may be found during pregnancy, in smokers, and in certain inflammatory diseases such as ulcerative colitis, Crohn's disease, and pulmonary infections. Raised levels may also be seen in association with some benign tumours. Grossly raised levels, in excess of $20\mu g/l$, are, however, strongly suggestive of malignancy.

As a tumour marker it suffers from low sensitivity (true positive rate) and poor specificity (true negative rate) and cannot, therefore, be used reliably as diagnostic agent for population screening or in the "at-risk" patient. Its value as a monitor of tumour elimination is hampered by a failure to define an acceptable biological half-life, estimates ranging from 6 to 60 days being reported [15]. This gross variation in biological half-life estimates is related to the molecular heterogeneity and to the more rapid elimination of deglycosylated components.

Regular and sequential assay of CEA may, however, have a role in the management of colorectal, breast, and bronchial carcinoma.

Oncofetal pancreatic antigen (OPA)

Oncofetal pancreatic antigen (OPA) [16,17] is one of a group of oncofetal antigens described in relation to carcinoma of the pancreas. OPA is described as having a molecular weight of about 40,000 daltons and to be relatively low in carbohydrate. As a marker of carcinoma of the pancreas, OPA has good sensitivity but only moderate specificity. Some overlap in assay values is seen in cases of chronic pancreatitis, and OPA synthesis is seen in cases of other foregut-derived tumours. The finding of postoperative decline in OPA values following successful resection of pancreatic carcinoma suggests that this antigen may have a place in the monitoring of this notoriously refractory malignancy.

Pregnancy-specific β-glycoprotein (SP1)

Pregnancy specific β-glycoprotein (SP1) is a glycoprotein of trophoblastic origin that has been examined as a potential second marker for choriocarcinoma and the trophoblastic elements of gonadal teratomas. The few cases where there is discordance between SP1 and HCG in relation to trophoblastic tumour load suggest that there may be differing responses to therapy within the metabolic pathways of the two markers [18]. The differences are, however, not sufficient to justify the inclusion of SP1 in the monitoring schedule at the present time.

Monoclonal immunoglobulins (MIg) and immunoglobulin fragments

Neoplastic proliferation of a single clone of immunoglobulin-producing cells leads to the production of a quantity of identical molecules that migrate on electrophoresis of serum or urine as a discrete abnormal band. This abnormal protein component has been variously termed "paraprotein," "M-component," or "monoclonal component." It is a true synthetic tumour marker in that it is the product of a neoplastic secretory cell line. Unbalanced immunoglobulin chain production by the neoplastic cell leads to an excess of free light chains that may appear in the urine, where they demonstrate the unique thermosolubility characteristics that have earned them the eponymic name of Bence Jones protein.

The neoplastic plasma cell proliferation is also associated with a reduction or paresis of the nonneoplastic immunoglobulin-producing cell lines. The protein abnormality required as one of the diagnostic criteria of myelomatosis [19] includes the presence of a serum or urine monoclonal component or an immune paresis.

Differentiation of the neoplastic from the benign monoclonal gammopathy is made by the relentless progression and increase in concentration of the neoplastic monoclonal component and the presence of the excess monoclonal free light chains. Monoclonal components may be seen as an age-related phenomenon with an increasing frequency after the age of 60 years [20]. Though many of them are benign, a proportion do have malignant potential [21].

Prostatic acid phosphatase (PAP)

The tartrate labile isoenzyme of acid phosphatase has long been used as a diagnostic test for carcinoma of the prostate [22]. Despite the long years of use, PAP is neither a sensitive nor a specific marker for carcinoma of prostate in its early stages. The advent of a specific radioimmunoassay [23] has done little to increase the sensitivity of the assay but has helped considerably in the specificity. Whilst with the enzymatic technique 50 to 70% of bony metastases [24] from carcinoma of prostate give elevated values, this proportion can be increased to better than 90% by the immunoassay [23].

Prostate-specific antigen (PSA)

Prostate-specific antigen (PSA) is a cell surface protein derived from the glandular element of the prostate and has been shown to have a molecular weight of 33,000 to 34,000 daltons with a marked propensity to polymerise or associate with normal plasma proteins [25]. Despite considerable reports of specificity for prostatic cancer, significant elevations may be seen in benign prostatic hypertrophy. There is, however, close correlation between plasma levels and both clinical stage and prognosis, with persistent elevation after prostatectomy signifying metastatic spread [26].

The specificity of this new marker for malignant disease of the prostate may be improved by simultaneous assay of PSA and PAP [27]. Although this demonstrates discordance between the two markers, the selection of relatively high cutoff values allows diagnosis of stage 1 disease in 60% of cases with only a 10% false positive rate in benign hypertrophy and no false positives in nonprostate disease. The positivity rate increases with the stage of disease to reach more than 90% in stage 4.

Acute phase reactant proteins (APRP)

The acute phase reactant proteins—α_1-acid glycoprotein, haptoglobin, ceruloplasmin, α_1-antitrypsin, and α_1-antichymotrypsin—are all known to rise in tumour-bearing patients [28]. The response is reactive on the part of the host and entirely nonspecific. Similar profile changes may also be seen in inflammatory and degenerative conditions and can never be taken as diagnostic of malignancy. They do, however, offer some small advantage in the long-term monitoring of patients treated for established malignant disease.

A linear discriminant function analysis involving concurrent assay of a profile of APRPs and CEA has been shown to have prognostic significance in relation to carcinoma of the colon [29]. Sequential analyses in the postoperative period could also demonstrate recurrence better than with CEA alone, but this system suffers from the stimulating effect of wounding on APRP synthesis, making many of the values totally unreliable in the first month after surgery.

A similar approach can be taken with carcinoma of prostate with the substitution of prostatic acid phosphatase as the specific marker in place of CEA [30]. This discriminant can satisfactorily identify extracapsular spread of the tumour with a greater sensitivity and accuracy than bone scanning and at less trauma to the patient than pelvic node biopsy. The value of local metastasis identification in patient management is, however, doubtful. Te Velde et al. [31] have shown a similar value of acute phase reactant proteins in identifying recurrence in patients with carcinoma of cervix. These workers claim a three-to-four-month lead time on the basis of serial estimations of α_1-antitrypsin, C1 esterase inhibitor, and C reactive protein.

Bradwell [32] showed a significant relationship between haptoglobin and α_1-acid glycoprotein levels and tumour mass in carcinoma of bronchus. There was also a significant relationship between α_1-acid glycoprotein concentrations and survival. This relationship was independent of the original concentration and tumour mass and may reflect silent metastatic disease at the time of primary surgery. Both haptoglobin and α_1-acid glycoprotein were shown to rise on average four months before the clinical appearance of metastatic disease

Table 4-2. Tumour markers of value in primary diagnosis

Marker	Diagnosis
Alphafetoprotein	Hepatoblastoma
Bence Jones protein	Plasmacytoma and myeloma
HCG	Choriocarcinoma

Table 4-3. Tumour markers unreliable in primary diagnosis

Carcinoembryonic antigen (CEA)
Casein
Fetal sulphaglycoprotein antigen (FSA)
Isoferritin (α_2H)
Noncross reacting antigen (NCA)
Pregnancy-associated macroglobulin (PAM, SP3)
Tennessee antigen
Tissue polypeptide antigen (TPA)

and with a greater reliability than CEA. The picture was, however, confused by the acute phase response in any episode of pulmonary infection (to which such patients are particularly prone).

Other reports have shown a close stage relationship between carcinoma of the bladder [33], carcinoma of the cervix [34], and non-Hodgkin's lymphoma [35], and the acute phase reactant profile. Whilst this relationship cannot be considered diagnostic, it can be of value in pretreatment assessment.

TUMOUR MARKERS AND PRIMARY DIAGNOSIS

The specificity of even the synthetic markers is in general too low to allow their reliable use as primary diagnostic aids. Although the initial studies with carcinoembryonic antigen (CEA) [36] suggested it to be both a sensitive and specific marker for adenocarcinoma of the colon, further studies have shown it to be produced by many tumour types and to be present in increased concentrations in a number of inflammatory or reactive states. There is now general agreement that only 40% of stage 1 adenocarcinoma of the colon is CEA positive and that any attempted screening programme would be faced with a similar 40% false positive rate. A similar situation can be found with most other tumour markers.

The relatively few markers that can be considered of proven value in primary diagnosis are listed in table 4–2; even here due consideration must be given to the clinical situation in which the assay is attempted. Alphafetoprotein (AFP) can be considered a diagnostic marker only in the situation of a possible hepatic tumour in the very young child. Human chorionic gonadatrophin (HCG) is similarly of diagnostic significance only in a woman who has previously had a hydatidiform mole and is known not to be pregnant.

Table 4–3 includes some of the more recently described markers that have no value in primary diagnosis, their specificity or sensitivity being such that the false negative and false positive results will significantly exceed the number of correct diagnoses made.

There is, however, a third group in which, under specific clinical circumstances, the presence of tumour markers may be a useful guide or indication to the primary diagnosis. Some of these are detailed in table 4-4. AFP, βHCG, and SP1 can all provide aids to diagnosis in a patient with a gonadal mass and, by virtue of their cytological origin, can give a guide to the histological appearance of the tumour and its prognosis.

Oncofetal pancreatic antigen (OPA), though being found in many tumours of the foregut derivatives, may be of considerable value in the differential diagnosis of an obstructive jaundice as will also the CEA level in pancreatic juice.

Gross excess of any marker may be considered diagnostic of the tumour-bearing state, but site of origin remains a clinical decision, although this may be considered as rather academic when the excessive marker levels are usually associated with stage 4 disease.

AFP in hepatoblastoma and hepatocellular carcinoma

AFP elevations above 50 to 100μg/l are seen in all cases of hepatoblastoma of childhood and in 80 to 90% of hepatocellular carcinoma in adults [37,38,39]. Sustained elevations of AFP can vary enormously in magnitude from the modest elevations of 100μg/l to several g/l [40].

The demonstration of AFP elevations prior to the development of liver tumours in genetically predisposed animals [41] and following ingestion of hepatic carcinogens [42] has raised the possibility of using AFP as a screening test for hepatocellular carcinoma in man. The temporal relationship between onset of hepatic malignancy and the elevation of measurable levels of AFP is however unclear. The situation is further confused by possible racial differences in reference values and the effect of endemic hepatitis-hepatic regeneration following hepatitis being associated with temporary elevations of AFP [43]. The incidence of hepatocellular carcinoma in Europe and the United States is too low to warrant population screening except in selected populations that have a recognised carcinogenic risk [44]. Repetitive testing in this situation is essential, as only sustained and increasing levels may be considered as indicative of malignancy.

One programme recorded [45] the mass screening of 500,000 individuals for the possible development of hepatocellular carcinoma. Several were detected and 10% showed a biphasic response on serial studies similar to that seen in chemical carcinogenesis [42].

AFP in other abdominal malignancy

In keeping with the synthesis of AFP by the fetal foregut, there are occasional reports of AFP elevations in association with tumours arising from foregut derivatives. Rare AFP-

Table 4–4. Tumour markers of value as a guide to diagnosis

Tumour marker	Diagnosis
Alphafetoprotein	Gonadal teratoma (yolk sac elements)
Carcinoembryonic antigen in pancreatic juice	Carcinoma of pancreas
Oncofetal pancreatic antigen	Carcinoma of pancreas
Thyrocalcitonin	Medullary carcinoma of thyroid
Pregnancy-specific β-glycoprotein (SP1)	Gonadal teratoma (trophoblastic elements)
β-subunit human chorionic gonadotrophin	Gonadal teratoma (trophoblastic elements)
Excessive levels of many markers	

producing tumours of the stomach, duodenum, and pancreas have been described [46]. Because of its rarity, this situation is more likely to introduce confusion into the diagnosis rather than be of assistance.

TUMOUR MARKERS IN THE MONITORING OF MALIGNANCY

The logical and appropriate use of tumour markers is in the field of monitoring therapy and the early detection of recurrent disease. In this role tumour markers have a valuable part to play in the modern management of malignant disease.

The three main lines of approach in relation to the use of tumour markers in the monitoring of malignant disease are listed in table 4–5. The serum level of the synthetic markers is related to the tumour load within fairly broad confines. In the teratoma group the AFP and βHCG levels will relate to the mass of yolk sac and trophoblastic tissue, respectively, rather than to the total tumour bulk. In the plasma cell malignancies the relationship of monoclonal component concentration to tumour bulk in different patients is much less marked unless the subclass of the monoclonal immunoglobulin is defined. Even with this proviso the relationship is weak, and estimates of tumour load are more reliably restricted to relative assessments within the one patient.

The rate of elimination of a marker after therapy is a complex calculation involving the doubling time of the tumour, the marker synthetic rate, and its biological half-life or catabolic rate.

Marker kinetics, where they can be calculated, offer an earlier indication of successful therapy than can be obtained by awaiting basal levels, which may never be achieved. This has been applied most satisfactorily to the decay of AFP levels following orchidectomy for testicular teratoma. The apparent half-life (AHL) after treatment should approximate biological half-life of the protein if there has been complete elimination of marker-producing tissue [47]. The slope of the marker regression curve derived from sequential sample analysis can be expressed as:

$$\text{AHL} = \frac{-0.693T}{\log_e \dfrac{(Ct)}{(Co)}}$$

where T is the interval in days between marker analyses, Ct is the concentration at time T, and Co the initial marker concentration. For AFP, with a biological half-life of 3.5 to 4

Table 4–5. The role of tumour markers in the monitoring of malignant disease

Indicators of residual tumours
  for second-look surgery
  selection for additional therapy

Early diagnosis of recurrent disease
  lead time for therapy
  early assessment of therapeutic trials

Response to therapy
  assessment of the effect of therapy
  indication for change of therapy

days, values for the AHL in excess of 5 days are indicative of residual disease that will eventually recur, and values in excess of 10 days carry an extremely bad prognosis with large volume residual disease and the probability of early overt recurrence. AHL values of less than 5 days are invariably associated with stage 1 disease and carry an excellent prognosis. This is essentially similar to, but rather simpler than, the Lange et al. [48] approach, where the expected AFP concentration X_t is compared with the observed level in the patient:

$$X_t = x_o e^{-0.139t}.$$

(X_o is the initial concentration, and X_t the concentration after t days.) Although most studies using this approach have concentrated on marker decay following primary surgical treatment, it can also be used following courses of cytotoxic therapy aimed at elimination of residual tumour load. The marker kinetics or rate of postoperative elimination of a marker are sensitive indicators of residual disease.

Marker recurrence after an initial fall is indicative of the need for further reassessment and/or treatment and a prolonged AHL indicates the need for additional therapy. Sequential monitoring over many weeks or months allows the early diagnosis of recurrent disease and may give a lead time of up to six months on the development of clinical symptoms. Marker kinetics, as opposed to clinical assessment, can also give an earlier indication of the effectiveness of a therapeutic regimen and allow earlier assessment of clinical trials of new chemotherapeutic agents.

This response to therapy can also be used to indicate the need to change a patient from one agent to another if marker elimination is not being achieved. Early assessment of the effectiveness or otherwise of a therapeutic regimen may considerably affect the eventual outcome in the individual patient and obviate the unnecessary use of toxic agents to no effect.

THE USE OF TUMOUR MARKERS IN THE MANAGEMENT OF SPECIFIC MALIGNANCIES

Choriocarcinoma

Serum levels of βHCG are measured routinely after uterine evacuation in all cases of hydatidiform mole and as a monitor of chemotherapy in choriocarcinoma [49]. In these situations, βHCG is an ideal marker, albeit of a relatively rare tumour. It can be used to good clinical effect both to monitor therapy and to diagnose recurrent disease. As the "at-risk" population is small and definable, it is also logistically possible to use the marker as a screening test for the development of the malignancy. The serum levels correlate closely with tumour load, and increased levels may be detected with a minimum of 10^5 cells [50]. Central nervous system involvement may be accurately predicted by estimation of βHCG levels in the CSF [51].

Germ cell tumours

Ninety percent of all testicular teratomas show elevations of either AFP or βHCG; in many instances both markers are elevated [52,53]. Similar elevations of either or both markers may be seen in malignant teratoma of ovary and extragonadal sites. βHCG elevations are also seen in a proportion of cases of seminoma usually associated with the presence of syncytial giant cells [54]. Some authors recommend the addition of CEA, SP1, and human placental lactogen (LPL) to the marker profile [55]. The proportion of positives for these markers is lower than for AFP and βHCG and the additional information gained is slight. CEA does, however, have a place in the monitoring of the rare Sertoli cell tumour. The combined use of both markers is crucial to the adequate management of germ cell tumours in all sites, both gonadal [56,57] and extragonadal [58].

Staging

Elevated levels of either marker prior to surgical excision will fall to normal in stage 1 disease within the biological half-life of the marker [47,53,59]. Falling marker levels and AHL estimates can be observed only if regular serum samples are taken for assay. Table 4-6 gives details of the recommended schedule for adequate monitoring of all germ cell tumours by regular assay of AFP and βHCG.

In testicular teratoma, marker decay with an AHL for AFP of greater than five days indicates residual disease and the need for cytotoxic chemotherapy. Elevated marker levels on follow-up without positive clinical or investigational findings are considered as minimal bulk metastatic disease [60]; the prognosis in this group is good after appropriate treatment. Rising levels after primary surgery indicate massive residual disease, and the overall prognosis is bleak. Whilst much of the available data refer to experiences with testicular germ tumours, the pattern of progression and prognosis is similar for germ cell tumours of ovarian and extragonadal origin [59,61].

Prognosis

Marker levels are a useful indicator of tumour load prior to surgery and can give a reliable prognostic indication for testicular teratoma. βHCG levels greater than 1×10^5 IU/litre and AFP greater than 1×10^3 IU/litre are associated with a one-year mortality of 40% [62,63]. In contrast, βHCG levels less than 5×10^4 IU/litre or AFP levels less than 0.5×10^3 IU/litre are associated with only a 10% mortality. Similar prognostic value can be gained from the AHL data: for AFP in endodermal sinus tumours, an AHL of less than 5 days has an excellent prognosis; for an AHL of 5 to 10 days the prognosis is guarded, with 75% recurrence inside two years; where the AHL exceeds 10 days the one-year mortality is almost total [59,61]. Evidence suggests that marker levels give a better prognostic index than can be achieved by assessment of tumour bulk [64].

Monitoring therapy

With current curative therapeutic regimens [56,65,66], it is imperative that adequate therapy be given. The assessment of adequate therapy is largely gauged by the serial

Table 4-6. Protocol for marker monitoring of germ cell tumour therapy

1.	Serum for AFP and βHCG on first examination (i.e., prior to surgery).
2.	Repeat serum prior to operation or primary treatment.
3.	Repeat serum twice weekly after primary treatment; continue for eight weeks or until marker levels become basal.
4.	Weekly samples for six months; if no clinical or marker recurrent, then
5.	Monthly samples; in the absence of clinical or marker recurrence, monitoring can cease after 3 years.

monitoring of marker levels for many months after the initial treatment (table 4–6). It has been suggested that therapy should continue for 12 weeks after marker levels have become basal [63] or for a total of six courses of combination therapy after that basal point is reached [61]; further maintenance therapy would seem to offer no benefit. Marker monitor should continue on a monthly basis for at least two years after therapy has been discontinued.

It should be remembered that AFP and βHCG are markers of specific cell types within the germ cell tumour. Advancing clinical disease in the absence of marker elevations indicates selection of nonmarker-producing elements and calls for a change in the therapeutic regimen. In this situation a nonspecific marker such as ferritin may be of value [67].

Colorectal carcinoma

Despite much work on the value of CEA in the diagnosis and monitoring of this group of malignancies, the picture remains unclear [68].

Staging

Elevated serum CEA levels are seen in only 20 to 30% of stage 1 or Dukes' A tumours compared with 75 to 80% of patients with hepatic metastases. Site of the tumour within the colorectal axis may also have an effect on CEA production, higher levels being seen in cases of left colonic and sigmoid tumours, and lower levels are seen in right colonic and rectal tumours [69].

Prognosis

Gross elevations usually indicate widespread disease with hepatic metastases and give a poor prognosis. Little further information can be gained that cannot be gleaned from clinical examination and histological examination of lymph node involvement in the operative specimen. The irregular and relatively low CEA positivity of some early colorectal tumours can be modified by the use of a combined CEA-APRP approach to staging and prognosis assessment.

A linear discriminant analysis utilising CEA, α_1-antitrypsin, and α_1-acid glycoprotein [29]

$$I = 6.2 - 2.6 \, (\log_{10} \text{CEA}) - 1.6 \, (\alpha_1 \text{AT}) + 1.3 \, (\alpha_1 \text{AGP})$$

allows both preoperative staging and an overall prognostic assessment. I values $+0.5$ indicate stage 1 or Dukes' A disease, and negative values indicate stage 3 (Dukes' C) or stage 4 disease. In an initial study 90% of those with a positive value for I showed no recurrence at two years after resection.

Monitoring

The use of CEA as an indicator for second-look surgery has been disappointing. Despite some enthusiastic claims with a clinical lead time of nine months [70], others have been less successful. In addition, a proportion of patients (20 to 50%) show clinical evidence of recurrent disease without concomitant elevations in CEA [71]. After complete surgical excision the CEA level should fall to normal within six weeks. Failure to observe such a fall in a case with preoperative CEA elevation is strong evidence for residual disease.

Falling CEA levels following chemotherapy or radiotherapy should be considered suggestive of a positive response, but rising levels are inconsistent with tumour regression and indicate the need to alter the therapeutic regimen.

Prostatic carcinoma

The assay of the prostatic isoenzyme of acid phosphatase (PAP) has long been used as a diagnostic test for carcinoma of the prostate. The advent of the radioimmunoassay for PAP [23] has increased only marginally the specificity and sensitivity of the test over the long-established enzymatic method [22]. As a diagnostic marker, PAP leaves much to be desired in that the probability of a positive marker elevation being associated with stage 1 disease in the symptomless population is less than 1%. In a patient with a palpable prostatic nodule, 30% of stage 1 or intracapsular lesions will give marker elevation. The sensitivity of PAP for extracapsular spread is much improved, and whilst the enzymatic method gave a positivity of 50 to 75% [24], the immunoassay can improve identification of distant metastasis to more than 90% [23].

The linking of acute phase proteins to the specific PAP marker can further improve metastasis identification [72]. In the discriminant function

$$I = -0.638 \log_e PAP + 0.767 \log_e PALB - 2.074 \log_e AAT +$$
$$0.605 \log_e AGP - 0.911 \log_e HPT + 4.996,$$

where PALB, AAT, AGP, and HPT (in g/l) are the serum concentrations of prealbumin, α_1-antitrypsin, acid glycoprotein, and haptoglobin, respectively, negative values for I indicate extracapsular spread and give better than 90% identification of bone and lymph node metastases. The profile does, however, suffer from the major problem that AAT is subject to genetic variation in concentrations, and AAT, AGP, and HPT are subject to variation in concentration with oestrogen administration. This latter phenomenon makes the profile unsuitable for use in the patient on standard treatment regimens.

Posttreatment monitoring with six-month immunoassay for PAP is an acceptable method of detecting late recurrence and the development of distant matastases. The linking of this with the concurrent assay of PSA will further improve the detection rate.

Ovarian carcinoma

Whilst AFP and βHCG are elevated in malignant teratoma of the ovary and βHCG may be elevated in some cases of dysgerminoma, the "germ cell marker profile" will serve only to monitor a small proportion of ovarian malignancies. Unlike in the male counterpart, the majority of ovarian tumours are of epithelial origin and have defied marker identification until the advent of monoclonal antibodies. A panel of such antibodies now exists that show considerable promise, not only for monitoring treatment but possibly also for diagnosis. Some of the antibodies even manage to discriminate between different types of epithelial ovarian malignancy (table 4–7).

Table 4-7. Marker specificity in ovarian carcinoma

Marker	Tumour type				
	Serous	Mucinous	Endometroid	Undifferentiated	Reference
CEA	−	+	−	+	
OVC-1	+	+	+	+	[73]
OVC-2	−	−	−	+	[73]
OCCA	+	+	−		[74]
OC-125	+	−	+	+	[75]

Myelomatosis and monoclonal gammopathies

The differentiation between benign and malignant monoclonal gammopathy depends on the former remaining at stable concentrations for at least three years and there being no evidence of associated immune paresis. Where a monoclonal serum component has been identified and bone marrow and radiological examinations are normal, the protein abnormality should be monitored by three-month examination of both serum and urine for at least three years before a firm diagnosis of benign monoclonal gammopathy can be made. Treatment of such an isolated protein abnormality is contraindicated.

The presence of a monoclonal serum or urinary protein abnormality is one of the cornerstones of the diagnosis of myelomatosis [19]. Serial estimates of the paraprotein concentration in serum and of Bence Jones protein in the urine are an excellent guide to tumour mass. Remission can be gauged by the degree or rate of reduction of the monoclonal component. Whilst two or three estimates prior to chemotherapy are useful to indicate growth rate of the tumour, serial estimates on treatment are not necessary more frequently than every three months unless marked clinical deterioration is noted.

Prognosis

Despite the excellent relationship between monoclonal component and tumour mass, the concentration is not a reliable indicator of prognosis. This is best achieved by attention to the serum albumin concentration [19] or to the haemoglobin and urea levels [76,77] and to the degree of immune paresis.

Increasing levels of serum paraprotein and/or urinary Bence Jones protein indicate escape from clinical control and require a change in therapeutic management. It should be remembered, however, that some cases of myelomatosis may revert to a more undifferentiated state and lose the ability to synthesise or secrete immunoglobulin. The total disappearance of the monoclonal component should not be taken as evidence of complete remission unless the immune paresis is also reversed.

REFERENCES

1. Bence Jones H. Papers in chemical pathology. Lancet 2: 88–92, 1847.
2. MacIntyre W. Case of mollities and fragilitas ossium. Med Chi Soc Trans 33: 211–232, 1850.
3. Dalrymple J. On the microscopic character of mollities ossium. Dublin J Med Sci 2: 85–95, 1846.
4. Bergstrand CG, Czar B. Demonstration of a new protein fraction in the serum from a human fetus. Scand J Clin Invest 8: 174, 1956.
5. Gitlin D. Normal biology of alphafetoprotein. Ann NY Acad Sci 259: 7–16, 1975.

6. Smith CJ, Kelleher RC. αfetoprotein: Separation of two molecular variants by affinity chromatography with concanavalin-A agarose. Biochim Biophys Acta 317: 231–235, 1973.
7. Abelev GI, Perova S, Khramkova NI, Postnikova ZA, Irlin I. Production of embryonal alphaglobulin by the transplantable mouse hepatomas. Transplant Bull 1: 174–180, 1963.
8. Tatarinov YS. Detection of embryospecific alphaglobulin in the blood serum of patients with primary liver tumour. Vopr Med Khim 10: 90–91, 1964.
9. Nørgaard-Pederson B, Albrechtsen R, Teilum G. Serum alphafetoprotein as a marker for endodermal sinus tumour (yolk sac tumour) or a vitelline component of teratocarcinoma. Acta pathol microbiol Scand 83: 573–589, 1975.
10. Talerman A, Haije WG. Alphafetoprotein and germ cell tumours: A possible role of yolk sac tumour in production of alphaprotein. Cancer 34: 1722–1726, 1974.
11. Teilum G. Endodermal sinus tumours of the ovary and testis. Comparative morphogenesis of the so-called mesonephroma ovarii (Schiller) and extra embryonic (yolk sac allantoic) structures of the rat placenta. Cancer 12: 1092–1105, 1959.
12. Rosen SW. Placental proteins and their subunits as tumour markers. Ann Int Med 82: 71–83, 1975.
13. Catalona WJ, Vaitukaitis JL, Fair WR. Falsely positive specific human chorionic gonadotrophin assays in patients with testicular tumours: Conversion to negative with testosterone administration. J Urol 122: 126–128, 1979.
14. Burtin B, Gold P. Carcinoembryonic antigen. Scand J Immunol 8, Suppl. 8: 27–38, 1978.
15. Goldenberg DM. Introduction to the international conference on the clinical applications of CEA, Lexington, Kentucky, 1977. Cancer 42: 1397–1398, 1978.
16. Banwo O, Versey J, Hobbs JR. New oncofetal antigen for human pancreas. Lancet 1: 643–645, 1974.
17. Knapp ML, Hobbs JR. Oncofetal pancreatic antigen. Protides of the biologic fluids 27: 63–66, 1980.
18. Searle F. New marker possibilities. In Anderson, Jones, and Milford Ward (eds.) Germ cell tumours. London: Taylor & Francis, 1981, pp. 233–249.
19. Medical Research Council. Myelomatosis: Comparison of melphalan and cyclophosphamide therapy. Br Med J 1: 640–641, 1971.
20. Axellson U, Hallan JA. A population study on monoclonal gammopathy. Acta Med Scand 191: 111–113, 1972.
21. Kohn J, Shrivastava PC. Paraproteinaemia in blood donors and the aged: Benign and malignant. Prot Biol Fluids 20: 257–261, 1972.
22. Gutman AB, Gutman EB. Acid phosphatase occurring in serum of patients with metastasising carcinoma of the prostate gland. J Clin Invest 17: 473–478, 1938.
23. Foti AG, Herschman H, and Cooper JT. A solid phase RIA for human prostatic acid phosphatase. Cancer Res 35: 2446–2452, 1975.
24. Huggins C, Hodges CT. Studies on prostatic acid phosphatase, I. The effect of castration, of oestrogen, and of androgen injection on serum acid phosphatase in metastatic carcinoma of prostate. Cancer Res 1: 293–297, 1941.
25. Wang MC, Papsidero LD, Valenzuela LA, Murphy GP, Chu TM. Prostate antigen: A new potential marker for prostatic cancer. Prostate 2: 89–96, 1981.
26. Pontes JE, Chu TM, Slack N, Karr J, Murphy GP. Serum prostatic antigen measurement in localised prostatic cancer: Correlation with clinical course. J Urol 128: 1216–1218, 1982.
27. Kuriyama M, Wang MC, Lee Ch, Killian CS, Papsidero LD, Inahi H, Loor RM, Lin MF, Nishiura T, Slack NH, Murphy GP, Chu TM. Multiple marker evaluation in human prostatic cancer with the use of tissue specific antigens. J Natl Cancer Inst 68: 99–105, 1982.
28. Cooper EH, Milford Ward A. Acute phase reactant proteins as aids to monitoring disease. Invest Cell Pathol 2: 293–301, 1979.
29. Milford Ward A, Cooper EH, Turner R, Anderson JA, Neville AM. Acute phase reactant protein profiles: An aid to the monitoring of large bowel cancer by carcinoembryonic antigen and serum enzymes.
30. Milford Ward A, Cooper EH, Houghton AL. Acute phase reactant proteins in prostatic cancer. Br J Urol 49: 411–418, 1971.
31. Te Velde ER, Faber JAJ, Roebersen W, Berghuys M, Zegers BJM, Ballieux RE. The predictive value of serial determinations of some acute phase reactants, complement components and immunoglobulins in patients with invasive carcinoma of the cervix. Prot Biol Fluids 27: 335–338, 1980.
32. Bradwell AR. Haptoglobin and orosomucoid in lung and breast tumours. In Milford Ward and Whicher (eds.), Immunochemistry in clinical laboratory medicine. Lancaster: MTP Press, 1979, pp. 197–215.
33. Bastable JRG, Richards B, Howarth S, Cooper EH. Acute phase reactant proteins in the management of carcinoma of the bladder. Br J Urol 51: 283–289, 1979.
34. Latner AL, Turner GA, Lamin MM. Plasma alpha$_1$ antitrypsin levels in early and late carcinoma of the cervix. Oncology 33: 12–14, 1976.

35. Child JA, Cooper EH, Illingworth S, Worthy TS. Biochemical markers in Hodgkin's disease and non-Hodgkin's lymphoma. Recent Results Cancer Res 64: 180–189, 1978.
36. Gold P, Freedman SO. Demonstration of tumour specific antigens in human colonic carcinomata by immunological tolerance and absorption techniques. J Exp Med 121: 439–462, 1965.
37. Abelev GI. αfetoprotein as a marker of embryo specific differentiations in normal and tumour tissues. Transplant Rev 20: 3–37, 1974.
38. McIntire KR, Vogel CR, Princler GL, Patel IR. Serum αfetoprotein as a biochemical marker for hepatocellular carcinoma. Cancer Res 32: 1941–1946, 1972.
39. Ruoslahti E, Salaspuro M, Pihko H, Anderson L, Seppala M. Serum αfetroprotein: Diagnostic significance in liver disease. Br Med J 2: 527–529, 1974.
40. Sizaret P, Tuyns A, Martel N, Jouvencaux A, Levin A, Ong YW, Rive J. αfetoprotein levels in normal males from seven ethnic groups with different hepatocellular carcinoma risks. Ann NY Acad Sci 259: 136–157, 1975.
41. Jalanko H, Engvall E, Virtanen I, Ruoslahti E. Early increase of serum αfetoprotein in spontaneous hepatocarcinogenesis in mice. Int J Cancer 21: 453–459, 1978.
42. Kroes R, Sontag JM, Sell S, Williams GM, Weisberger JH. Elevated concentrations of serum alphafetoprotein in rats with chemically induced liver tumours. Cancer Res 35: 1214–1217, 1975.
43. Murray Lyon IM, Orr AH, Gazzard B, Kohn J, Williams R. Prognostic value of serum alphafetoprotein in fulminant hepatic failure including patients treated by charcoal haemoperfusion. Gut 17: 576–580, 1976.
44. Okuda K, Kotoda K, Obata H, Hayashi N, Hisamitsu T, Tamiya M, Kubo Y, Yakushiji F, Nagata E, Jinnouchi S, Shimokawa Y. Clinical observations during a relatively early stage of hepatocelluar carcinoma with special reference to αfetoprotein levels. Gastroenterology 69: 226–234, 1975.
45. Co-ordinating Group for the Research on Liver Cancer Studies on human αfetoprotein I. αfetoprotein assay in primary hepatocellular carcinoma. Mass survey and followup studies. The Peoples Republic of China, 1974.
46. McIntire KR, Waldmann TA, Moertel CG, Go VLW. Serum αfetoprotein as a biochemical marker for the gastrointestinal tract. Cancer Res 35: 991–996, 1975.
47. Kohn J. The dynamics of serum alphafetoprotein in the course of testicular teratoma. Scand J Immunol 8 (Suppl. 8): 103–108, 1978.
48. Lange PH, Fraley EE. Serum alphafetoprotein and testicular tumours. N Eng J Med 296: 694, 1977.
49. Bagshawe KD. Choriocarcinoma. London: Edw. Arnold, 1969.
50. Bagshawe KD. Recent observations related to the chemotherapy and immunology of gestational choriocarcinoma. Ad Cancer Res 18: 231–263, 1973.
51. Bagshawe KD, Harland S. Immunodiagnosis and monitoring of gonadotrophin producing metastases in the central nervous system. Cancer 38: 112–118, 1976.
52. Newlands ES, Dent J, Kardona A, Searle F, Bagshawe KD. Serum αfetoprotein and HCG in patients with testicular tumours. Lancet 2: 744–745, 1976.
53. Milford Ward A. Markers in germ cell tumours: The current state of the art: AFP, βHCG and AHL kinetics. In Anderson, Jones, and Milford Ward (eds.), Germ cell tumours. London: Taylor and Francis, 1981, pp. 207–215.
54. Javadpour N. Management of seminoma based as tumour markers. Urol Clin North Am 7: 773–780, 1980.
55. Szymendera JJ, Zborzil J, Sikorawa L, Leuko J, Kaminska JJ, Gradek A. Evaluation of five tumour markers (AFP, CEA, LCG, LPL, and SP) in monitoring therapy and follow-up of patients with testicular germ cell tumours. Oncology 40: 1–10, 1983.
56. Jones WG. Germ cell tumours—The current state of the art and problems in clinical management. In Anderson, Jones, and Milford Ward (eds.), Germ cell tumours. London: Taylor and Francis, 1981, pp. 3–14.
57. Wiltshaw E. Germ cell tumours in females. In Anderson, Jones, and Milford Ward (eds.), Germ cell tumours. London: Taylor and Francis, 1981, pp. 179–188.
58. Corbett PJ. Extragonadal germ cell tumours: Biological and clinical relevance. In Anderson, Jones, and Milford Ward (eds.), Germ cell tumours. London: Taylor and Francis, 1981, pp. 165–168.
59. Milford Ward A, Bates GE. Serum AFP and apparent half-life estimates in the management of endodermal sinus tumours. Prot Biol Fluids 27: 356–368, 1979.
60. Javadpour N. Improved staging for testicular cancer using biologic tumour markers: A prospective study. J Urol 124: 58–59, 1980.
61. Scott IV, Milford Ward A, Bradwell AR, Wilson A. αfetoprotein, HCG apparent half-life in the clinical management of malignant ovarian teratoma. In Anderson, Jones, and Milford Ward (eds.), Germ cell tumours. London: Taylor and Francis, 1981, pp. 189–191.
62. Germa-Lluch JR, Begent RHJ, Bagshawe KD. Tumour marker levels and prognosis in malignant teratoma of the testis. Br J Cancer 42: 850–855, 1980.
63. Newlands ES, Begent RHJ, Kaye SB, Rustin GJS, Bagshawe KD. Chemotherapy of advanced malignant teratoma. Br J Cancer 42, 378–384, 1980.

64. Begent RHJ, Newlands ES, Germa-Lluch JK, Bagshawe KD. Tumour marker levels and prognosis in malignant teratoma of the testis. In Anderson, Jones, and Milford Ward (eds.), Germ cell tumours. London: Taylor and Francis, 1981, pp. 227–229.

65. Einhorn LH, Donohue JP. Cisdiammine-dichloroplatinum, vinplastine, and bleomycin combination chemotherapy in disseminated testicular cancer. Ann Int Med 87: 293–298, 1977.

66. Newlands ES, Begent RHJ, Rustin GJS, Bagshawe KD. The development of modern chemotherapy for malignant teratomas and results of sequential chemotherapy at Charing Cross Hospital. In Anderson, Jones, and Milford Ward (eds.), Germ cell tumours. London: Taylor and Francis, 1981, pp. 359–367.

67. Hancock BW, Grail A, Bates GE, Jones WG, Milford Ward A. Serum ferritin as a third marker in malignant germ cell tumours. In Anderson, Jones, and Milford Ward (eds.), Germ cell tumours. London: Taylor and Francis, 1981, pp. 253–255.

68. National Institutes of Health, Consensus Development Conference Statement. CEA: Its role as a marker in the management of cancer. Tum Diagn 2: 59–61, 1981.

69. Livingston AS, Hampson LG, Shuster J, Gold P, Hinchley EJ. Carcinoembryonic antigen in the diagnosis and management of colorectal carcinoma. Arch Surg 109: 259–264, 1974.

70. Neville AM, Patel S, Lawrence DJR, Cooper EH, Tuberville C, Coombes RC. The monitoring role of plasma CEA alone and in association with other tumour markers in colorectal and mammary carcinoma. Cancer 42: 1448–1451, 1978.

71. Sugarbaker PH, Zamcheck N, Moore FD. Assessment of serial carcinoembryonic assays in postoperative detection of recurrent colorectal carcinoma. Cancer 38: 2310–2315, 1976.

72. Milford Ward A, Cooper EH, Houghton AL. Acute phase reactant proteins in prostate cancer. Br J Urol 49: 411–418, 1977.

73. Immamura N, Takahashi U, Lloyd KO, Lewis JL, Old H. Analysis of human ovarian tumour antigens using heterologous antisera: Detection of a new antigenic system. Int J Cancer 21: 570–577, 1978.

74. Battacharya M, Barlow JJ. Tumour specific antigens associated with human ovarian cystadenocarcinoma. In Waters H. (ed.), Handbook of cancer immunology. New York: Garland Publishing, 1978, pp. 277–295.

75. Kabawat SE, Bast RE, Welch WR, Knapp RC, Colvin RB. Immunopathologic characterisation of a monoclonal antibody that recognises common surface antigens of human ovarian tumours of serous, endometrioid, and clear cell types. Am J Clin Pathol 79: 98–104, 1983.

76. MRC Working Party. Report on the second myelomatosis trial after five years follow-up. Br J Cancer 42: 813–822, 1980.

77. MRC Working Party. Prognostic features in the third MRC myelomatosis trial. Br J Cancer: 42: 831–840, 1980.

5. THE USE OF RADIOLABELED ANTIBODIES FOR THE LOCALISATION OF TUMOURS

A.R. BRADWELL

INTRODUCTION

Tumour diagnosis is becoming increasingly dependent on the use of serum and tissue markers. These are usually proteins produced in excess by malignant cells that may be used to identify malignant tissue. It was soon realised that antibodies against these proteins could specifically identify tumour tissue in histological sections and more recently, with attached radiolabels, could be used for in vivo tumour localisation (known as radioimmunodetection—RAID—or radioimmunolocalisation—RIL). The appeal of the technique is that tumours are localised on the basis of specific biochemical substances rather than on general characteristics such as density (CT scanning, etc.). RAID has been particularly applied to tumours of the gastrointestinal tract and other organs producing carcinoembryonic antigen, germ cell tissues producing alphafetoprotein or chorionic gonadotrophin, and a variety of rarer tumours. Although at present there is no definitive use for RAID, new developments suggest that its sensitivity will improve and its application will become important. This chapter describes the theory and development of the technique, clinical results to date, and future areas of development.

HISTORY

The concept of antibodies that might specifically localise and destroy tumours was popular even before the turn of the century. In 1895 Hericourt and Richet [1] prepared antisera

The collaborative research work of Drs. D.S. Fairweather and P.W. Dykes and the financial support of the Cancer Research Campaign are gratefully acknowledged.

B.W. Hancock and A.M. Ward (eds.), Immunological Aspects of Cancer. Copyright © 1985, Martinus Nijhoff Publishing, Boston/Dordrecht/Lancaster.

against a human osteogenic sarcoma in animals and claimed they were successful in reducing the size of a fibrosarcoma of the chest wall and a tumour of the stomach. Subsequently, 50 cases were treated and successful results claimed. For a variety of reasons, which are now obvious, subsequent investigators were unable to confirm these results, and it was not until the work of Pressman in 1953 [2] that progress was made. By making use of developments in the purification of antibodies and isotopic labeling techniques, they showed that iodinated antibodies directed against certain animal tumours gave in vivo localisation. In a series of experiments these results were confirmed by Bale et al. [3], but both the lack of suitable animal models and of the identification of human tumour antigens hindered further advances. In the 1970s purified preparations of several human tumour products became available, such as carcinoembryonic antigen (CEA), human chorionic gonadotrophin (HCG), and alphafetoprotein (AFP). Initial studies were performed with xenografts of human tumours in hamster cheek pouches. Quinones et al. [4] demonstrated specific localisation of antibodies to HCG in xenografts of choriocarcinoma; soon after this Goldenberg et al. [5] in a similar fashion showed specific localisation of anti-CEA in transplanted human colon tumours. This was soon followed by similar work in nude mice [6]. These encouraging results culminated in the clinical studies of CEA-radiolocalising antibodies by Goldenberg et al. [7] and others [8,9]. Reports since 1980 have attempted to improve the sensitivity of the technique or to study tumours where other scanning procedures have limitations.

THEORETICAL CONSIDERATIONS

Many parameters are involved in RAID; whilst some have an obvious relationship to the outcome of the scan, others may have a more subtle influence. Thus, a theoretical understanding of the potential and limitations of the technique allows the most useful avenues to be explored. With this in mind Rockoff et al. [10] defined the major factors involved and used a computer model to show the likely limitations of RAID. We have further adapted this to determine the practical limitations in relationship to the present state-of-the-art [11]. Figure 5-1 indicates the eleven parameters that we used.

Three of the parameters are patient dependent and therefore fixed. These are (1) the tumour area (as seen by the camera), (2) the tumour depth, and (3) the patient depth at the site of the tumour. The signal to noise ratio (4) is also fixed, and it is generally considered that the minimum value that can be reliably visualised is three.

The uptake ratio (5) of antibody onto the tumour compared with the surrounding normal tissue is the most important single determinant of scan sensitivity. Unfortunately, there are a host of factors that reduce antibody uptake in vivo and some of these are discussed later. Reported values in patients vary between one and ten (see table 5-1), although animal results have been considerably better [12]. The influence of the uptake ratio in detecting different sized lesions at various depths as determined by the model is shown in figure 5-2.

Calculations indicate that, next to uptake ratios, the most important factor is the absolute count rate of the tumour locating isotope (6). When using ^{131}I, count rates are usually low compared with other methods using isotopes and in our hands often less than 100 per cm^2 in the image. A trebling of this rate would be equivalent to doubling the uptake ratio and a tenfold increase equivalent to a threefold rise in uptake ratio (figure 5-3). The ques-

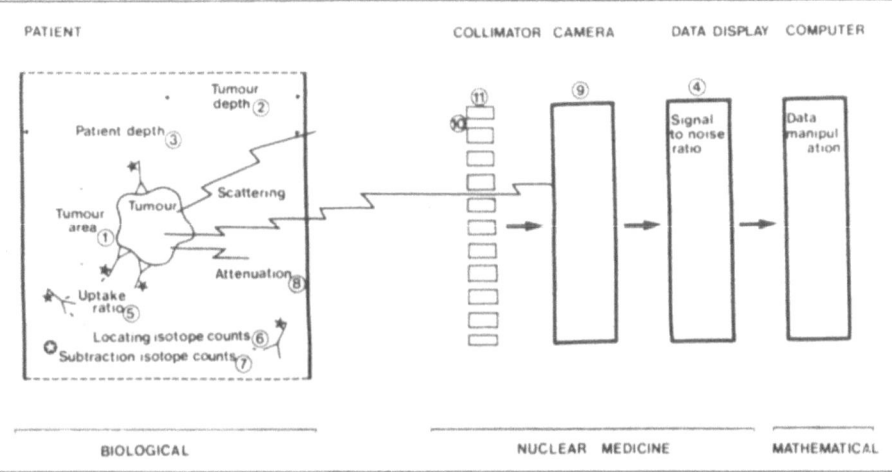

Figure 5-1. Parameters used in the model for the radioimmunodetection of tumours. (Units: 1, 2, and 3 in cm². 4, signal-to-noise ratio. 5, uptake ratio. 6 and 7, counts/cm². 8, per cm. 9, camera resolution; FWHM in mm. 10, hole diameter in mm. 11, hole depth in mm). (From Bradwell AR, Fairweather DS, Dykes PW. Radioimmunodetection of endocrine tumours. In Saunders KB (ed.), Advanced medicine 19. London: Pitman, 1983, pp. 76-98.)

Table 5-1. Comparison of ^{111}In- and ^{131}I-labeled anti-CEA for tumour detection in 5 patients with CEA-producing tumours

	Number of sites revealed	
Scan result	^{111}In	^{131}I
+ +	10	4
+	3	4
−	2	7

tion of the value of a subtraction isotope has caused considerable controversy and attempts have been made to avoid its use [9,13]. On theoretical grounds such a process must add noise [11]. However, its advantage is that it masks the variation in vascular supply to different tissues, thereby allowing small tumours, with low uptake ratios, to be detected (discussed later in the chapter). Indeed, it was the use of this subtraction scanning procedure that enabled Goldenberg et al. to obtain the first convincing results in patients [7].

With regard to the nuclear medicine aspects (figure 5-1) the computer model does not suggest that marked benefit is likely to follow from improvements in conventional gamma cameras although, for specific areas such as the neck, magnifying collimators may be of value. Computerised tomography would potentially be advantageous. Most other factors, such as gamma ray scattering in the body, camera blurring, and sensitivity, are physical limitations inherent in the present systems.

Several techniques of data manipulation have been studied. To reduce subjectivity, scans can be thresholded to display only significant counts, and nonlinear deconvolution techniques should improve the signal-to-noise ratio [14] over the established techniques. Scans

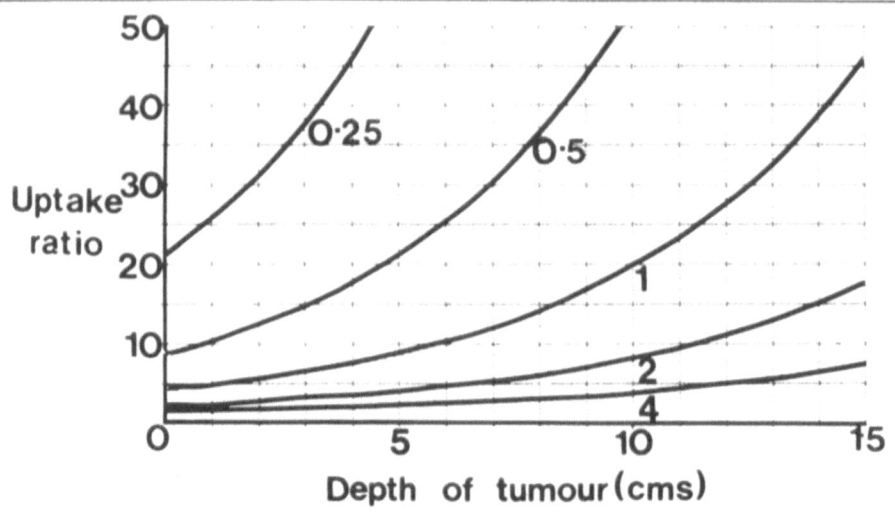

Figure 5-2. Relationship between uptake ratio (5) and tumour depth (2) with contours on tumour area (1). Other parameters from figure 5-1: 3 = 20; 4 = 3; 6 = 300; 7 = 300; 8 = 0.127 ([111]I); 9 = 4.8; 10 = 4.3; 11 = 50.

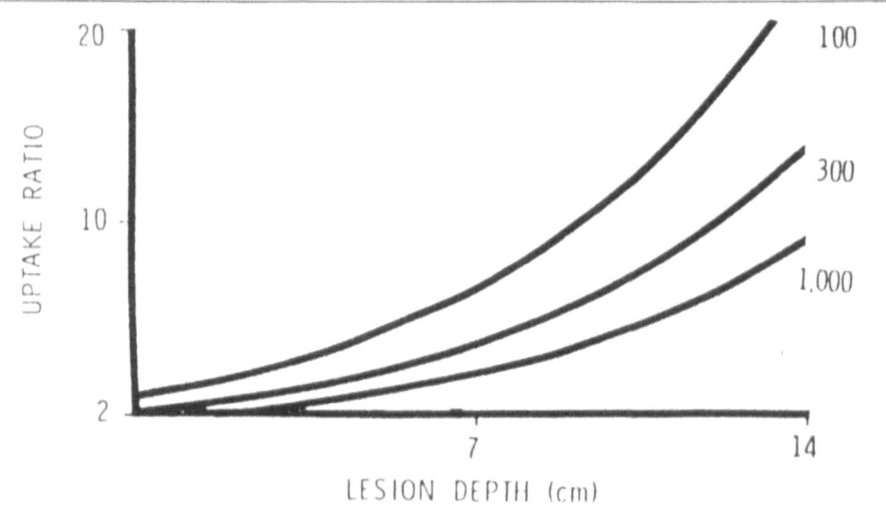

Figure 5-3. Demonstrates the relationship between count rates and uptake ratio in detecting a 2-cm-diameter tumour at different depths. Parameters from figure 5-1: 3 = 20; 4 = 3; 7 = 1000; 8 = 0.11 (^{131}I); 9 = 4.8; 10 = 4.3; 11 = 50.

should therefore be quantitatively assessed with due regard to the statistical significance of different areas. These techniques are discussed later.

As with other new techniques, there are no accepted normal limits for antibody scans. Poor count rates and a low uptake ratio both contribute to an image containing artifacts and the distinction between true signal and the noise can seem arbitrary.

RADIOIMMUNODETECTION PROCEDURES

Antisera

The relevant antigen (e.g., CEA) is purified and an antiserum raised in a suitable animal (e.g., sheep, goat, mouse, etc.). The specificity of the antiserum is then checked against the antigen and normal serum [15] and by the staining of various tissue sections (normal and tumour) using a sensitive method such as the peroxidase-antiperoxidase reaction [16]. If these tests reveal cross-reacting antibodies, they should be solid phase adsorbed with polymers of serum and tissues. An immunoglobulin fraction is then prepared by ion-exchange chromatography. We have tended to label the antiserum without further processing, although most workers have added an affinity purification step [7]. This latter process may, however, have some undesirable effects (see below). In the case of most monoclonal antibodies, protein A is a useful material for effecting separation of the immunoglobulin subclasses [17]. After purification, the antibody is sterilised by filtration and checked for acute toxicity in animals [18] and stored frozen or freeze-dried for future use.

Radiolabeling

Until recently, only iodine isotopes have been suitable for simple attachment to proteins and appropriate for external scanning with gamma cameras. The chloramine-T method is usually employed for iodination [19], since it can be shown that this causes little or no detectable change in the biological behaviour of immunoglobulin molecules. The most frequently used iodine isotope has been ^{131}I although studies with ^{123}I have been successful [20]. In addition [124]I has been used for positron tomography but is unlikely to find wide application [21].

[111]In has been suggested as a useful alternative to ^{131}I for several reasons: (1) because of its lower energy (247 and 173 keV) but higher abundance, photons; (2) the lack of high-radiation beta particles; and (3) the half-life (2.83 days) is ideal for antibody scanning. There are several technical difficulties in preparing ^{111}In-labeled antibodies of high specific activity but these have recently been overcome [22,23], and the results indicate greater sensitivity than comparable ^{131}I-labeled antibodies [24]. The details are discussed later.

Most workers have attempted to remove aggregated immunoglobulin after labeling because it may cause false-positive localisation in the liver and other reticuloendothelial sites. Gel-filtration or centrifugation may be used, but we have favoured the latter because it is simple and sterility is easy to maintain.

Preparation of the patient

Uptake of radioactive antibody by the thyroid and stomach is blocked by giving potassium iodide (KI), 420 mg, and potassium perchlorate (KClO$_3$), 400 mg, 30 minutes before the

[131]I-labeled antibody; followed by 120 mg KI, 6 hourly, and 200 mg $KC10_3$, 6 hourly, for two days. After the second scan, only the KI is continued at 120 mg eight hourly [25].

Prior to injecting the labeled antibody, a small amount is given intravenously via a "butterfly" needle. Providing there is no reaction, the remainder is given slowly. The documented side effects are remarkably few. Out of 80 patients scanned only two have had a pyrexia, which required no treatment. Approximately 15 patients have had two or more scans and have had no adverse reactions. This experience is similar to that reported by other investigators [26].

Nuclear medicine techniques

When ^{131}I is used as the radiolabel, at least 18.5 MBq (0.5 mCi) must be injected to obtain sufficient counts for imaging. In general the higher the dose the better and 37 to 74 MBq is preferable. In our experience, the whole body absorbed dose from ^{131}I-labeled sheep IgG is 0.135 mSv/MBq (500 mRem/mCi). This compares favourably with other imaging techniques (e.g., 1 Rem/CT examination).

Images are obtained with a large field of view (LFOV) gamma camera (although rectilinear scanners have been used) usually 24 and 48 hours postinjection. As mentioned previously less than 1% of the injected antibody accumulates in any one tumour site [9] and the distribution of antibody in the body is not uniform (about 50% remaining in the vascular compartment). With experience, it is possible to gauge the expected background pattern and therefore pick out small abnormal areas but this is very subjective.

COMPUTER SUBTRACTION

The subtraction technique described by Goldenberg made use of a second isotope to mimic the distribution of normal immunoglobulin [7]. This is illustrated in figure 5–4. In practice 20 MBq each of [99m]Technetium (^{99m}Tc) labeled pertechnetate and ^{99m}Tc-albumin are injected 30 and 5 minutes, respectively, before each scan. A camera and computer with a dual-isotope facility are required to record the 141KeV ^{99m}Tc photons and 364Kev ^{131}I photons simultaneously and effect the subtraction.

Although this improves contrast, it does so at the expense of adding artifacts and introducing further statistical fluctuations without increasing the signal, that is, reducing the signal-to-noise ratio [11]. Goldenberg used the blood pool (the heart) for normalisation and although this is reported to improve contrast twofold [27], it is subject to bias on exactly which area is taken. An alternative approach is to correlate the ^{99m}Tc and ^{131}I image pixels using the "least squares" method where the normalising factor is given by the slope of the regression line [14].

Other problems with subtraction are that the technetium pharmaceuticals do not distribute in exactly the same way as normal IgG and the large difference between ^{99m}Tc and ^{131}I gamma energies leads to differences in attenuation and scattering, dependent on the area being scanned. These effects can be compensated for, to some extent, by the use of local subtraction [28] where the factor is calculated separately for each organ of interest. This may improve contrast 20-fold, but it is both time consuming and open to greater bias.

Noise (random fluctuation in the background) is a feature of all nuclear medicine techniques but especially antibody scans when ^{131}I is used, since count rates are usually low (typically less

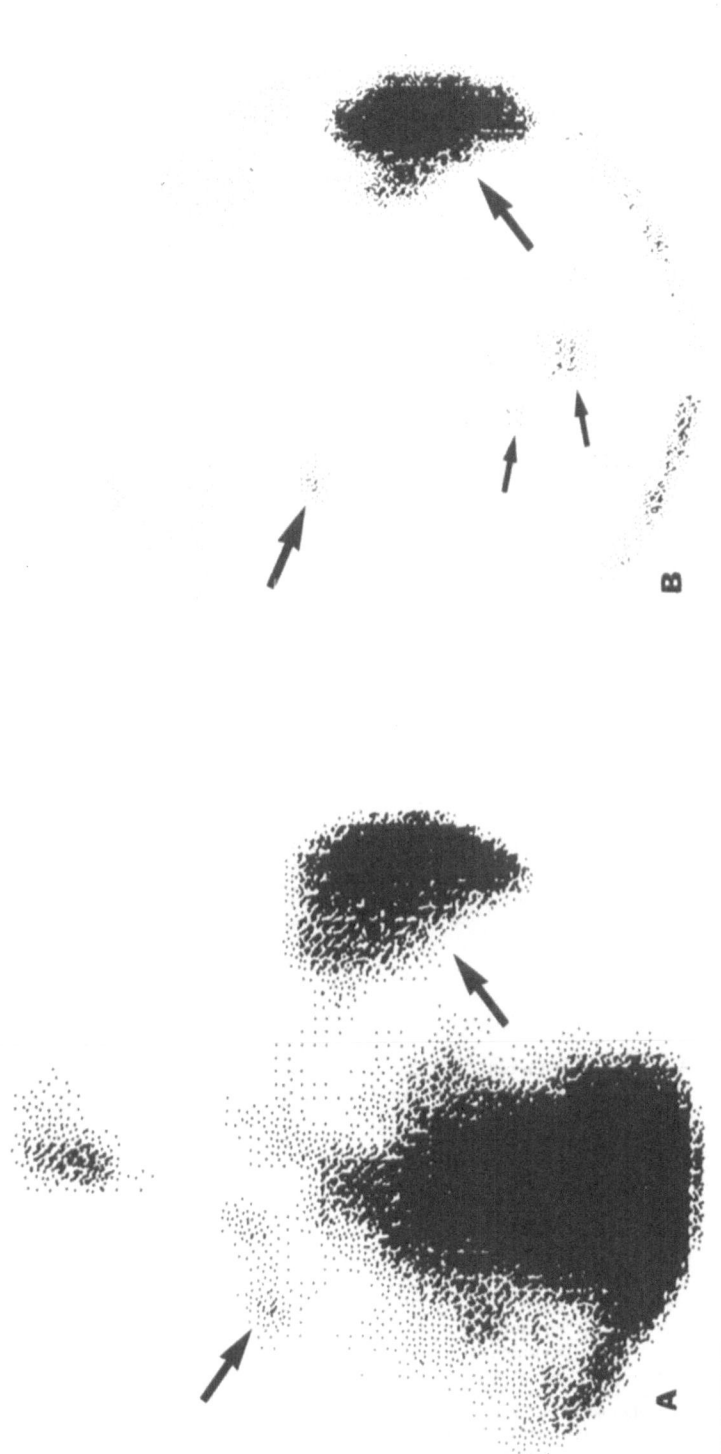

Figure 5-4. Antibody scan of a patient with a thyroid follicular tumour 24 hours after injection with ^{131}I labeled antithyroglobulin.

(A) Total ^{131}I counts with left shoulder and clavicle lesion arrowed.

(B) Subtraction scan showing the enhanced lesions plus pulmonary deposits but also a ring artifact and a silhouette.

(From Fairweather DS, Bradwell AR, Watson-James SF, Dykes PW, Chandler S, Hoffenberg R. Detection of thyroid tumours using radiolabelled antithyroglobulin. Clin Endocrinol 18:563–570, 1983.)

than 200/cm²). Since this fluctuation is given by a Poisson distribution, the variance for each pixel in the subtraction picture can be calculated and the significance of counts in the subtraction picture assessed by replotting after subtracting two standard deviations from each pixel, any counts remaining being regarded as highly significant [14]—see figure 5–4 where the lesion arrowed in (a) is shown to be highly significant (b).

However, regardless of the subtraction technique used, it is not possible to equalise the counts in all areas. Thus the bladder always contains an excess of free iodine or technetium, as may other parts of the urinary tract, which leads to hot or cold areas. Inequalities may also occur around the heart or stomach although the latter can usually be blocked with KI and $KC10_3$. Thus, intelligent assessment of the scans is always required.

CLINICAL RESULTS

Overall results of published series are given in table 5–2. In general > 70% positivity rate is achieved with a low (approximately 10%) false positive rate. It is interesting that similar results are reported by different groups using different antisera and in different situations.

Table 5–2. Clinical studies with radiolabeled antibodies

Antigen detected and authors [ref]	Antibody type*	Tumour type	No. of lesions scanned	Positive rate %	Uptake ratio U	Smallest lesion found-cm
CEA						
Goldenberg 1978 [7]	AP	mixed	40	85	2.5	?
Dykes 1980 [8]	PC	colon	14	80	2.5	2
Mach 1980 [9]	AP	colon	21	58	3.6	?
Mach 1981 [30]	Mab	mixed	28	50	4	?
Deland 1982 [31]	AP	mixed	156	75	?	?
Berche 1982 [32]	Mab	mixed	17	94	?	1+
Smedley 1983 [33]	Mab	mixed	27	60	?	?
Fairweather 1983 [24]	PC	mixed	31	90	?	?
Goldenberg 1983 [34]	AP	colon	65	88	?	?
AFP						
Goldenberg 1980 [35]	PC	mixed	13	85	?	?
Halsall 1981 [36]	PC	germ cell	15	80	?	2
HCG						
Begent 1980 [37]	AP	germ cell	21	72	?	0.5
Goldenberg 1980 [38]	PC	germ cell	18	100	40£	?
THYROGLOBULIN						
Fairweather 1983 [25]	PC	thyroid	40	85	?	1.7
INSULIN						
Fairweather 1982 [39]	PC	insulinoma	3	66	2.2	2
UNKNOWN						
Ghose 1980 [40]	Mab	renal	28	95	2.3	2
Farrands 1982 [41]	Mab	colon	10	90	2.3	?
Epenetos 1982 [20]	Mab	mixed	32	75	?	?
Larson 1983 [42]	Mab	melanoma	25	88	4.3	1.5
Rainsbury 1983 [43]	Mab	breast	102	52	4	?

*PC = polyclonal. AP = Affinity purified polyclonal. Mab = Monoclonal.
U = Tumour to normal tissue ratio in surgically resected samples.
+ = Using photon emmission tomography. £ = One sample only. ? = unknown.

Although tumour-to-normal-tissue ratios in surgically excised specimens have not been routinely measured, those available indicate similar localising abilities in vivo for all types of antisera—conventional, affinity-purified, and monoclonal. Apart from one group [32] who used single-photon-emission tomography (SPET), most claim that the smallest tumours detectable are 1.5 to 2 cm in diameter, depending on the site. This may in part be related to the difficulty in confirming smaller areas by conventional tests. However, most patients scanned have had lesions much bigger than this, and large masses are easy to localise by many techniques.

A number of recurring problems have emerged. First, as with any new technique, interpretation of the image may be subjective and difficult to quantify, and the "picture quality" is poor. Second, there is always some difficulty in establishing the true extent of patients' disease in order to define false positives and false negatives. Third, because different centres pursue conventional investigations with varying vigour, comparisons with established techniques may be difficult.

It is too early, as yet, to determine the role of RAID in tumour detection because of rapid progress, but some authors suggest its use as a routine procedure and most claim to detect a substantial number of lesions not detected by other imaging techniques. Goldenberg et al. [34] are keen protagonists and claim that in colorectal cancer, for example, RAID can (1) contribute to the preoperative staging of the patients, (2) assist in the postoperative evaluation of tumour recurrence or spread, (3) complement other methods used to assess tumour response to therapy, (4) support the indication for second-look surgery in the presence of a rising CEA titre, and (5) confirm the findings of other detection measures that are less tumour specific.

We are less enthusiastic [44] and feel that the main consideration is whether it helps in patient management. There is limited value in locating tumours that cannot be removed or do not respond to therapy, and, unfortunately, this is true for most tumours producing CEA. AFP- and HCG-producing tumours are usually treated with polychemotherapy based on monitoring the serum concentration so, again, accurate localisation is of restricted use. Many of the other studies described also fall into these categories. Furthermore, RAID has to compete with other techniques in terms of sensitivity and cost. It is unlikely that it will ever compare favourably with CAT scanning of the lungs where density contrast is high. However, in the abdomen the opposite is true, and many workers have detected lesions missed by other methods. One potential advantage of RAID over all other techniques is that it can determine the tissue type of a known mass. We have scanned a few patients with anti-AFP who had residual masses, after uncertain chemotherapy, of viability. Results were consistent with the subsequent clinical progress and may have prevented a rather more risky biopsy. If the sensitivity improves sufficiently to reliably detect lesions half a centimeter in diameter, then a variety of tumours could be usefully located; in particular, relatively benign endocrine tumours could be located prior to surgical excision. This level of sensitivity would also allow accurate staging of a host of tumours prior to surgery or chemotherapy.

RECENT DEVELOPMENTS

The tantalising feature of RAID is that antibodies are highly specific probes for in vitro use and in some animal/tumour models. What, therefore, are the promising avenues that might be explored to help realise the potential indicated by the experimental data and the theoretical considerations?

Uptake ratios

A small lesion receives only a minute proportion of the cardiac output and this limits the percentage uptake, since antibody will inevitably be catabolised elsewhere. A good analogy is the detection of differentiated thyroid carcinoma with ^{131}Iodide where a very high dose may have to be given to disclose small lesions, despite a specific and high-affinity uptake mechanism. Access may also be limited by circulating antigen that can form complexes and block antibody binding sites. Further restrictions are the slow rate of immunoglobulin diffusion out of the normal vascular tree (50% always remains intravascular), and antigenic sites in the tumour may be limited.

Evidence regarding the actual site of antibody binding is conflicting [30,45,46]. Antigen may be present within or on the surface of the cells or externally (either soluble or immobilised on cell debris) or in phagocytic cells. Accumulation in any, or more, of the above areas will contribute to a positive scan [47].

Even when antibody has attached to antigen on the tumour cell surface, it may be rapidly lost. Cross-linking of cell surface components may induce movements in the membrane [48], which can lead to the shedding of the antibody-antigen complexes (antigenic modulation) or rapid endocytosis and catabolism (patching and capping). CEA is known to cap [49], and there is circumstantial evidence that cell surface bound anti-CEA is lost rapidly [50].

Potential areas for improvement include increasing the titre and affinity of the antisera and finding tumour antigens of greater specificity. Monoclonal antibodies (Mabs) may seem the ideal answer. There is impressive in vitro and animal work to show they can be superior to polyclonal antisera, and uptake ratios of over 200—more than ten times those achieved with conventional antisera—have been achieved [12]. However, human studies have been disappointing (see table 5-2). Some aspects of Mabs that should be born in mind follow:

1. Their extreme specificity may reduce tumour accumulation if the quantity of antigen is limited, especially if the Mabs can recognise only one binding site (epitope) per antigen molecule. In contrast, several polyclonal antibody molecules may attach to each antigen.
2. An apparently specific Mab may bind unexpectedly to other antigens; for example, a Mab against a segment of CEA may recognise a similar segment in a quite different antigen.
3. The affinity of the antiserum may have to be high (as well as the titre). This has not been easy to achieve.
4. Mouse immunoglobulins may interact with human Fc receptors and produce false positive localisation unless fragments are prepared. Again, this has been problematical.

Nevertheless, it is likely that further studies will show considerable improvements.

There are also problems associated with affinity purified antisera: it is likely that the highest affinity antibodies are not eluted from the affinity column, and it is known that agents capable of breaking the antibody antigen bond may disrupt the whole molecule sufficiently to alter its biological properties [51]. These factors may explain why it is has proved difficult to improve on high-grade polyclonal antisera.

An alternative approach to increasing the uptake ratio is to use a second antibody to clear the circulation of the unbound first (radiolabeled) antibody. This was initially proposed encapsulated in a liposome, with good results [13], but it has since been shown that this may be unnecessary. A sevenfold increase in clearance of unbound localising antibody has been achieved in animals by using a second antibody [52]. In patients given second antibody, blood counts have fallen more than twice as quickly as in control subjects, yet tumour counts have been maintained [53].

This second antibody technique could be applied to whatever antibody system is being used providing it does not generate spurious uptake in reticuloendothelial sites. The optimal system has yet to be evaluated.

A further refinement is the use of immunoglobulin fragments that may gain access to tumours more easily than the whole molecule, but results were not strikingly better in one careful in vivo study [30].

Regarding the relevence of the antigen location, it is logical to aim the antibody at a cell surface antigen, although we have successfully scanned patients with antibodies directed against antigens that are not primarily cell surface components, i.e., AFP [36] and thyroglobulin [25]. By this means, particularly with antithyroglobulin, we hoped to avoid the "capping" and loss of cell surface bound antibody (modulation) that occurs with divalent antibodies. Overall, the results were similar to those obtained with anti-CEA (table 5–2), perhaps reflecting the multiple factors that determine scanning success in patients. Studies are presently underway to investigate the value of a monovalent antibody that is known to have enhanced tumour binding because modulation does not occur [54]. Mabs also may not induce modulation, but this needs to be investigated. Alternatively, use may be made of modulation by labeling the protein with an isotope that is retained within cells.

Count rates

Higher count rates with iodine labels can obviously be achieved by giving a larger dose to the patient and/or counting for longer. Both are subject to practical limitations. A dose of 74 MBq of ^{131}I-labeled antibody gives similar absorbed radiation to x-ray CT (1 Rem) and a scanning time of 5 to 10 minutes per view is comparable to other nuclear medicine techniques.

^{131}I, in particular, is not a good isotope for these studies. First, the high photon energy (364 KeV) is poorly detected by present gamma cameras and requires the use of a high-energy collimator, which reduces sensitivity still further. Second, the beta emmission contributes to a high radiation dose to the patients and this limits the activity that can be injected. ^{123}I has a more suitable photon energy for detection and delivers a radiation dose only one-tenth that from ^{131}I. Unfortunately, the short half-life (13 hours) is not ideal, and it cannot be used with ^{99m}Tc for background subtraction due to overlapping photon energies. ^{123}I-labeled antibodies have been used successfully [20], but in this study only large tumours were visualised.

^{111}In has suitable characteristics for gamma camera imaging and also gives a threefold to eightfold higher count rate than ^{131}I with our gamma camera (SEARLE LFOV) for a similar administered dose. We have labeled anti-CEA with ^{111}In using a bifunctional chelating agent [22,23]. A strong chelating group, DTPA (diethylenetriamine pentaacetic acid), was covalently attached to the antibody [24]. This modified antiserum is then radiolabeled with ^{111}In by mixing the two in solution, when a chelate bond is formed spontaneously. Although this bond is reversible, it is sufficiently stable for in vitro studies.

We have studied five patients with CEA containing tumours with both ^{111}In labeled anti-CEA and ^{131}I-labeled anti-CEA for comparison (see table 5–1). Not only did ^{111}In show more sites than the ^{131}I-labeled antibody but did so with greater certainty. This advantage of ^{111}In appears to be due to two factors: first, the improved count rates (the patients received the same dose of each isotope and were scanned for equal times) and second, the greater retention of ^{111}In by tumours [24]. It appears that since the isotope is a trivalent metal ion, once it has entered the cell it is retained for long periods. This is in contrast to iodine that is rapidly excreted. Thus, modulation may be an advantage with indium-labeled antibodies. This is illustrated in figure 5–5 where the higher contrast with ^{111}In is clearly visible at day 5, whereas with ^{131}I an adequate image could not be obtained after two days.

Unfortunately, the long biological half-life of indium contributes to an absorbed dose equal to that of [131]I (which has a shorter biological half-life), but nevertheless it is clearly a superior isotope for scanning.

Alternative imaging methods

As indicated, improvements to the conventional gamma camera are unlikely to yield strikingly better results. The greatest improvement is likely to come from tomographic methods. There are two different types of emission tomography, single photon (SPET) and positron (PET). There are important differences between the two techniques [56]. SPET can be implemented with a conventional gamma camera detector and established isotopes but is subject to the limitations inherent in collimated cameras. PET utilises the paired gamma rays produced from the interaction of positrons with electrons in the body. These rays are emitted at 180 degrees to each other, and can be accurately located by two linked detectors opposite one another and without using a collimator.

Berche et al. [32] have applied SPET and ^{131}I-labeled monoclonal antibodies to patients with apparently successful results. However, tomographic reconstruction is heavily dependent upon good count statistics which perhaps reflect their need to scan for 40 minutes. Furthermore they did not compare SPET with a conventional LFOV gamma camera and technetium subtraction.

We have investigated a prototype positron camera [56] that shows promise and have been able to demonstrate hepatic metastases with a very small injected dose (1 MBq). [123]I or ^{111}In would appear ideal for SPET, particularly ^{123}I because of its favourable dosimetry and because with tomography the inability to use technetium subtraction may be less of a drawback.

Data manipulation

The original subtraction method for scan enhancement improved the contrast in the image about twofold [7]. If an organ-specific pharmaceutical is used for local subtraction (e.g., ^{99m}Tc-sulphur colloid for the liver), the contrast can be improved twentyfold [31].

To improve objectivity in the subtraction picture, the variance can be calculated and each point represented as standard deviations above background. Alternatively, statistical noise can be assessed for each point (pixel) in the picture and removed by using a Weiner filter [14] for

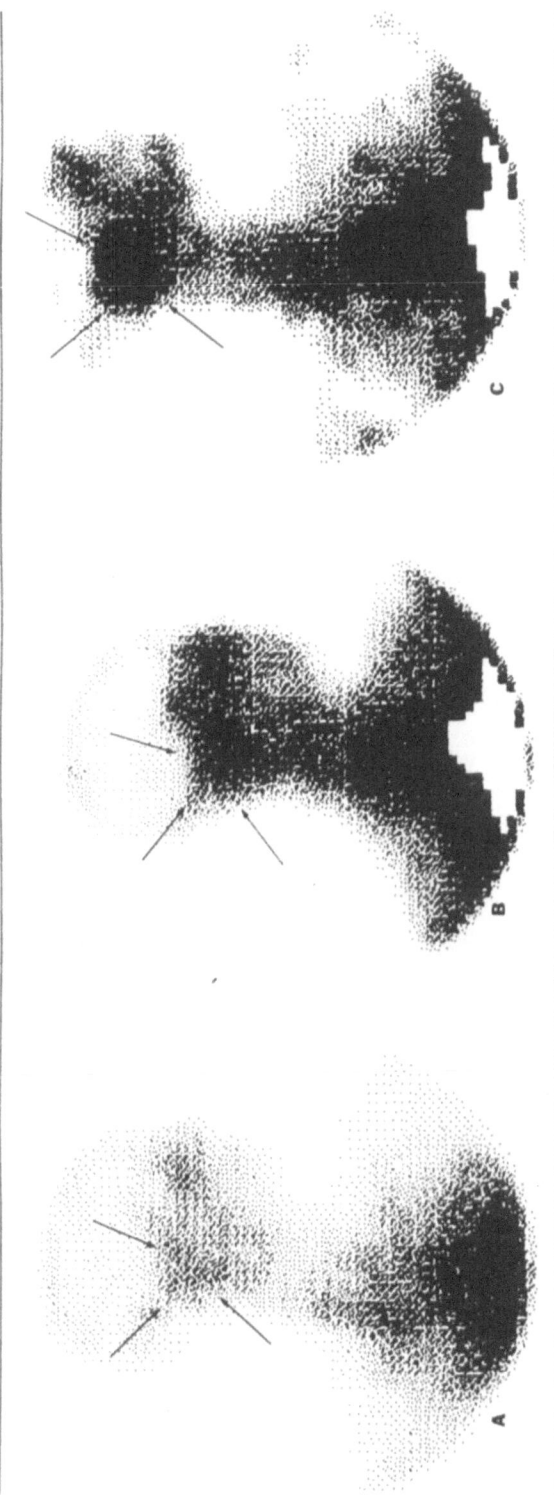

Figure 5-5. Comparison of ^{131}I- and ^{111}In-labeled anti-CEA in the same patient. All scans are unsubtracted and the arrows indicate a deposit of CEA producing squamous carcinoma near the right submandibular joint.

(A) ^{131}I scan at 24 hours.

(B) ^{111}In scan at 24 hours.

(C) ^{111}In scan at 5 days. The greater count rates from ^{111}In are seen together with its gradual accumulation in the tumour.

(From Fairweather DS, Bradwell AR, Dykes PW, Vaughan AT, Watson-James SF, Chandler S. Improved tumour localisation using 111-indium labeled antibodies. Br Med J 287:167–170, 1983.)

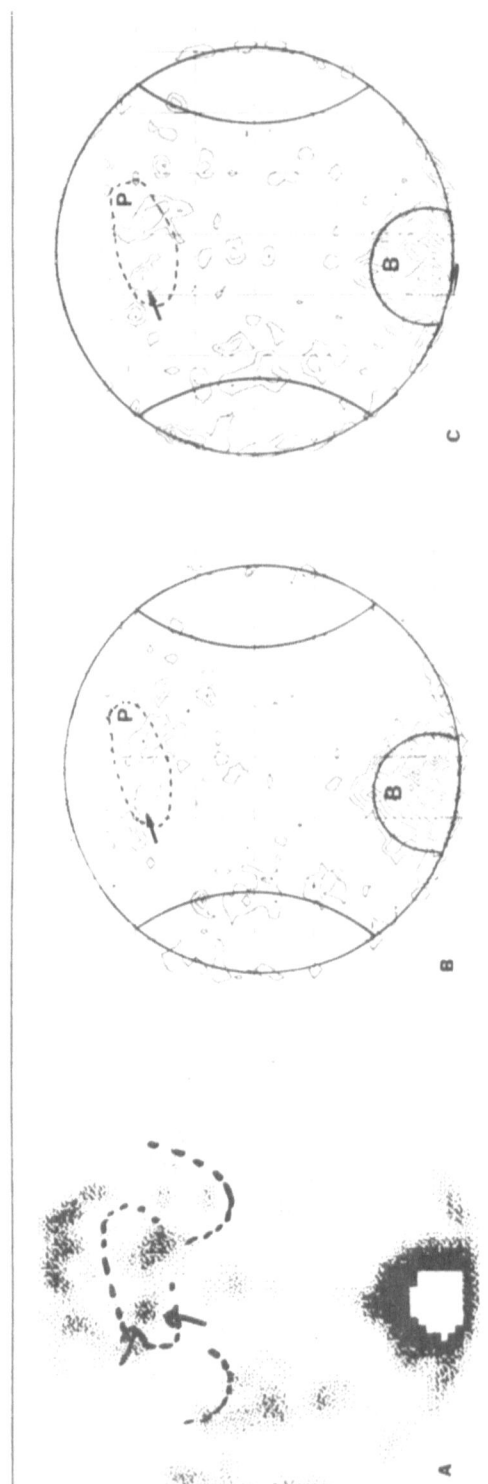

Figure 5-6. Data manipulation. Scans of a patient with a malignant insulinoma (arrowed) after injection of ^{131}I-labeled anti-insulin.

(A) Subtracted image.

(B) The same data processed through a Wiener filter to remove artifact.

(C) Same data after deconvolution. Each contour is one standard deviation above the background noise. P = Pancreas. B = Bladder.

(From Bradwell AR, Fairweather DS, Dykes PW. Radioimmunodetection of endocrine tumours. In Saunders KB (ed.), Advanced medicine 19. London: Pitman, 1983, pp. 76–98.)

each image before subtraction. Figure 5–6 shows a resulting image plotted in contours, each step representing one standard deviation above background. The data can be further improved by deconvolution and contouring in standard deviations above background noise.

Initial results indicate that this improves contrast a further twofold. Furthermore, this approach avoids arbitrary scaling of the image and enables a rapid and quantitative assessment of each area of the scan.

CONCLUSION

Antibody scanning is an exciting new method that brings together techniques from several disciplines. Although RAID may seem attractive, clinical relevance should not be overlooked. Accurate localisation of tumours is important only if local therapy is contemplated. If local therapy cannot be offered, it is usually sufficient to know whether tumour is present and the total tumour burden. For this purpose, measurement of tumour markers in the serum may prove more sensitive and certainly more convenient. Thus, it seems unlikely that antibody scanning can have a major impact on the management of the common malignant tumours, at least until more effective therapy can be devised. However, such scans may be useful research tools by helping in the assessment of new surgical or drug regimens. Furthermore, present absorbed radiation doses from antibody scanning are too high for this to be used as a routine screening procedure.

It must not be forgotten that antibodies can locate normal as well as malignant tissue [58]. Endocrine tissue is characterised by the production of specific substances to which antisera can be raised. The products are highly organ specific, e.g., thyroglobulin for thyroid tissue. We have already shown that antibodies to thyroglobulin and insulin can locate sites of production, and it is probable that other endocrine sites can be imaged as well. Myocardial infarcts have also been imaged by antibodies [58], as have parasite cysts [59].

Antibody scans provide functional information (the production and presence of an antigen and its quantity) rather than just structural information. Imaging, combined with the great variety of antisera that can be produced, is likely to find application in diverse fields.

REFERENCES

1. Hericourt J, Richet C. Traitment d'un case de sarcome par la serotherapie. CR Acad Sci 120: 948–950, 1895.
2. Pressman D. The development and use of radiolabelled anti-tumour antibodies. Cancer Res 40: 2960–2964, 1980.
3. Bale WF, Spar IL, Goodland RL, Wolfe DE. In vivo and in vitro studies of labelled antibodies against rat kidney and Walker carcinoma. Proc Soc Biol Med 89: 564–568, 1955.
4. Quinones J, Mizejewski G, Bierwaltes WH. Choricocarcinoma scanning using radiolabelled antibody to chorionic gonadotrophin. J Nucl Med 12: 69–75, 1971.
5. Goldenberg DM, Preston DF, Primus FJ, Hansen HJ. Photoscan localisation of GW-39 tumours in hamsters using radiolabelled anticarcinoembryonic antigen immunoglobulin G. Cancer Res 34: 1–9, 1974.
6. Mach J-P, Carrel S, Merenda C, Sordat B, Cerottini J-C. In vivo localisation of radiolabelled antibodies to carcinoembryonic antigen in human colon carcinoma grafted into nude mice. Nature 248: 704–706, 1974.
7. Goldenberg DM, Deland F, Kim E, Bennett, S Primus FJ, Van Nagell JR Jr, Estes N, Rayburn P. Use of radiolabelled antibodies to carcinoembryonic antigen for the detection and localisation of diverse cancers by external photoscanning. N Engl J Med 298: 1384–1388, 1978.
8. Dykes PW, Hine KR, Bradwell AR, Blackburn JC, Reeder TA, Drolc Z, Booth SN. Localisation of tumour deposits by external scanning after injection of radiolabelled anti-carcinoembryonic antigen. Br Med J 280: 220–222, 1980.

9. Mach JP, Carrel S, Forni M, Ritschard J, Donath A, Alberto P. Tumour localisation of radiolabelled antibodies against carcinoembryonic antigen in patients with carcinoma, a critical evaluation. N Eng J Med 303: 5–10, 1980.

10. Rockoff SD, Goodenough DJ, McIntire KR. Theoretical limitations in the immunodiagnostic imaging of cancer with computed tomography and nuclear scanning. Cancer Res 40: 3054–3058, 1980.

11. Bradwell AR, Taylor JR, Dykes PW, Fairweather DS. Model for the radioimmunodetection of tumours. Prot Biol Fluids 31: 1983, in press.

12. Hedin A, Wahren B, Hammerstrom S. Tumour localisation of CEA-containing human tumours in nude mice by means of monoclonal anti-CEA antibodies. Int J Cancer 30: 547–552, 1982.

13. Begent RHJ, Keep PA, Gren AJ, Searle F, Bagshawe KD, Jewkes RF, Jones BE, Barratt GM, Ryman BE. Liposomally entrapped second antibody improves tumour imaging with radiolabelled (first) anti tumour antibody. Lancet 2: 739–742, 1982.

14. Fairweather DS, Irwin M, Bradwell AR, Dykes PW, Flinn RM. Computer analysis of antibody scans. Prot Biol Fluids 31: 1983, in press.

15. Stanworth DR, Turner MW. Immunochemical analysis of immunoglobulins and their subunits. In DM Weir (ed.), Handbook of experimental immunology. Oxford: Blackwell Scientific Publications, 1978, vol. 1, chapter 6.

16. Sternberger L. The unlabelled antibody peroxidase-antiperoxidase (PAP) method. In Immunocytochemistry, 2nd ed. New York: J Wiley and Sons, 1979, pp. 104–169.

17. Ey PL, Prowse SJ, Jenkin CR. Isolation of pure IgGl, IgG2a and IgG2b immunoglobulins from mouse serum using protein A-Sepharose. Immunochemistry 15: 429–436, 1978.

18. European Pharmacopoeia. Tests for pyrogens 3: 58–60, 1971.

19. Watson-James SF, Fairweather DS, Bradwell AR. A shielded, sterile apparatus for iodinating proteins. Med Lab Sci 40: 67–68, 1981.

20. Epenetos AA, Britton KE, Mather S, Shepherd J, Granowska M, Taylor-Papadimitriou J, Nimmon CC, Durbin H, Hawkins LR, Malpas JS, Bodmer WF. Targetting of iodine-123-labelled tumour-associated monoclonal antibodies to ovarian, breast and gastrointestinal tumours. Lancet 2: 999–904, 1982.

21. Bateman JE, Flesher AC, Fairweather DS, Bradwell AR. Positron tomography of the thyroid gland. Clin Sci Mol Med 65: 18p, 1983.

22. Sundberg MW, Mears CF, Goodwin DA, Diamanti CI. Selective binding of metal ions to macromolecules using bifunctional analogs of EDTA. J Med Chem 17: 1304–1307, 1974.

23. Krejcarek GE, Tucker KL. Covalent attachment of chelating groups to macromolecules. Biochem Biophys Res Commun 77: 581–585, 1977.

24. Fairweather DS, Bradwell AR, Dykes PW, Vaughan AT, Watson-James SF, Chandler S. Improved tumour localisation using 111-indium labelled antibodies. Br Med J 287: 167–170, 1983.

25. Fairweather DS, Bradwell AR, Watson-James SF, Dykes PW, Chandler S, Hoffenberg R. Detection of thyroid tumours using radiolabelled anti-thyroglobulin. Clin Endocrinol 18: 563–570, 1983.

26. Begent RHJ, Boultbee J, Jewkes R, Katz D, McIvor J. Radioimmunolocalisation. Clin Oncol 2: 144–158, 1983.

27. Deland FH, Kim EE, Simmons G, Goldenberg DM. Imaging approach in radioimmunodetection. Cancer Res 40: 3046–3049, 1980.

29. Goldenberg DM, Kim EE, DeLand FH. Human Chorionic gonadotrophin radioantibodies in the radioimmunodetection of cancer and for disclosure of occult metastases. Proc Natl Acad Sci (USA) 78: 7754–7758, 1981.

30. Mach JP, Buchegger F, Forni M, Ritschard J, Berche C, Lumbroso JD, Schreyer M, Girardet C, Accola RS, Carrel S. Use of radiolabelled monoclonal anti-CEA antibodies for the detection of human carcinomas by external photoscanning and tomoscintigraphy. Immunol Today 2: 239–249, 1981.

31. DeLand FH, Kim EE, Goldenberg DM. In vivo radioimmunodetection of cancer. In Wilson CG, Hardy JG, Frier M and Davis SS (eds.), Radionuclide imaging in drug research. London: Croom Helm, 1982, 181–202.

32. Berche C, Mach JP, Lumbroso, JD, Langlais C, Aubrey F, Buchegger F, Carrel S, Rougier P, Parmentier C, Tubiana M. Tomoscintigraphy for detecting gastrointestinal and medullary thyroid cancers: First clinical results using radiolabelled monoclonal antibodies against carcinoembryonic antigen. Br Med J 285: 1447–1451, 1982.

33. Smedley HM, Finan P., Lennox ES, Ritson A, Takei F, Wraight P, Sikora K. Localisation of metastatic carcinoma by radiolabelled monoclonal antibody. Br J Cancer 47: 253–259, 1983.

34. Goldenberg DM, Kim EE, Bennett SJ, Nelson MO, DeLand FH. Carcinoembryonic antigen radioimmunodetection in the evaluation of colorectal cancer and in the detection of occult neoplasms. Gastroenterology 84: 524–532, 1983.

35. Goldenberg DM, Kim EE, DeLand FH, Spremulli E, Nelson MO, Cockerman JP, Primus FJ, Corgan RL, Alpert E. Clinical studies on the radioimmunodetection of tumours containing alphafetoprotein. Cancer 45: 2500–2505, 1980.

36. Halsall AK, Fairweather DS, Bradwell AR, Blackburn JC, Dykes PW, Howell A, Reeder A, Hine KR. Localisation of malignant germ cell tumours by external scanning after injection of radiolabelled anti alpha-fetoprotein. Br Med J 283: 942–944, 1981.

37. Begent RHJ, Searle F, Stanway G, Jewkes RF, Jones BE, Vernon P, Bagshawe KD. Radioimmunolocalisation of tumours by external scintigraphy after administration of ^{131}I antibody to human chorionic gonadotrophin. J Soc Med 73: 624–630, 1980.

38. Goldenberg DM, Kim EE, DeLand FH, Van Nagell JR, Javadpour N. Clinical radioimmunodetection of cancer with radioactive antibodies to human chorionic gonadotrophin. Science 208: 1284–1286, 1980.

39. Fairweather DS, Bradwell AR, Dykes PW. Monoclonal antibodies for in vivo localisation. Lancet 2: 660, 1982.

40. Ghose T, Norvell ST, Aquino J, Belitsky P, Tai J, Guclu A, Blair AH. Localisation of I-131-labelled antibodies in human renal cell carcinomas and in a mouse hepatoma and correlation with tumour detection by photoscanning. Cancer Res 40: 3018–3031, 1980.

41. Farrands PA, Perkins AC, Pimm MV, Hardy JD, Embleton MJ, Baldwin RW, Hardcastle JD. Radioimmunodetection of human colorectal cancers by anti-tumour monoclonal antibody. Lancet 2: 397–400, 1982.

42. Larson SM, Brown JP, Wright PW, Carrasquillo JA, Hellstrom I, Hellstrom KE. Imaging of melanoma with I-131-labelled monoclonal antibodies. J Nucl Med 24: 123–129, 1983.

43. Rainsbury RM, Ott RJ, Westwood JH, Kalirai TS, Coombes RC, McCready VR, Neville AM, Gazet J-C. Location of metastatic breast carcinoma by a monoclonal antibody chelate labelled with Indium-111. Lancet 2: 934–938, 1983.

44. Dykes PW, Bradwell AR. Carcinoembryonic antigen radioimmunodetection. Gastroenterology 84: 651–653, 1983.

45. Lewis JCM, Bagshawe KD, Keep PA. The distribution of parenterally administered antibody to CEA in colorectal xenografts. Onco Develop Biol Med 3: 161–168, 1982.

46. Moshakis V, Bailey MJ, Ormerod MG, Westwood JH, Neville AM. Localisation of human breast-carcinoma xenografts using antibodies to carcinoembryonic antigen. Br J Cancer 43: 575–581, 1981.

47. Fairweather DS, Bradwell AR, Dykes PW. Localisation of malignant germ cell tumours. Br Med J 284: 1478, 1982.

48. Unanue ER, Karnovsky MJ. Ligand-induced movement of lymphocyte membrane macromolecules. V. Capping, cell movement and microtubular function in normal and lectin-treated lymphocytes. J Exp Med 140: 1207–1220, 1974.

49. Hirai T, Yamamoto H, Hamoaka T. Relationship between carcinoembryonic antigen and major histocompatibility antigens in cultured human carcinoma cells. J Immunology 124: 2765–2771, 1980.

50. Stern P, Hagan P, Halpern S, Chen A, David G, Adams T, Desmond W, Brautigam K, Royston I. The effect of the radiolabel on the kinetics of monoclonal anti-CEA in a nude mouse-human colon tumour model. In Mitchel MS, Oettgen HF, (eds.), Hybridomas in cancer diagnosis and treatment. New York: Raven Press 1982, 245–253.

51. Searle F. Boden J, Lewis JCM, Bagshawe KD. A human choriocarcinoma xenograft in nude mice; a model for the study of antibody localisation. Br J Cancer 44: 137–144, 1981.

52. Bradwell AR, Vaughan A, Fairweather DS, Dykes PW. Improved radio-immuno-detection of tumours using a second antibody. Lancet 1: 247, 1983.

53. Bradwell AR, Fairweather DS, Keeling A, Watson-James S, Vaughan A, Dykes PW. Antibody interactions in the radioimmunodetection of tumours. Clin Sci Mol Med 65: 31p, 1983.

54. Glennie MJ, Stevenson GT. Univalent antibodies kill tumour cells in vitro and in vivo. Nature 295: 712–713, 1982.

55. Brownell GL, Budinger TF, Lauterbur PL, Megeer PL. Positron tomography and nuclear magnetic resonance imaging. Science 215: 619–626, 1982.

56. Bateman JE, Flescher AL, Fairweather DS, Bradwell AR, Wilkinson R. In vivo imaging of the human thyroid with the Rutherford positron camera using [124]I. Science and Engineering Research Council Rutherford Laboratory Report RL: 8L–36, 1982.

57. Brault JW, White OR. The analysis and restoration of astronomical data via the fast fourier transform. Astr Astrophys 13: 169–189, 1971.

58. Khaw BA, Fallon JT, Strauss HW, Harbe E. Myocardial infarct imaging of antibodies to canine cardiac myosin with indium-111-diethylene triamine pentaacetic acid. Science 209: 295–297, 1980.

59. Skromne-Kadlubik G, Celis C, Ferez A. Cysticerosis of the nervous system: Diagnosis by means of specific radioimmunoscan. Ann Neurol 2: 343–344, 1977.

6. IMMUNODEFICIENCY, AUTOIMMUNITY, AND MALIGNANCY

M.A.H. FRENCH

INTRODUCTION

Much of our current knowledge about the normal physiology of the immune system has been derived from the study of primary immunodeficiency diseases in the context of "experiments of nature." Not surprisingly, therefore, a similar approach has been taken as one way of testing the hypothesis that immune responses are part of the normal homeostatic mechanism for controlling malignancy ("immune surveillance"). The demonstration of an increased incidence of malignancy in patients with primary immunodeficiency diseases might provide evidence in support of this view. Furthermore, the association of malignancy with particular types of immune defects might provide insight into which parts of the normal immune response are involved with tumour immunity.

Studies performed over the last two decades have, indeed, demonstrated an increased incidence of malignancy in primary immunodeficiency diseases. However, it has become clear that the concept of immune surveillance cannot be fully accepted on the evidence available from these studies.

It, therefore, becomes necessary to explain malignancy as a complication of primary immunodeficiency in other terms. The types of malignancy that occur as a complication of some immunodeficiency diseases are similar to those that may complicate some autoimmune diseases, particularly connective tissue diseases. It is perhaps in this common ground that some mechanisms operating in the development of malignancy in these immunological diseases, and perhaps in general, can be studied. To this end this chapter will discuss the malignant complications of various primary immunodeficiency diseases and connective tissue diseases, particularly in relation to the immunological abnormalities. It will become clear that the risk of

B.W. Hancock and A.M. Ward (eds.), Immunological Aspects of Cancer. Copyright © 1985, Martinus Nijhoff Publishing, Boston/Dordrecht/Lancaster.

developing malignancy in different diseases is variable and that the mechanisms underlying oncogenesis are heterogeneous.

PRIMARY IMMUNODEFICIENCY AND MALIGNANCY

An early survey by Gatti and Good [1] indicated marked increase in the incidence of malignancy in all types of primary immunodeficiency disease. There was a particularly high incidence of lymphoreticular malignancy. However, the data were obtained from a literature survey, a data collection method that Asherson and Webster [2] argued may have overestimated the true incidence. There are also potential problems in the description and classification of the malignancy and in the classification of the immunodeficiency disease [2].

To study the association in more depth, the World Health Organisation Committee on Primary Immunodeficiencies [3] established the Immunodeficiency-Cancer Registry (ICR). Although this is also a retrospective analysis of cases, the method of case collection probably allows for a more accurate estimate of the incidence of malignancy in immunodeficiency diseases than do literature surveys. It has also provided valuable information on the types of malignancy that occur. The first report [4] confirmed an increased incidence of malignancy, but subsequent reports have shown that the risk is different for different types of immunodeficiency syndrome.

Sex-linked hypogammaglobulinaemia

This prototype antibody deficiency syndrome was the first immunodeficiency syndrome to come under close scrutiny for an increased incidence of malignancy [5]. Patients with this condition are abnormally prone to infections, particularly pyogenic infections of the respiratory tract, because of an inability to produce systemic and secretory antibody responses. There is an absence of plasma cells and consequently hypogammaglobulinaemia. B-cells in peripheral blood, lymph nodes, and spleen are absent or very low, but the number of pre-B-cells in the bone marrow is normal. It would appear that there is a defect of the maturation of pre-B-cells to B-cells. The number and function of T-cells are normal, as is "natural killer" (NK) cell function [6].

Early reports [5] were followed by more extensive surveys [4], indicating an increased incidence of malignancy, particularly leukaemias, amongst patients with sex-linked hypogammaglobulinaemia. However, this is now disputed [7,2], and a good prognosis about malignancy can be anticipated in patients with this type of immunodeficiency syndrome.

Common variable immunodeficiency

Hypogammaglobulinaemia and defective antibody production, resulting in an abnormal susceptibility to pyogenic infections, are also characteristic of this syndrome, but the immunological and clinical findings differ from sex-linked hypogammaglobulinaemia. Common variable immunodeficiency (CVID) is a heterogeneous group of conditions, with hypogammaglobulinaemia common to all [8]. Other names for this condition are common variable hypogammaglobulinaemia and late-onset hypogammaglobulinaemia. Some cases present in early childhood and may be cases of congenital hypogammaglobulinaemia without evidence of a sex-linked inheritance. Other cases present in later life, sometimes in old age.

Hypogammaglobulinaemia, by definition, is universal, but the extent is more variable than in the congenital form. There is a deficiency of plasma cells but B-cells are usually present and may be increased in numbers. In most cases, however, there is evidence of B-cell immaturity [9,10]. A minority of cases have abnormalities of regulator T-cell function (excess T-suppression or impaired T-help), probably accounting for failure of antibody production [9]. Abnormalities of T-cell immunity are present in approximately one-third of patients [11] manifesting as absent-delayed hypersensitivity on skin testing and/or depressed lymphocyte transformation to mitogens such as phytohaemagglutinin (PHA). T-cell numbers are usually normal but may be low. Despite the presence of T-cell abnormalities in many patients, susceptibility is not increased to the types of infection seen in patients with T-cell immunodeficiency syndromes. NK-cell function is normal [6].

The incidence of malignancy amongst patients with CVID appears to have increased, although the validity of some reported cases has been questioned [2]. Filipovich et al. [12] have reported 74 cases from the ICR with CVID and malignancy. Half of these had lymphoreticular malignancies, but only 5% had leukaemias. Lymphoreticular malignancies included lymphocytic lymphomas, histiocytic lymphomas, and Hodgkin's disease [7]. Epithelial malignancies were also common, occurring in 44% of collected cases; these were almost all cases of carcinoma of the stomach. This confirms the findings of others [13].

Although the incidence of lymphoreticular malignancy has increased, it is probably not as high as once thought [2], and lymphoma is a rare cause of death. Splenomegaly as a complication of the immunodeficiency syndrome is more common than as a manifestation of complicating lymphoma. Unless there are good indications, splenectomy for diagnostic purposes should be discouraged because of the added risks of infection it would incur. Although splenomegaly is a relatively common finding in patients with CVID, lymphadenopathy is not and the presence of significant lymphadenopathy requires the exclusion of lymphoma.

In some cases, at least, lymphoproliferation probably results from persistent antigenic stimulation of the immune system by infective agents, and in the gut by food antigens. Progression to monoclonal proliferation results in the development of lymphoma. Although uncommon, cases of nodular lymphoid hyperplasia of the gut have progressed to immunoblastic B-cell lymphomas [14].

The relationship between CVID and carcinoma of the stomach is not understood but could be of great interest. Other gastrointestinal complications are common in patients with CVID who develop carcinoma of the stomach. These include nodular lymphoid hyperplasia, malabsorption, giardiasis, atrophic gastritis, and pernicious anaemia [7,13]. Pernicious anaemia occurs at a younger than expected age in patients with CVID [15]. Whether the development of carcinoma of the stomach is related to any of these complications is difficult to determine. Possibly, however, secretory antibody deficiency adds to the risk of bacterial colonisation of the stomach in patients with achlorhydria. Bacterial colonisation and the production of nitrosamines by bacteria is a possible aetiological mechanism in the development of carcinoma of the stomach in patients with pernicious anaemia [16].

Thymoma and immunodeficiency

Some patients with a late onset immunodeficiency syndrome have an associated thymoma that may be benign or malignant. Late onset hypogammaglobulinaemia and chronic mucocutaneous candidiasis are the most common syndromes, but other immune defects may also be found [17].

Autoimmune diseases are also a well-recognised complication of a thymoma [18] and may occur in patients with thymoma and immunodeficiency. Possibly the immunodeficiency results from an autoimmune process. There is little doubt that the thymoma is an aetiological factor in the development of immunodeficiency rather than a complication of it. Evidence in support of this is the absence of thymoma as a complication of congenital immunodeficiency syndromes and the fact that thymoma and hypogammaglobulinaemia is distinct from other cases of late-onset hypogammaglobulinaemia in terms of immunological and clinical features [19].

Malignancy may be a cause of death in patients with malignant thymoma, but the prognosis is good in those patients with a benign thymoma provided the immunodeficiency and any other complications can be treated. Thymectomy is indicated in the management of the thymoma but does not lead to improvement of the hypogammaglobulinaemia.

Selective IgA deficiency

Selective deficiency of IgA in serum and secretions is the commonest type of primary immunoglobulin deficiency syndrome. The deficiency, which may be congenital or acquired, probably reflects a defect of B-cell maturation [20]. The majority of individuals with selective IgA deficiency are healthy, whereas others may suffer from abnormal susceptibility to infections, autoimmune disease, allergies, immune complex disease, and gluten enteropathy [21]. Infections can vary in severity from viral upper respiratory tract infections to bacterial infections of the lower respiratory tract complicated by bronchiectasis. Apparently healthy individuals with IgA deficiency have compensatory mechanisms, such as secretory IgM and IgG antibody, whereas symptomatic individuals may have additional immune defects, such as low serum concentrations of IgG_2 [22]. T-cell function is normal.

Patients with IgA deficiency have been suggested to have an increased risk of developing malignancy [7]. Interestingly, there seems to be a particular risk of developing carcinoma of the stomach [7,23], as is the case in patients with CVID. However, the association is not as strong for IgA deficiency as with some other immunodeficiency syndromes, and further studies are required to establish a definite link.

A study in which serum immunoglobulin concentrations were measured in a large group of patients attending a cancer-orientated hospital [23] showed that selective IgA deficiency was more common than in a normal population but that the incidence was not significantly different from a hospital population. However, the incidence of IgA deficiency was increased above expected in patients with lymphoreticular and gastric malignancy. Lymphoreticular malignancies included lymphoma, lymphosarcoma, immunoblastic lymphadenopathy, and myeloma.

The data showing a link between IgA deficiency and lymphoreticular malignancy must be interpreted with caution, as the immunoglobulin deficiency may be secondary to the lymphoproliferative process and/or the treatment of it. Should the link with carcinoma of the stomach be established, further support will be provided for a link between absent secretory IgA and the development of gastric carcinomas as is seen in patients with CVID and ataxia telangiectasia. However, other factors must be important, as patients with sex-linked hypogammaglobulinaemia do not have an increased risk of developing carcinoma of the stomach.

Selective IgM deficiency

Patients with this type of primary immunoglobulin deficiency are abnormally susceptible to infections, particularly septicaemia and meningococcal meningitis [24]. A small number of cases with associated malignancy have been described [12]. Again, caution must be exercised in the interpretation of this finding, as 75% of malignancies were lymphoreticular and selective IgM deficiency may antedate more extensive immunoglobulin deficiency in patients with lymphoproliferative disease.

Severe combined immunodeficiency syndrome

Severe combined immunodeficiency syndrome (SCID) is a heterogeneous group of disorders that result in severe defects of T-cell and antibody-mediated immunity [8]. The inheritance may be X-linked or autosomal recessive. Some cases with an autosomal recessive mode of inheritance are due to a deficiency of an enzyme in the lymphocyte purine salvage pathway [25]. One variant, Nezelof's syndrome, is characterised by normal or increased concentrations of one or more classes of serum immunoglobulin but antibody production is usually defective. Children with SCID are prone to infections because of defective antibody and cell-mediated immunity and, therefore, suffer from repeated bacterial, viral, fungal, and protozoal infections. Most patients do not survive past the age of two years unless treated by bone marrow transplantation.

Thirteen cases of malignancy and SCID have been collected by the ICR [12]. All were cases of lymphoreticular malignancy or leukaemia. As many patients die from infection or from the complications of bone marrow transplantation, death probably occurs in many patients before malignancy has had time to develop. Malignancy has not been reported in patients successfully treated by bone marrow transplantation [7].

Immunodeficiency involving T-cells, phagocytes, or NK-cells

In view of the experimental evidence that T-cells, macrophages, and NK-cells are involved in tumour immunity, it is surprising that malignancy is not a well-recognised complication of immunodeficiency involving these types of cell. Severe deficiencies of T-cell immunity as present in the DiGeorge syndrome (thymic hypoplasia and thereby absent T-cells, due to embryonic maldevelopment of the third and fourth branchial arches) and more selective defects as present in patients with chronic mucocutaneous candidiasis do not appear to be associated with an increased risk of malignancy. Indeed, not one case has been reported by the ICR [12].

Similarly, if natural monocyte- or macrophage-mediated immunity is an important mechanism in the immune response against malignancy, an increased incidence of malignant disease might be expected in patients with primary defects of phagocytic cell function. In one such disease, chronic granulomatous disease (CGD), there is a defect involving the generation of bactericidal oxidising agents that affects the function of polymorphonuclear leucocytes, monocytes, and macrophages. This intracellular mechanism, as well as others, may be a mechanism of monocyte- and macrophage-mediated tumour cell cytotoxicity [26].

There is, however, no reported increase in the incidence of malignancy in patients with CGD or other primary phagocytic cell defects.

Patients with the Chediak-Higashi syndrome [27] have defects of polymorphonuclear cell function leading to immunodeficiency but are particularly interesting because there is also marked impairment of NK-cell function [28]. The beige mouse provides an animal model for this disease. In this model there does appear to be a relationship between NK-cell deficiency and susceptibility to transplantable tumours [29,30]. Patients with the Chediak-Higashi syndrome frequently develop a "lymphomalike" accelerated phase [27], but whether this is true lymphoma is debatable. There does not appear to be an increased incidence of other malignancies. At present, therefore, these "model" immunodeficiency diseases cannot be said to have demonstrated a definite relationship between NK-cell deficiency and malignancy, in humans at least.

Wiskott-Aldrich syndrome

The Wiskott-Aldrich syndrome (WA syndrome) provides some of the strongest evidence for a link between malignancy and primary immunodeficiency. Unlike the immunodeficiency syndromes discussed so far, immunodeficiency in the WA syndrome is one manifestation of a generalised fundamental metabolic defect. The characteristic clinical features of this X-linked recessive condition are thrombocytopaenia, eczema, and immunodeficiency [31].

Thrombocytopaenia is due to a shortened platelet half-life and frequently leads to problems with haemorrhage. The platelets are small and show abnormal function in vivo, a condition that may be related to a defect of cell energy metabolism [32]. Eczema occurs early in the course of this disease and often resembles infantile eczema. The serum IgE concentration is elevated, which may be related to defective T-cell regulation, and patients frequently have allergic disease.

Immunodeficiency is due to defects of cell-mediated and antibody-mediated immunity. The latter are of greatest clinical importance and result in recurrent pneumonia, meningitis, skin infections, and otitis media. There is a particular susceptibility to infections with encapsulated bacteria such as pneumococci and meningococci that reflects defective antibody responses against polysaccharide antigens, a characteristic feature of this syndrome [33,34]. Consequently, the serum IgM concentration is often low. Serum IgA is high or normal, and serum IgG is usually normal but occasionally low. Defects of cell-mediated immunity are variable and often become progressively worse with time. When present, these manifest as depressed delayed hypersensitivity to skin test antigens, low in vitro lymphocyte transformation responses to antigens and mitogens, and low numbers of peripheral blood T-cells. NK-cell function is impaired [35]. It is presumed that the defects of immunity and the platelet abnormalities are related in terms of an underlying biochemical defect, but this has not yet been defined.

Although infections and haemorrhagic complications are the major causes of death, accounting for 59% and 27% of deaths, respectively [36], malignancy is a significant cause of morbidity and mortality. Early reports suggesting an increased risk of malignancy in the WA syndrome [4,34] have been confirmed [36]. There is an age- and sex-adjusted relative risk of well in excess of 100 compared with the general population. This risk increases with age. Lymphomas, leukaemias, and Hodgkin's disease account for the great majority of cases [table 6–1]. Extranodal spread of lymphoreticular malignancies is common, in particular intracranial involvement by histiocytic lymphoma and reticulum cell sarcoma [36,37]. In this respect the malignant disease of the WA syndrome resembles that found in immunosuppressed patients.

Malignancy is treated in a conventional manner. It is difficult to know whether correction of the immunological defects would prevent the development of malignancy, as a definitive cure is difficult to achieve—although bone marrow transplantation might provide some hope [38].

Immunodeficiency in "chromosome breakage syndromes"

Immunodeficiency and an increased susceptibility to malignancy are common to three syndromes—ataxia telangiectasia (AT), Bloom's syndrome (BS), and Fanconi's anaemia (FA)—all having the characteristic cytogenetic abnormality of a DNA repair defect and/or overt chromosome damage. All have an autosomal recessive mode of inheritance. These syndromes have been studied in some detail from the point of view of a relationship between the cytogenetic defects and malignancy [39], the development of which might also be related to the immunodeficiency. Xeroderma pigmentosum is a syndrome with similar cytogenetic defects and an increased susceptibility to malignancy, but immunodeficiency is not a complication.

Ataxia telangiectasia

The clinical syndrome of ataxia telangiectasia consists of a progressive neurological disorder with ataxia of early onset, choreoathetosis, oculomotor signs, and postural anomalies; pro-

Table 6–1. Distribution of 36 malignancies in 301 WA syndrome patients by histology

Histology	No. of cases
Lymphoreticular tumours	23[*]
Malignant histiocytosis/reticulosis/	
microgliomatosis	9
Histiocytic lymphoma/reticulum cell sarcoma	6
Lymphoma not otherwise specified	7
Lymphocytic lymphoma/lymphosarcoma	1
Leukaemias	7
Myelogenous	5
Acute, not otherwise specified	1
Type not specified	1
Hodgkin's disease	3
Other	3
Pinealoma	1
Leiomyosarcoma	1
Encephalomatous tumour	1
Total	36

[*]Of these, 13 were extranodal primary tumours of the brain (8), digestive system (3), lung (1), and skin (1).
Source: Reproduced from [36] with the permission of the authors.

gressive telangiectasia; and recurrent sinopulmonary infections due to a combined immuno-deficiency syndrome affecting cell-mediated and antibody-mediated immunity [40]. Other clinical abnormalities include retarded growth, pigmentary skin changes, actinic skin damage, absent or hypoplastic ovaries, and an abnormal susceptibility to malignancy.

Spontaneous chromosome damage is a characteristic finding but differs from that found in BS and FA. There is an increase in structural chromosome changes in lymphocytes and fibroblasts, and approximately 20 to 30% of cultured lymphocytes show chromosome breaks. Cells are susceptible to X- and γ-irradiation, which induces increased chromosome damage at early G1 and G2 stages of the cell cycle. Susceptibility to the effects of ultraviolet (uv) radiation is not increased, although chromosome damage may be induced by some chemicals. The chromosome damage probably occurs because there is a DNA repair defect.

Immunodeficiency is very common, occurring in approximately 80% of patients, and is the commonest cause of death. This is usually a combined immunodeficiency but varies in severity from patient to patient [41]. Selective IgA deficiency is the most common finding and may be associated with a deficiency of IgE and of IgG_2 in some cases. Hypogamma-globulinaemia is occasionally present. Systemic antibody responses are usually detectable but reduced in quantity. Reduced immunoglobulin synthesis, particularly of IgA, has been demonstrated in vitro; it would appear that there is a defect of terminal differentiation of B-cells into IgA- and IgE-secreting plasma cells with a disorder of T-helper cells being a contributory factor in some patients. Disorders of cell-mediated immunity are also common. Thymic hypoplasia is a frequent finding and there may be absent delayed hypersensitivity to skin test antigens, reduced numbers of peripheral blood T-cells, and impaired in vitro lymphocyte transformation in response to mitogenic, antigenic, and allogeneic cell stimulation. The capacity to produce cytotoxic T-cells against virally infected cells is reduced [42], and NK-cell function is impaired [35].

A unifying hypothesis for the various abnormalities in AT is that a single gene defect results in abnormal DNA repair mechanisms so that environmental agents such as X- and γ-irradiation and some chemicals cause chromosomal instability and breakage. The consequences of this might be, first, impaired development and proliferation of lymphocytes resulting in restricted diversity of immune responses and, second, cellular degeneration, for example, in the nervous system.

Ataxia telangiectasia is an interesting model in which to study the relationship between cytogenetic abnormalities, immunodeficiency, and malignancy. However, the complexity of the cytogenetic and immunological disturbances makes it difficult to determine to what extent any one abnormality is related to the development of malignant disease. Since the description of malignancy in one of eight patients in the series described by Sedgwick and Boder [43], it has become apparent that about 10% of patients will develop this complication. The incidence is similar, therefore, to that in the WA syndrome.

At least 108 patients with AT and malignancy have been collected by the ICR [44]. Six of these cases had multiple tumours. Lymphoreticular malignancies and leukaemias were most common, as seen in most other immunodeficiency syndromes, but carcinomas also occurred. Non-Hodgkin's lymphomas (NHL) were present in 45%, leukaemias in 24%, Hodgkin's disease in 11%, and carcinomas in 20%. Regarding the types of malignancy, AT lies between the congenital immunodeficiency syndromes such as SCID, X-linked hypogammaglobulinaemia, and WA syndrome, in which lymphoreticular malignancies predominate, and late-onset immunodeficiency syndromes, such as CVID and IgA deficiency, in which lymphomas and carcinomas occur together.

Carcinoma of the stomach is the most common carcinoma, with carcinoma of the uterus and ovary occurring less frequently. NHL are predominantly of B-cell type as found in patients without immunodeficiency. However, there is an unexpected predominance of T-cell leukaemias. In patients with acute lymphocytic leukaemia the leukaemic cells have T-cell markers in 62.5% of cases, "non-T non-B" in 37.5%, and none has B-cell surface markers. This is in contrast to patients who are not immunodeficient, amongst whom "non-T non-B" acute lymphocytic leukaemias are most common [45]. Similarly, although chronic lymphocytic leukaemia (CLL) is present in only a small number of patients with AT, it is interesting that all cases are T-cell CLL [12]. Approximately 98% of cases of CLL are of B-cell origin in nonimmunodeficient patients.

CLL in patients with AT is of interest in other respects. Three of seven such patients had abnormalities of chromosome 14 [12]. In some patients chromosome-14 abnormalities have been markers of proliferative clones of lymphocytes [46,47]. Of the various cytogenetic abnormalities present in AT-cells, chromosome-14 abnormalities are particularly common [48] and may be related to the development of lymphoproliferative disease.

It seems most likely that malignancy in AT is a complication of the cytogenetic abnormalities rather than a direct consequence of the immunodeficiency, although immunodeficiency may have some effect. Where a relationship between the type and severity of the immune defect and the development of malignancy has been sought, no direct relationship could be demonstrated [44]. There is, however, a lack of data on NK-cell and cytotoxic T-cell function in relation to the development of malignancy. A prospective study of the relationship between immunodeficiency and malignancy in AT is clearly needed.

The cytogenetic abnormalities in AT have some practical as well as theoretical importance. Because of the sensitivity of cells to ionising radiation and some chemicals, there may be adverse effects from radiotherapy or chemotherapy used to treat malignancies. Radiation dermatitis is common [49], and basal cell carcinoma of the scalp has been reported following the use of radiotherapy [50].

Bloom's syndrome

Although Bloom's syndrome (BS) is much less common than AT, valuable data on the relationship between "chromosome breakage syndromes" and malignancy have been obtained because of the thorough collection, documentation, and study of cases by German et al. [51] through the Bloom's syndrome registry. BS is particularly common amongst Ashkenazic Jews, although a small number of cases have been reported in the United Kingdom. The characteristic clinical features are growth retardation leading to a short stature, sensitivity to uv light, resulting in actinic erythema of the face (figure 6–1), and immunodeficiency. An increased incidence of malignancy is now well recognised. The basic defect in BS is unknown. Structural chromosome anomalies tend to occur, and the characteristic cytogenetic finding, which is of greatest diagnostic value, is an increase in sister chromatid exchanges [52].

Abnormal susceptibility to respiratory tract infections is a problem in many patients. There is a limited amount of data on immune function testing [53,54], but this does indicate

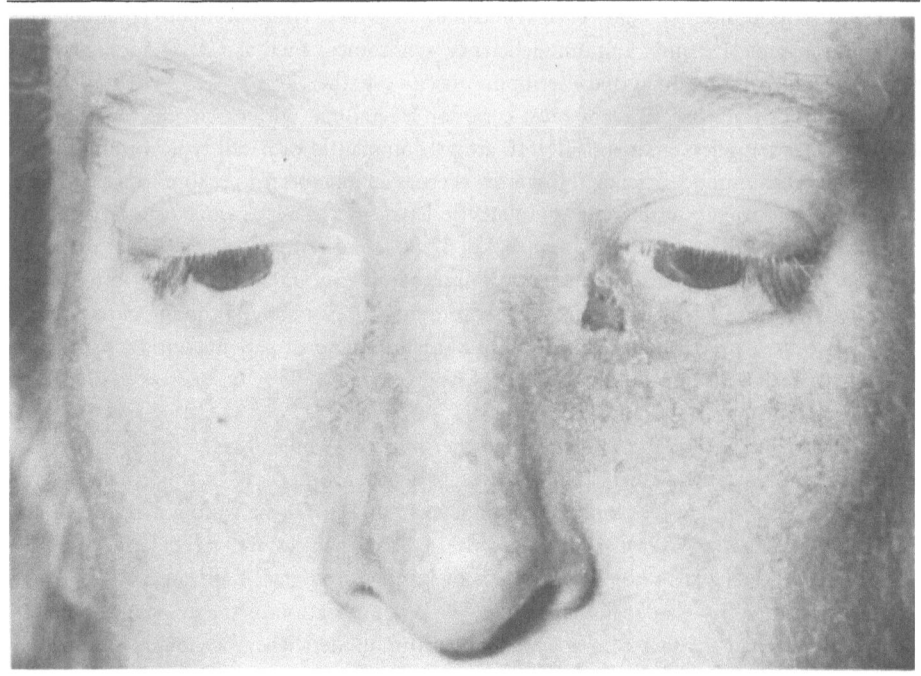

Figure 6-1. Typical actinic malar erythema in a patient with Bloom's syndrome. There is, in addition, a left chronic dacryocystitis due to the immunodeficiency syndrome.

defects of antibody-mediated and cell-mediated immunity. Serum immunoglobulin concentrations are often low but rarely is there hypogammaglobulinaemia. Systemic antibody responses following immunisation may be low or normal. Peripheral blood T- and B-cell numbers are normal, but there is reduced mitogen-induced lymphocyte transformation in vitro. Similarly, in mixed lymphocyte cultures the lymphocytes of BS patients are poor responders but are normal stimulators. There is a general disorder of cellular proliferation in BS, and defective lymphocyte proliferation is probably a reflection of this. With regard to defective immune responses in vivo, the aforementioned disorder probably results in impairment of B-cell differentiation and impaired function of regulator T-cells [55].

Malignancy has occurred in 21% of the 77 well-documented cases [51]. Acute leukaemias predominate with equal numbers of lymphocytic and nonlymphocytic types. NHL, including lymphosarcoma and reticulum cell sarcoma, are also frequent. Carcinomas have occurred in five patients, and all but one have been of the gastrointestinal tract.

Fanconi's anaemia

Patients with FA are known to have problems similar to patients with AT and BS, including immunodeficiency and an increased incidence of malignancy. Documentation however is limited. The characteristic clinical findings [56] are growth retardation; hyperpigmentation including cafe-au-lait patches; multiple malformations including skeletal abnormalities, renal disease, microcephaly with mental retardation and hypogonadism; and pancytopaenia due to a failure to produce functioning stem cells. One of the consequences of the latter complication is immunodeficiency.

Chromosomal instability is present in cultured cells from FA patients including bone marrow cells, lymphocytes, and skin fibroblasts. Cells are abnormally susceptible to ionising radiation. The exact defect is not known, but it results in chromosome breaks, gene mutation, and impaired cell division with prolongation of the cell cycle. There may be a defect of DNA replication or repair. One finding of particular interest is that FA cells demonstrate an increased tendency to transform in vitro when exposed to the oncogenic hamster virus SV 40 [57]. This correlates with the patient's risk of developing malignancy. Few data are available on the immune defects in FA, but abnormalities of cell-mediated immunity and serum immunoglobulins have been reported [58,59].

The increased incidence of malignancy is due mainly to leukaemias, squamous cell carcinomas, and hepatocellular carcinoma [60]. Hepatocellular carcinoma may be related to androgen therapy given for the aplastic anaemia. Unlike AT and BS, the risk of developing malignancy is poorly documented.

The nature of the relationship between "chromosome breakage syndromes" and malignancy

As previously discussed, the available evidence indicates that malignant disease in AT, BS, and FA does not result directly from the immunodeficiency but rather that malignancy and immunodeficiency are both a manifestation of the fundamental cytogenetic abnormalities. Other evidence supports this finding. First, the carrier state for AT and FA is associated with an increased risk of developing malignancy [61], and, second, patients with xeroderma pigmentosum who have cytogenetic abnormalities similar to AT, BS, and FA are prone to the development of malignancies but do not have immunodeficiency.

The chromosome abnormalities in these syndromes might result in spontaneous oncogenesis, but it is more probable that defective DNA repair and chromosomal instabilty following damage by ionising radiation or chemicals are the crucial factors. It is also possible that chromosome breaks might allow oncogenic viruses to integrate into DNA.

X-linked lymphoproliferative syndrome

The X-linked lymphoproliferative syndrome is a recently described immunodeficiency disease with a sex-linked recessive mode of inheritance. It is a potentially interesting model to study the role of virus infections, particularly Epstein-Barr virus (EBV) infection, in the development of lymphoproliferative disease in immunodeficient individuals. Following the first descriptions of the syndrome in isolated families [62,63], further cases and detailed descriptions of the clinical features, pathology, and immunology have been described [64].

Affected males have a subtle immunodeficiency syndrome with particular susceptibility to EBV infection. Variable disease expression with four major manifestations follows infection with EBV: variable degrees of serum immunoglobulin deficiency including hypogammaglobulinaemia, acute fatal or chronic infectious mononucleosis, aplastic anaemia, and B-cell lymphoproliferative disease.

The susceptibility of these patients to EBV infection is fundamental to the various manifestations of the syndrome. It would appear that this susceptibility is due to a preexisting immunodeficiency state. Some patients have partial IgA deficiency or mild hypogammaglobulinaemia prior to the EBV infection. Even more convincing evidence is the finding of defective antibody responses to EBV, particularly EB nuclear antigen, in patients and carrier females [65].

Malignant lymphoma is very common, occurring in approximately 40% of patients. Various B-cell lymphoproliferative disorders may be found, including immunoblastic sarcoma and Burkitt's lymphoma. Immunoblastic sarcoma with extranodal involvement is the most common finding. Lymphoma frequently follows infectious mononucleosis but may occur without any antecedent history of this. The B-cell lymphoproliferative disease appears to be a direct consequence of EBV infection. Continued EBV infection of B-cells in the absence of a protective immune response against it induces polyclonal B-cell proliferation. Monoclonal proliferation might result from B-cell cytogenic defects occurring spontaneously or as a result of the immune response against viral antigens expressed on B-cell surface membranes [66].

Acquired immunodeficiency syndrome

In recent years there has been a substantial increase in the number of cases of Kaposi's sarcoma (KS) in certain parts of America. This has been linked with the recently described acquired immunodeficiency syndrome (AIDS) [67]. This syndrome is distinct from other acquired immunodeficiency syndromes such as acquired hypogammaglobulinaemia. Patients with AIDS are also prone to opportunistic infections, particularly *Pneumocystis carinii* pneumonia.

The first cases were described in American male homosexuals amongst whom three probable risk factors for the development of the syndrome were identified: sexual promiscuity, the use of sexual stimulant drugs, such as amyl nitrite, and sexually transmitted viral infections, particularly cytomegalovirus and EBV. It is now apparent that the syndrome does present in countries other than America, including the United Kingdom, and that it is not restricted to homosexuals. Other groups of people at risk of developing AIDS are intravenous drug abusers who are not homosexual, Haitian immigrants to America who are not homosexuals or drug abusers, haemophiliacs, and perhaps female prostitutes. Because the development of AIDS cannot always be linked with sexual promiscuity or the use of drugs, an infectious aetiology seems most likely. Recent evidence that the disease may be transmitted by blood products [68] and from affected males to their female partners [69] supports this hypothesis.

The immune defect is predominantly of cell-mediated immunity. Immunological investigation of patients usually demonstrates lymphopenia, anergy to skin test antigens, and reduced in vitro proliferative responses of lymphocytes to mitogens. A common finding, and that of greatest diagnostic value, is a reversal of the ratio of T-helper/inducer (OK T4+) cells to T-suppressor/cytoxic (OK T8+) cells, which reflects a reduction of the T-helper/inducer subset. Other abnormalities that have been described include impaired NK-cell and monocyte function and decreased production of α-interferon. Serum immunoglobulin concentrations are normal or raised and serum complement is normal.

Awareness of AIDS and subsequent investigation of "at-risk" groups have shown that less severe disease is even more common. A syndrome of fever, weight loss, and generalised lymphadenopathy occurring in homosexual males may be a prodrome of AIDS. Immunological investigations in asymptomatic homosexual males have demonstrated T-cell abnormalities similar to those of AIDS patients but to a lesser degree. Similarly, low OK T4+/OK T8+ ratios have been demonstrated in approximately one-third of asymptomatic haemophiliacs and are even more common (57%) in those patients using factor VIII concentrates.

The nature of the relationship between AIDS and KS is not completely understood but is presumably similar to that in other immunosuppressed patients. Any patient who is found to have KS that is not due to immunosuppressant therapy, particularly those in an at-risk group and/or with opportunistic infections, must be suspected of having this syndrome.

AUTOIMMUNE DISEASE AND MALIGNANCY

Malignancy has been recognised as a possible complication of autoimmune disease for many years. In 1967 Oleinick [70] presented data suggesting an increased incidence of leukaemias and lymphomas in patients with autoimmune disease, but the findings were inconclusive because data were not available on sufficient numbers of patients. Since then there have been several surveys of malignancy rates in patients with various autoimmune diseases, particularly connective tissue diseases. Although malignancy has been associated with other autoimmune diseases, such as pemphigus [71], only the connective tissue diseases will be discussed here.

In most instances the increase in tumours is due to lymphoreticular malignancy, presumably reflecting the involvement of the immune system in disease pathogenesis. In dermatomyositis the relationship is different and malignancy is apparently involved in pathogenesis rather than a complication of it. For the sake of completeness, a discussion of this will be included.

Sjögren's syndrome

The evidence that a persistent autoimmune response may cause lymphoreticular malignancy is strongest in Sjögren's syndrome (Sicca syndrome) (SS). This autoimmune exocrinopathy may occur alone (primary SS) or in association with another autoimmune disease (secondary SS). There is evidence of an autoimmune response against exocrine glands in both types, but there are differences between them in terms of the serum autoantibodies present and the association with major histocompatibility antigens [72]. Although not an absolute finding, primary SS is associated with autoantibodies to extractable nuclear antigens, in particular SS-A (Ro) and SS-B (La), and with the HLA haplotype B8, DR3, whereas SS secondary to rheumatoid arthritis is associated with salivary duct antibodies and the HLA antigen DR4.

A universal finding in SS is focal lymphoid proliferation in exocrine glands, particularly the salivary and lacrimal glands. Approximately one-quarter of patients develop lymphoproliferation in extraglandular sites in addition to this. In some patients this may develop the characteristics of a pseudolymphoma, most often involving lymph nodes, liver, spleen, and lung. The pseudolymphomatous changes consist of aggregates of lymphoid tissue with the appearances of tumour but do not meet the criteria for malignancy.

Considering the degree to which lymphoproliferation occurs in SS, it is not surprising that an increased incidence of lymphoreticular malignancies has been reported. Early reports indicating an increased incidence of NHL and Waldenström's macroglobulinaemia in SS

[73] were followed by others and the increased risk was definitely established in an epidemiological survey of 136 patients [74]. This survey demonstrated that there was a relative risk of 43.8 for developing NHL in SS. Three histological types of NHL were found: diffuse histiocytic, diffuse mixed lymphocytic and histiocytic with epithelial cell reaction (Lennert's lymphoma), and poorly differentiated lymphocytic lymphoma. There was an increased incidence of Waldenström's macroglobulinaemia, but the relative risk for nonlymphoid tumours was only very slightly increased.

The lymphoproliferation is of B-cells [75]. Where intracytoplasmic immunoglobulin is present it is always IgM, and when malignant lymphoma develops monoclonal IgM is frequently found, interestingly always IgMk. The malignant lymphoma cells of some patients do not express intracytoplasmic IgM, and it is possible that this represents a stage of B-cell dedifferentiation. Apparently, therefore, a progression of lymphoproliferative changes occurs, from benign polyclonal lymphoepithelial infiltration of the salivary glands through to pseudolymphoma with extraglandular involvement, monoclonal proliferation, sometimes with plasmacytoid cells, and, finally, possible B-cell dedifferentiation.

NHL occurs with equal frequency in primary and secondary SS. Risk factors for the development of malignant lymphoma are parotid swelling, lymphadenopathy, and splenomegaly, all manifestations of localised or systemic lymphoid hypertrophy. Patients with the benign polyclonal lymphoproliferative phase usually have increased serum immunoglobulin concentrations and a high incidence of serum rheumatoid factor and other autoantibodies. These abnormalities may revert if monoclonal lymphoproliferation develops. Concurrent with this may be the development of a serum monoclonal ·IgM paraprotein. The serial measurement of serum immunoglobulins, rheumatoid factor, and other autoantibodies may therefore be of value in predicting the progression of benign lymphoproliferation to a malignant phase.

Systemic lupus erythematosus

The occurrence of malignancy in patients with systemic lupus erythematosus (SLE) might be expected. There are several potential risk factors. First, chronic stimulation of the immune system occurs, related to the persistent production of autoantibodies against diverse nonorgan-specific autoantigens. Antinuclear antibodies are most important but other autoantibodies are also involved in disease pathogenesis. There appears to be an underlying propensity of B-cells to proliferate excessively [76]. Second, secondary immunodeficiency occurs in many patients including defects of T-cell-mediated immunity [77] and NK-cell function [78]. These abnormalities are probably epiphenomena, which in the case of T-cells are due, in part, to lymphocytoxic antibodies [76]. Finally, most cases of SLE are treated with steroid therapy, often in association with immunosuppressant drugs, thereby increasing the likelihood of malignancy from this cause.

There were many early reports, often anecdotal, suggesting that patients with SLE were more likely than normals to develop lymphoreticular malignancy [reviewed in 79]. Later, two controlled studies of large patient groups [80,81] found malignancy to be increased in general but found no increase in lymphoreticular malignancies. The most common malignancies in these two studies were carcinoma of the cervix and the uterus. These findings presumably reflect the preponderance of females with SLE. More recently, attention has again been drawn to the development of lymphoreticular malignancy in SLE [82].

Lymphoreticular malignancies may be encountered more frequently now than previously because of current trends to use high-dose steroids and immunosuppressant therapy. In the New Zealand black mouse model of SLE, intensive therapy with azathioprine frequently results in the development of malignant lymphoma [83]. In addition, prolonged patient survival resulting from earlier diagnosis and more effective treatment could increase the chances of malignancy occurring so that it is a more common cause of death than previously.

The data are insufficient to determine the risk of developing malignancy in the SLE. There appears to be a propensity to lymphoreticular malignancy. Further studies of this are required, in particular to determine the role of immunosuppressant therapy.

Rheumatoid arthritis

The evidence for an increase in malignancy amongst patients with rheumatoid arthritis (RA) is conjectural. Indications of an increased incidence, in the main based on case reports [reviewed in 81], were not substantiated by analyses of malignancy rates in larger groups of patients [81,84]. Indeed, one study [81] demonstrated a lower than expected incidence. However, a recent survey of 11,483 male and 34,618 female RA patients in Finland [85] has demonstrated an increased incidence of lymphoreticular malignancies in males but not in females. These malignancies included leukaemias, NHL, Hodgkin's disease, and myelomas. It is not known how many of these patients had SS in which the development of lymphoreticular malignancy would be expected. Of importance is the consideration of modes of therapy, as treatment of RA patients with immunosuppressant drugs may lead to an increase in acute leukaemia [86].

Progressive systemic sclerosis

The aetiology of this connective tissue disease is unknown, but, no doubt, immunological mechanisms are involved and progressive systemic sclerosis (PSS) is related to the other connective tissue diseases [87]. Serum antinuclear antibodies are present in 95% of patients [88]. Decreased numbers of peripheral blood T-cells and reduced lymphocyte transformation by mitogens have been described in patients with PSS in several but not all studies [reviewed in 87]. Reduced antibody-dependent-cell-mediated cytotoxicity [89] and NK-cell activity [90] are present in some patients, apparently related to disease severity. Whether these abnormalities are an epiphenomenon of the disease or are related to disease pathogenesis is yet to be established.

The views on the occurrence of malignancy in PSS are conflicting. Whereas some authors have presented data interpreted to show increased incidence of carcinoma, mainly of the lung [91,92], others have disputed this [93]. These differences presumably reflect different methods of data collection and analysis. Those surveys showing an increased incidence of carcinoma presented data derived predominantly from literature surveys inevitably leading to a bias toward overestimation. There was, however, a predominance of cases of carcinoma of the lung and it has been suggested that the pulmonary fibrosis of PSS may be a predisposing factor in this. A survey of 2,141 patients with PSS [93] demonstrated that the relative frequency of malignancies was similar to that in the general population. Carcinomas of the breast and the uterus were most common, reflecting the predominance of female patients. Lymphomas and leukaemias were also common. There was no apparent increase in the incidence of carcinoma of the lung. Further surveys are needed.

Dermatomyositis and polymyositis

In both dermatomyositis (DM) and polymyositis (PM) there is a diffuse inflammatory myopathy of skeletal muscle, which in the former is associated with a characteristic skin rash. Both occur in diverse clinical settings and it has been possible to classify cases into five groups (table 6–2) based on clinical characteristics. Immunological factors are involved in the pathogenesis. There is evidence of cell-mediated immunity to skeletal muscle [95], and the incidence of serum antinuclear antibodies is increasing with the improving definition of new nuclear antigen/antibody systems [96].

A relationship between myositis and malignancy has been noted on many occasions [reviewed in 97]. However, the validity of these observations has been questioned [94] on the grounds that, first, the relationship has been demonstrated by analysis of cases reported in the literature and that adequate epidemiological data were unavailable and, second, in most studies the diagnostic criteria for DM or PM were not defined adequately. Where retrospective analyses of large patient groups have been performed, using strict criteria for the diagnosis of DM or PM, the prevalence of malignancy has been found to be 8.5% of all cases of myositis [98] and 26% of cases of DM or PM excluding patients in groups IV and V [99].

Therefore, an increased risk of malignancy is found in patients presenting with DM or PM, but the risk is not as great as some authors have suggested. Patients over the age of 40 are more likely to have malignancy, but this finding presumably reflects the fact that the age of presentation of patients in groups I to III is older than those in groups IV and V [98]. It has been suggested that malignancy occurs predominantly in patients with DM [99] but this is disputed [98].

There is no particular cell type or site of malignancy associated with DM or PM though adenocarcinomas, particularly of breast, uterus, and cervix seem most common [99]. The tumour may present before, at the time of, or after the diagnosis of myositis. In most cases the myositis presents before the tumour, which may take up to seven years to develop.

In general, malignancy is not associated with type IV or V myositis. Adults presenting with DM or PM who do not have another connective tissue disease should have a detailed clinical and routine laboratory examination. It has been argued that extensive invasive investigations beyond this are unnecessary [100]. Some clinical and laboratory features may help to predict the risk of associated malignancy. Arthralgia, myalgia, Raynaud's phenomenon, and sclerodactyly are uncommon in patients with DM or PM associated with malignancy. They are found mainly in patients with a connective tissue disease "overlap syndrome." The presence of serum antinuclear antibodies might argue against group III myositis [98], but it has been shown that the presence of serum DNA antibodies and antibodies to extractable

Table 6–2. Classification of PM and DM into groups of I through V according to clinical characteristics

I	Polymyositis
II	Dermatomyositis
III	Polymyositis or dermatomyositis associated with malignancy
IV	Childhood polymyositis or dermatomyositis
V	Polymyositis or dermatomyositis that 'overlaps' with another connective tissue disease

Source: Data from Bohan et al. [94].

nuclear antigens, mainly antibodies to nuclear ribonucleoprotein, does not discriminate between cases with and without malignancy [101]. However, titres of antibody are low in those patients with malignancy. Muscle histology is probably not useful in predicting the presence of malignancy [98]. The relationship between myositis and malignancy is obviously different from that occurring in other connective tissue diseases. The nature of this relationship is yet to be determined.

GENERAL COMMENTS ON THE OCCURRENCE OF MALIGNANCY IN IMMUNODEFICIENCY AND AUTOIMMUNE DISEASE

Although there can be little doubt that malignancy is a complication of some primary immunodeficiency diseases and some autoimmune diseases, that the nature of the relationship is heterogeneous is clear. It is, therefore, misleading to consider malignancy incidence figures for immunodeficiency diseases or for autoimmune diseases as a whole. Figures for each condition must be analysed separately, as has been done here. From the findings in the diseases discussed, several comments can be made concerning the nature of the relationship between malignant disease and the immune system.

There is a lack of evidence in support of the concept of immunological surveillance [102]. Two findings are of particular note. First, the increase in malignancy is restricted to certain types, predominantly lymphoreticular malignancy. Of 292 patients collected by the ICR, 58% had lymphoid tumours. If primary immunodeficiency results in a breakdown of immunological surveillance, an increase in all types of tumours would be expected. Possibly, of course, immunological surveillance mechanisms are principally involved in controlling the development of lymphoreticular malignancy. Second, immunodeficiency specifically involving T-cells, macrophages, and NK-cells, cells that are fundamental to proposed immunological surveillance mechanisms, is not associated with an increased risk of developing malignancy. Defects of T-cell-mediated immunity and NK-cell function are present in a proportion of patients with various immunodeficiency diseases and autoimmune diseases, but it is not possible to directly relate these abnormalities with the development of malignancy. However, further studies in this area are clearly required.

An increased tendency for malignant changes to occur, rather than a decreased capacity to eliminate malignant cells through immunological surveillance mechanisms, seems the most likely mechanism of oncogenesis in patients with immunodeficiency disease or autoimmune disease. Several mechanisms are possible.

There is strong evidence that intrinsic cellular defects are operating in the "chromosome breakage" syndromes. Cytogenetic abnormalities themselves, or in association with extrinsic factors such as radiation, chemicals, or viruses, may lead to the development of malignant clones of cells. Rapidly dividing cells would be most at risk, which might explain the predominance of lymphoreticular tumours and leukaemias. This might be one explanation for the relatively high incidence of gastrointestinal malignancy. Immunodeficiency in these syndromes may compound the intrinsic cellular defects by, for example, increasing the risks of virus infection.

Chronic antigenic stimulation of the immune system can cause lymphoproliferation, which may become neoplastic. This has been studied in animal models [103]. Repeated and persistent infections in patients with immunodeficiency, and chronic autoimmune responses in patients with autoimmune disease, may be sufficient stimuli for this to occur. Certainly, this appears to be the case in SS.

The evidence for an effect of oncogenic viruses is becoming increasingly apparent. EBV infection may induce lymphoproliferative disease in immunodeficient and immunosuppressed individuals [66], and it is possible that other viruses linked with human tumours could also be important agents. Several factors may be relevant to the establishment of an oncogenic virus infection [104]. Immunodeficiency would allow repeated and persistent virus infections to occur. Some virus infections, for example, by C type RNA viruses, may induce both malignancy and autoimmune disease. It is also possible that autoimmune responses may activate latent virus infections.

One final mechanism, for which there is little experimental or clinical support, is that defective immunoregulation might result in uncontrolled lymphoproliferation. Although defects of immunoregulation are present in some autoimmune diseases, particularly SLE, this is not a general feature of immunodeficiency diseases. Indeed, increased suppressor cell activity is found in some.

REFERENCES

1. Gatti RA, Good RA. Occurrence of malignancy in immunodeficiency diseases. Cancer 28: 89–98, 1971.
2. Asherson GL, Webster ADB. Malignancy and immunodeficiency disease. In Diagnosis and treatment of immunodeficiency diseases. Oxford: Blackwell Scientific Publications, 1980, pp. 274–281.
3. Fudenberg H, Good RA, Goodman HC, Hitzig W, Kunkel H, Roitt I, Rosen F, Rowe D, Seligmann M, Soothill J. Primary immunodeficiencies, report of a World Health Organisation Committee. Paediatrics 47: 927–946, 1971.
4. Kersey JH, Spector BD, Good RA. Primary immunodeficiency diseases and cancer: The immunodeficiency-cancer registry. Int J Cancer 12: 333–347, 1973.
5. Page AR, Hansen AE, Good RA. Occurrence of leukaemia and lymphoma in patients with agammaglobulinaemia. Blood 21: 197–206, 1963.
6. Koren HS, Amos DB, Buckley RH. Natural killing in immunodeficient patients. J Immunol 120: 796–799, 1978.
7. Spector BD, Perry GS, Good RA, Kersey JH. Immunodeficiency diseases and malignancy. In Twomey JJ, Good RA (eds.), Comprehensive immunology, vol. 4. New York: Plenum, 1978, pp. 203–222.
8. Report of a WHO scientific group. Immunodeficiency. Clin Immunol Immunopathol 13: 296-359, 1979.
9. De Gast GC, Wilkins SR, Webster AD, Rickinson A, Platts-Mills TA. Functional immaturity of isolated B cells from patients with hypogammaglobulinaemia. Clin Exp Immunol 42: 535–544, 1980.
10. Platts-Mills TAE, de Gast GC, Pereira RS, Webster ADB, Wilkins SR. The significance of immature B cells found in the peripheral blood of patients with late onset hypogammaglobulinaemia. In Seligman M, Hitzig WH (eds.), Primary immunodeficiencies. Inserm symposium no. 16. Amsterdam: Elsevier/North Holland Biomedical Press, 1980, pp. 39–48.
11. Webster ADB, Asherson GL. Identification and function of T cells in the peripheral blood of patients with hypogammaglobulinaemia. Clin Exp Immunol 18: 499–504, 1974.
12. Filipovich AH, Spector BD, Kersey J. Immunodeficiency in humans as a risk factor in the development of malignancy. Prev Med 9: 252–259, 1980.
13. Hermans PE, Diaz-Buxo JA, Stobo JD. Idiopathic late-onset immunoglobulin deficiency. Clinical observations in 50 patients. Am J Med 61: 221–237, 1976.
14. Gonzalez-Vitale JC, Gomez LG, Goldblum RM, Goldman AS, Patterson M. Immunoblastic lymphoma of small intestine complicating late-onset immunodeficiency. Cancer 49: 445–449, 1982.
15. French M, Dawkins R, Jackson M. Primary immunoglobulin deficiency and haematological disorders. Postgrad Med J 59: 32–36, 1983.
16. Ruddell WSJ, Bone ES, Hill MJ, Blendis LM, Walters CL. Gastric juice nitrate: A risk factor for cancer in the hypochlorhydric stomach? Lancet 2: 1037–1039, 1976.
17. Asherson GL, Webster ADB. Thymoma and immunodeficiency. In Diagnosis and treatment of immunodeficiency diseases. Oxford: Blackwell Scientific Publications, 1980, pp. 78–98.
18. Sonadjian JV, Enriquez P, Silverstein MN, Pépin J. The spectrum of diseases associated with thymoma: Coincidence or syndrome. Arch Intern Med 134: 374–379, 1974.

19. Asherson GL, Johnson S, Platts-Mills TAE, Webster ADB. Pathogenesis of hypogammaglobulinaemia with thymoma and late-onset hypogammaglobulinaemia. J Clin Path 32: Suppl (Roy Coll Path) 13: 5–9, 1979.

20. Cassidy JJ, Oldham G, Platts-Mills TAE. Functional assessment of a B-cell defect in patients with selective IgA deficiency. Clin Exp Immunol 35: 296–305, 1979.

21. Asherson GL, Webster ADB. Selective IgA deficiency. In Diagnosis and treatment of immunodeficiency diseases. Oxford: Blackwell Scientific Publications, 1980, pp. 99–128.

22. Oxelius VA, Laurell AB, Lindquist B, Golebiowska H, Axelsson U, Björkander J, Hanson LA. IgG subclasses in selective IgA deficiency: Importance of IgG_2-IgA deficiency. N Eng J Med 304: 1476–1477, 1981.

23. Cunningham-Rundles C, Pudifin DJ, Armstrong D, Good RA. Selective IgA deficiency and neoplasia. Vox Sang 38: 61–67, 1980.

24. Hobbs J. IgM deficiency. In Bergsma D (ed.); Immunodeficiency in man and animals. Birth defects original article series XI. Sunderland, MA: Sinauer Associates, 1975, pp. 112–116.

25. Webster ADB. Metabolic defects in immunodeficiency diseases. Clin Exp Immunol 49: 1–10, 1982.

26. Nathan CF, Murray HW, Cohn ZA. The macrophage as an effector cell. New Eng J Med 303: 622–626, 1980.

27. Blume RS, Wolff SM. The Chediak-Higashi syndrome: Studies in four patients and a review of the literature. Medicine 51: 247–280, 1972.

28. Roder JC, Haliotis T. A selective natural killer cell deficiency in man and a mouse model. In Seligmann M, Hitzig WH (eds.), Primary immunodeficiencies. Inserm symposium no. 16. Amsterdam: Elsevier/North Holland Biomedical Press, 1980, p. 207–217.

29. Karre K, Klein GO, Kiessling R, Klein G, Roder JC. Low natural in vivo resistance to syngeneic leukaemias in natural killer-deficient mice. Nature 284: 624–626, 1980.

30. Talmadge JE, Meyers KM, Prieur DJ, Starhey JR. Role of NK cells in tumour growth and metastasis in beige mice. Nature 284: 622–624, 1980.

31. Blaese RM, Strober W, Waldmann TA. Immunodeficiency in the Wiskott-Aldrich syndrome. In Bergsma D (ed.), Immunodeficiency in man and animals. Birth defects original article series. Sunderland, MA: Sinauer Associates, 1975, pp. 250–254.

32. Shapiro R, Gerrard JM, Perry GS, White JG, Krivit W, Kersey JH. A metabolic abnormality in platelets from Wiskott-Aldrich syndrome heterozygotes. Lancet 1: 121–123, 1978.

33. Blaese RM, Strober W, Brown RS, Waldmann TA. The Wiskott-Aldrich syndrome: A disorder with a possible defect in antigen processing or recognition. Lancet 1: 1056–1060, 1968.

34. Cooper MD, Chase HP, Lowman JT, Krivit W, Good RA. Wiskott-Aldrich syndrome: An immunologic deficiency disease involving the afferent limb of immunity. Am J Med 44: 499–513, 1968.

35. Lipinski M, Virelizier JL, Tursz T, Griscelli C. Natural killer and killer cell activities in patients with primary immunodeficiencies or defects in immune interferon production. Eur J Immunol 10: 246–249, 1980.

36. Perry GS, Spector BD, Shuman LM, Mandel JS, Aderson E, McHugh RB, Hanson MR, Fahlstrom SM, Krivit W, Kersey JH. The Wiskott-Aldrich syndrome in the United States and Canada (1892–1979). J Paediatrics 97: 72–78, 1980.

37. Heidleberger KP, Le Golvan DP. Wiskott-Aldrich syndrome and cerebral neoplasia: Report of a case with localised reticulum cell sarcoma. Cancer 33: 280–284, 1974.

38. Parkman R, Rappeport J, Geha R, Belli J, Cassady R, Levey R, Nathan DG, Rosen RS. Complete correction of the Wiskott-Aldrich syndrome by allogeneic bone marrow transplantation. New Eng J Med 298: 921–927, 1978.

39. Polani PE. DNA repair defects and chromosome instability disorders. In Ciba Foundation Symposium 66 (new series), Human genetics: Possibilities and realities. Amsterdam: Excerpta Medica, 1979, pp. 81–133.

40. McFarlin DE, Strober W, Waldmann TA. Ataxia telangiectasia. Medicine 51: 281–314, 1972.

41. Waldmann TA. Immunological abnormalities in ataxia telangiectasia. In Bridges BA, Harriden DG (eds.), Ataxia telangiectasia—A cellular and molecular link between cancer, neuropathology and immune deficiency. Chichester: John Wiley, 1982, pp. 37–51.

42. Nelson DL. Lymphocyte-mediated cytotoxicity in immunodeficiency patients. In Seligmann M, Hitzig WH (eds.), Primary immunodeficiencies. Inserm symposium no. 16. Amsterdam: Elsevier/North Holland Biomedical Press, 1980, pp. 141–149.

43. Sedgwick RP, Boder E. Ataxia telangiectasia. In Vinken PJ, Bruyn GW (eds.), Handbook of clinical neurology 14. Amsterdam: North Holland Publishing, 1972, pp. 267–339.

44. Spector BD, Filipovich AH, Perry GS, Kersey JH. Epidemiology of cancer in ataxia telangiectasia. In Bridges BA, Harden DG (eds.), Ataxia telangiectasia—A cellular and molecular link between cancer, neuropathology and immune deficiency. Chichester: John Wiley, 1982, pp. 103–138.

45. Brouet JC, Seligmann M. The immunological classification of acute lymphoblastic leukaemias. Cancer 42: 817–827, 1978.

46. Hecht F, McCaw B, Koler RD. Ataxia telangiectasia: Clonal growth of translocation lymphocytes. New Eng J Med 289: 286–291, 1973.
47. McCaw BK, Hecht F, Harnden DG, Teplitz R. Somatic rearrangement of chromosome 14 in human lymphocytes. Proc Natl Acad Sci (USA) 72: 2071–2075, 1975.
48. Oxford JM, Harnden DG, Parrington JM, Delharty JD. Specific chromosome aberrations in ataxia telangiectasia. J Med Genet 12: 251–262, 1975.
49. Cunliffe PN, Mann JR, Camerson AH, Roberts KD. Radiosensitivity in ataxia telangiectasia. Br J Radiol 48: 374–376, 1975.
50. Levin S, Perlov S. Ataxia telangiectasia in Israel with observations on its relationship to malignant disease. Isr J Med Sci 7: 1535–1541, 1971.
51. German J, Bloom D, Passarge E. Bloom's syndrome. VII. Progress report for 1978. Clin Genet 15: 361–367, 1979.
52. Chaganti RSK, Schonberg S, German J. A manyfold increase in sister chromatid exchanges in Bloom's syndrome lymphocytes. Proc Nat Acad Sci (Wash) 71: 4508–4512, 1974.
53. Hütteroth TH, Litwin SD, German J. Abnormal immune responses of Bloom's syndrome lymphocytes in vitro. J Clin Invest 56: 1–7, 1975.
54. Weemaes CMR, Bakkeren JAJ, Ter Haar BGA, Hustinx TWJ, van Munster PJJ. Immune responses in four patients with Bloom's syndrome. Clin Immunol Immunopath 12: 12–19, 1979.
55. Taniguchi N, Mukai M, Nagaoki T, Miyawaki T, Moriya N, Takahashi H, Kondo N. Impaired B-cell differentiation and T-cell regulatory function in four patients with Bloom's syndrome. Clin Immunol Immunopathol 22: 247–258, 1982.
56. Beard MEJ, Young DE, Bateman CJT, McCarthy GT, Smith ME, Sinclair L, Franklin AW, Scott RB. Fanconi's anaemia. Q J Med 42: 403–422, 1973.
57. Miller RW, Tedaro GJ. Viral transmission of cells from persons at high risk of cancer. Lancet 1: 81–82, 1969.
58. Karup-Pederson F, Hertz H, Lundsteen C, Platz P, Thomsen M. Indication of primary immune deficiency in Fanconi's anaemia. Acta Paediatr Scand 66: 745–751, 1977.
59. Abels D, Reed WB. Fanconi-like syndrome. Immunologic deficiency, pancytopaenia and cutaneous malignancies. Arch Dermatol 107: 419–423, 1973.
60. Sarna G, Tomasulo P, Lotz MJ, Bubinak JF, Shulman RN. Multiple neoplasms in two siblings with a variant form of Fanconi's anaemia. Cancer 36: 1029–1033, 1975.
61. Swift M. Malignant neoplasms in heterozygous carriers of genes for certain autosomal recessive syndromes. In Mulvill JJ (ed.), Genetics of human cancer, progress in cancer research and therapy, vol. 3. New York: Raven Press, 1977, pp. 209–221.
62. Provisor AJ, Iacuone JJ, Chilcote RR, Neiburger RG, Crussi FG, Baehner RL. Acquired agammaglobulinaemia after a life-threatening illness with clinical and laboratory features of infectious mononucleosis in three related male children. New Eng J Med 293: 62–65, 1975.
63. Purtilo DT, Cassel CK, Yang JPS, Harper R, Stephenson SR, Landing BJ, Vawter GF. X-linked recessive progressive combined variable immunodeficiency (Duncan's disease). Lancet 1: 935–941, 1975.
64. Purtilo DT, Paquin L, De Florio D, Virzi F, Sakhuja R. Immunodiagnosis and immunopathogenesis of the X-linked recessive lymphoproliferative syndrome. Sem Haematol 16: 309–343, 1979.
65. Sakamoto K, Freed HJ, Purtilo DT. Antibody responses to Epstein-Barr virus in families with the X-linked lymphoproliferative syndrome. J Immunol 125: 921–925, 1980.
66. Purtilo DT. Epstein-Barr virus-induced oncogenesis in immune-deficient individuals. Lancet 1: 300–303, 1980.
67. Waterson AP. Acquired immune deficiency syndrome. Br Med J 286: 743–746, 1983.
68. Menitove JE, Aster RH, Casper JT, Lauer SR, Gottschall JL, Williams JE, Gill JC, Wheeler DV, Piaskowski V, Kirchner P, Montgomery RR. T-lymphocyte subpopulations in patients with classic hemophilia treated with cryoprecipitate and lyophilised concentrates. N Eng J Med 308: 83–86, 1983.
69. Masur H, Michelis MA, Wormser GP, Lewin S, Gold J, Taper ML, Giron J, Lerner CW, Armstrong D, Setia U, Sender JA, Siebken RS, Nicholas P, Arlen Z, Maayan S, Ernst JA, Siegal FP, Cunningham-Rundles S. Opportunistic infections in previously healthy women. Initial manifestations of a community-acquired cellular immunodeficiency. Ann Intern Med 97: 533–539, 1982.
70. Oleinick A. Leukaemia or lymphoma occurring subsequent to an autoimmune disease. Blood 29: 144–153, 1967.
71. Krain LS, Bierman SM. Pemphigus vulgaris and internal malignancy. Cancer 33: 1091–1099, 1974.
72. NIH Conference. Sjögren's syndrome (Sicca syndrome): Current issues. Ann Intern Med 92: 212–226, 1980.
73. Talal N, Bunim JJ. The development of malignant lymphoma in the course of Sjögren's syndrome. Am J Med 36: 529–540, 1964.

74. Kassan SS, Thomas TL, Montsopoulous HM, Hoover R, Kimberly RP, Budman DR, Costa J, Decker JL, Chused TM. Increased risk of lymphoma in Sicca syndrome. Ann Intern Med 89: 888–892, 1979.
75. Zulman J, Jaffe R, Talal N. Evidence that the malignant lymphoma of Sjögren's syndrome is a monoclonal B-cell neoplasm. New Eng J Med 299: 1215–1220, 1978.
76. Steinberg AD. Studies of immune regulation, 587–592. In Decker JL, moderator. Systemic lupus erythematosus: Evolving concepts. Ann Intern Med 91: 587–604, 1979.
77. Paty JG, Sienknecht CW, Townes AS, Hanissian AS, Miller JB, Masi AT. Impaired cell-mediated immunity in systemic lupus erythematosus (SLE): A controlled study of 23 untreated patients. Am J Med 59: 769–779, 1975.
78. Neighbour PA, Grayzel AI, Miller AE. Endogenous and interferon-augmented natural killer cell activity of human peripheral blood mononuclear cells in vitro. Studies of patients with multiple sclerosis, systemic lupus erythematosus or rheumatoid arthritis. Clin Exp Immunol 49: 11–21, 1982.
79. Caldwell DS. Musculoskeletal syndromes associated with malignancy. Sem Arthr Rheum 10: 198–223, 1981.
80. Canoso JJ, Cohen AS. Malignancy in a series of 70 patients with systemic lupus erythematosus. Arthritis Rheum 17: 383–390, 1974.
81. Lewis RB, Castor CW, Kinsley RE, Bole GG. Frequency of neoplasia in systemic lupus erythematosus and rheumatoid arthritis. Arthritis Rheum 19: 1256–1260, 1976.
82. Green JA, Dawson AA, Walker W. Systemic lupus erythematosus and lymphoma. Lancet 2: 753–756, 1978.
83. Casey TP. Azathioprine (Imuran) administration and the development of malignant lymphomas in NZB mice. Clin Exp Immunol 3: 305–312, 1968.
84. Owens DS, Waller M, Toone E. Rheumatoid disease and malignancy. Arthritis Rheum 10: 302–303, 1967 (abstr.).
85. Isomaki H, Hakulinen T, Joutsenlahti U. Lymphoma and rheumatoid arthritis. Lancet 1: 392, 1979 (letter).
86. Kahn MF, Arlet J, Bloch-Michel H, Caroit M, Chaonat Y, Renier JC. Leúcemies aigües après traitement par agents cytotoxiques en rheumatologie. 19 observations chez 2006 patients. Nouv Presse Med 8: 1393–1397, 1979.
87. Haynes DC, Gershwin ME. The immunopathology of progressive systemic sclerosis (PSS). Sem Arthritis Rheum 11: 331–351, 1982.
88. Bernstein RM, Steigerwald JC, Tan EM. Association of antinuclear and antinucleolar antibodies in progressive systemic sclerosis. Clin Exp Immunol 48: 43–51, 1982.
89. Wright JK, Hughes P, Rowell NR, Sneddon IB. Antibody dependent and phytohaemagglutinin-induced lymphocyte cytotoxicity in systemic sclerosis. Clin Exp Immunol 36: 175–182, 1979.
90. Wright JK, Hughes P, Rowell NR. Spontaneous lymphocyte-mediated (NK cell) cytotoxicity in systemic sclerosis: A comparison with antibody-dependent lymphocyte (K cell) cytotoxicity. Ann Rheum Dis 41: 409–413, 1982.
91. Talbott JH, Barrocas M. Progressive systemic sclerosis (PSS) and malignancy, pulmonary and non-pulmonary. Medicine 58: 182–207, 1979.
92. Talbott JH, Barrocas M. Carcinoma of the lung in progressive systemic sclerosis: A tabular review of the literature and a detailed report of the roentgenographic changes in two cases. Sem Arthritis Rheum 9: 191–217, 1980.
93. Duncan SC, Winkelmann RK. Cancer and scleroderma. Arch Dermatol 115: 950–955, 1979.
94. Bohan A, Peter JB. Polymyositis and dermato-myositis. New Eng J Med 292: 344–347, 1975.
95. Dawkins RL, Mastaglia FL. Cell-mediated cytotoxicity to muscle in polymyositis: Effect of immunosuppressive therapy. New Eng J Med 288: 434–438, 1973.
96. Tan EM. Autoantibodies to nuclear antigens (ANA): Their immunobiology and medicine. In Kunkel HG, Dixon FJ (eds.), Advances in immunology vol 33. London: Academic Press, 1982, pp. 167–240.
97. Barnes BE. Dermatomyositis and malignancy: A review of the literature. Ann Intern Med 84: 68–76, 1976.
98. Bohan A, Peter JB, Bowman RL, Pearson CM. A computer-assisted analysis of 153 patients with polymyositis and dermatomyositis. Medicine 56: 255–286, 1977.
99. Callen JP, Hyla JF, Bole GG, Kay DR. The relationship of dermatomyositis and polymyositis to internal malignancy. Arch Dermatol 116: 295–298, 1980.
100. Callen JP. The value of malignancy evaluation in patients with dermatomyositis. J Am Acad Dermatol 6: 253–259, 1982.
101. Venables PJW, Mumford PA, Maini RN. Antibodies to nuclear antigens in polymyositis: Relationship to autoimmune "overlap syndromes" and carcinoma. Ann Rheum Dis 40: 217–223, 1981.
102. Penn I. Depressed immunity and the development of cancer. Clin Exp Immunol 46: 459–474, 1981.
103. Armstrong MYK, Ruddle NH, Lipman MB, Richards FF. Tumour induction by immunologically activated murine leukaemia virus. J Exp Med 137: 1163–1179, 1973.
104. Hirsch MS, Proffitt MR, Black PH. Auto-immunity, oncornaviruses and lymphomagenesis. Contemp Top Immunobiol 6: 209–227, 1977.

7. IMMUNOSUPPRESSION IN CANCER

B.W. HANCOCK

INTRODUCTION

The association between cancer and immunosuppression has long been recognised. Which condition precedes the other, however, is still not established. Based on "immunosurveil-lance" theory, defective immunological control of potentially neoplastic cells allows their proliferation and development into a cancer [1]. Immunosurveillance remains a controversial subject, but, undoubtedly, as the cancer becomes more widespread immunity becomes progressively more defective; in addition, radiotherapy and cytotoxic chemotherapy are known to have profound effects on many aspects of the immune system.

IMMUNOLOGICAL ASSESSMENT

The recognition of the importance of immunosuppression in cancer and its therapy has led to attempts at monitoring the immunological status in the preliminary management and in the follow-up of patients. Many tests are available but, unfortunately, they usually measure in vitro immunoreactivity, which may not necessarily reflect the immunocompetence or proneness to infection of the patient. Certainly, in the assessment of an individual's immunity it is important to measure as many indices as possible to get an overall assessment of the situation; even then great care must be taken in extrapolating such findings to the clinical situation.

Well-established tests of cellular immunity include the in vivo assessment by delayed hypersensitivity skin testing with multiple recall antigens, such as tuberculin, mumps, and candida, or by direct challenge with dinitrochlorobenzene (DNCB); the in vitro assessment

B.W. Hancock and A.M. Ward (eds.), Immunological Aspects of Cancer. Copyright © 1985, Martinus Nijhoff Publishing, Boston/Dordrecht/Lancaster.

of lymphocyte transformation responses with T-cell mitogens (for example, phytohaemag-glutinin, concanavalin A), where the uptake of tritiated thymidine in stimulated lymphocyte cultures is measured; and the various indirect methods of assessing lymphokine production, for example, by macrophage migration inhibition, leucocyte migration inhibition, or leucocyte-adherence inhibition techniques. The overall T-cell population may be assessed by the sheep cell rosetting (E-rosette) technique; individual subpopulations, such as suppressor and helper T-cells, can now be defined by the use of monoclonal antisera. Natural killer (NK) and natural cytotoxic (NC) cells are assessed using isotope release assays dependent on the ability of these cells to exhibit cytotoxicity to susceptible target cell lines.

Humoral immunity may be assessed by measurement of immunoglobulin levels in the serum by immunodiffusion methods; by studying antibody production (in vivo) after antigenic challenge by vaccination with, for example, tetanus toxoid or the Vi antigen of *E.coli*; by measuring lymphocyte transformation with pokeweed mitogen; by detection of surface immunoglobulin using fluorescein-labeled antiglobulin preparations; by B-cell rosetting techniques (erythrocyte, antibody, complement-EAC-rosettes); and by using monoclonal antisera.

Macrophage function is usually assessed by testing peripheral blood monocytes, which are separated and assessed for phagocytosis, motility, or adherence following nonspecific stimulation. Reticuloendothelial macrophage function can be crudely assessed by determining the in vivo clearance of particulate antigens. Neutrophil leucocyte function may be assessed by the nitroblue tetrazolium (NBT) test or by in vitro phagocytosis killing tests using microorganisms.

IMMUNE STATUS IN MALIGNANCY

The effects on different components of the immune system seen in various malignancies and therapeutic modalities are summarized in table 7–1.

Leukaemia and myeloma

Chronic B-cell lymphatic leukaemia (CLL) may be associated with marked immunosuppression, partly from suppression of immunologically competent B-cells and T-cells by their malignant counterparts and partly by the commonly seen association of hypogamma-

Table 7-1. Immunosuppression in cancer

	Neutrophil function	Cellular immunity	Humoral immunity
Leukaemia	↓ +	↓ +	↓ +
Myeloma Non-Hodgkin's lymphoma	N	↓ +	↓ + +
Hodgkin's disease	N	↓ + + +	N
Solid tumours	N	↓ +	N or ↓ +
Radiotherapy	↓ +	↓ + +	↓ +
Chemotherapy	↓ + +	↓ + + +	↓ + +

globulinaemia. IgM is usually the first class of immunoglobulin to be affected. Deficient NK-cell activity has also been demonstrated in patients with CLL [2]. Acute and chronic myeloid leukaemia may be associated with defects in neutrophil function. Such defects will be compounded by the effects of chemotherapy. Surprisingly, in acute lymphoblastic leukaemia, humoral and cellular immunity are initially intact, and only during intensive chemotherapy or with relapse of the leukaemia are such defects found, usually in association with profound myelosuppression.

In multiple myeloma, levels of normal immunoglobulins are depressed though the level of the characteristic monoclonal antibody is raised; this paraprotein is of course immunologically incompetent.

Malignant lymphoma

The classical deficiency in Hodgkin's disease is of cellular immunity, and in non-Hodgkin's lymphoma of humoral immunity. Such defects may be found when the patient first presents but are generally more severe with extensive disease. However, as with other cancers the effects of surgery, radiotherapy, and chemotherapy further complicate the situation so that any or all aspects of a patient's immunity may be affected. Neutrophil function is usually normal or enhanced [3].

Hodgkin's disease

Whilst it is acknowledged that cellular immune defects predominate in Hodgkin's disease [4,5,6], the actual cause(s) of these defects is not fully elucidated [see 7 for review]. The putative malignant cell in Hodgkin's disease has not yet been positively identified as having T-lymphocyte, B-lymphocyte, or macrophage origin. Immunological defects may persist for some years. Such defects appear to be in specific components of immunoreactivity testing; Kun and Johnson [8] were able to show no evidence of residual haematological or immunological depression in 71 consecutive patients treated successfully for Hodgkin's disease by radiotherapy five years previously, by assessment of delayed hypersensitivity reactions and quantitative immunoglobulin levels, whereas Fuks et al. [9], in a study of 26 patients in complete remission from 12 to 111 months after radiation therapy, showed T-cell lymphocytopenia and significant impairment of in vitro lymphocyte transformation responses. Other studies have also demonstrated persistent defects months and many years after radiotherapy [10,11]. Likewise, significant reductions in E-rosette and mitogen-induced proliferation have been observed in 47 long-term survivors of Hodgkin's disease successfully treated with MOPP chemotherapy [12]; the defects continued for up to 11 years. Many patients in these studies had of course had diagnostic laparotomy with splenectomy, and it is generally accepted that serious infections, for example, septicaemia, occur more frequently after splenectomy, particularly in patients who have had aggressive treatment of the underlying Hodgkin's disease [13,14]. Impaired humoral defense mechanisms against Haemophilus influenzae type B and low levels of IgM have been found in patients having chemotherapy and prior splenectomy [15]. In our own study [16], where immunological indices were reassessed in 27 patients in remission from Hodgkin's disease for five years following treatment, cellular immunity (as assessed by leucocyte migration inhibition and lymphocyte transformation) was depressed and progressive falls in serum immunoglobulins were noted. Low values in IgG and IgM were particularly a feature of patients who had had splenectomy and chemotherapy. As in many other studies we were unable to show any increased incidence of infections in patients showing depressed immunoreactivity.

The findings of such prolonged abnormalities in T-lymphocyte function may favour the hypothesis of a constitutional rather than just a disease- and/or treatment-mediated defect. Such a defect may be related to the presence of certain serum factors [17,18] or to the presence of either suppressor T-cells or suppressor monocytes [19,20]. Certainly, increased sensitivity to normal monocyte suppressor cells regulating mixed lymphocyte culture responses has been observed [20]. In our own study using Sephadex column passage to deplete monocytes from peripheral leucocyte suspensions, we have shown interactions between monocyte and lymphocytes in Hodgkin's disease; lymphocyte transformation was particularly inhibited by prostaglandin-secreting monocyte suppressor cells [21].

The picture is further complicated by the finding that spontaneous natural killer cell responses are depressed in patients with malignant lymphoma, particularly Hodgkin's disease; peripheral blood NK-cells also show defective responses to interferon augmentation [22].

Non-Hodgkin's lymphoma

It is well known that untreated B-cell non-Hodgkin's lymphoma may be associated with humoral immune defects; paraproteins and hypogammaglobulinaemia may be found, as in myeloma. Widespread disease is also accompanied by cellular immunosuppression, which, of course, is exacerbated by therapy, particularly chemotherapy [23]. Defects in natural killer cell activity, with failure to enhance such activity with interferon, have also been demonstrated [22]. Studies on non-Hodgkin's lymphoma in remission are few, but it seems that prolonged defects in immunity are not usually found in such patients after aggressive chemotherapeutic regimes [11].

Solid tumours

In the majority of solid tumours, immune function is normal during early stages of the disease, and neutrophil and macrophage function may in fact be enhanced [24,25]. If the cancer becomes widely metastatic, progressive failure of humoral and particularly cellular immunity may occur and, of course, be exaggerated by the further effects of treatment. Defects in natural killer cell activity [26] and macrophage function [25] are also found in advanced cancer.

Immunity may return to normal following successful treatment of a tumour, resulting from improvement in the patient's general condition and from reduction of tumour burden with the resultant clearance of the various immunosubversive factors that have been described in malignancy. Nevertheless, several studies have suggested that defects in immunoreactivity may persist for months and even years after treatment [27,28,29]. There is no evidence in the clinical setting, however, that these abnormalities are associated with an increased incidence of infection.

Radiotherapy and chemotherapy

Little is known about the precise mechanisms of action of individual cancer treatment agents on the immune system, although certain broad principles are recognised (see also chapter 1). Lymphocytes are extremely radiation sensitive; they undergo intermitotic death, and their numbers in the peripheral blood may fall after only one to two days of large field conventional radiotherapy. B-cells recover more rapidly than T-cells, which may remain depressed for several months or even years. Antibody responses, however, tend to be relatively well maintained.

Antitumour agents can have profound effects on all aspects of cellular and humoral immunity—antigen uptake and recognition, lymphocyte transformation and proliferation, antibody production, and effector cell reactions [30]. Alkylating agents affect cells in all phases of the immune response, whereas antimetabolites affect mainly the proliferative phase: the timing and duration of chemotherapy in relation to the antigen exposure are of obvious importance. For example, cyclophosphamide, an alkylating agent that acts throughout the cell cycle on resting and proliferating cells, inhibits cellular and primary and secondary humoral immune responses; its action is independent of its time of administration in relationship to antigenic challenge. However, methotrexate and other cell cycle phase-specific agents (e.g., 6-mercaptopurine) prevent lymphoblastic development and proliferation, and secondary antibody responses are generally maintained; maximal immunosuppression is observed if drug administration is within 48 hours of antigen challenge. It is worthwhile emphasizing that the degree of immunosuppression does not necessarily correlate with bone marrow status.

Radiotherapy

The depressive effects of different radiotherapy regimens for different tumours are clearly variable, though radiotherapy seems to have less immunosuppressive effects than intensive cytotoxic chemotherapy. Improved skin hypersensitivity has been noted following radiotherapy [31], though some reports suggest that both deterioration and improvement in skin responses may be seen [32]. In our experience neutrophil function is essentially unchanged by treatment [24], though absolute neutrophil and lymphocyte counts fall and may remain depressed for up to 12 months [33]. Cellular immunity on in vitro assessments is depressed by treatment and may remain subnormal for up to five years in patients attaining remission [34,35]. Several studies also seem to confirm that defects in immunoreactivity may persist after treatment [9,10,11,27,28,29], whereas others have shown no gross defects in overall immunity [8,36].

Chemotherapy

Intensive chemotherapy undoubtedly suppresses immune function [37]. Short intensive courses of chemotherapy may be followed by a rebound recovery [38], and some authors have claimed that even after prolonged continuous chemotherapy, immunity may be only slightly depressed and may even recover to normal [39,40]. Again this is a somewhat controversial area; for example, in Hodgkin's disease, as we have seen, cellular immunity may remain depressed for years after chemotherapy [12,16], though this may be a disease rather than a treatment association.

Obviously, as with radiotherapeutic regimens, different forms of cancer will have been treated by a multitude of regimens, and, quite clearly, differing schedules will have varying immunosuppressive effects.

Assessing immune status

The picture during and following treatment is complicated by the fact that the patient's immunity will be deranged by the behaviour of the tumour itself, differing types and burdens of tumour altering the host immune environment in diverse ways. Where persistent defects have been demonstrated after successful treatment of the tumour, it is still unclear whether these are a manifestation of the host-tumour interaction or are sequelae of the intensive therapy.

Clearly, individual tests of immunity may be variably affected by both disease and therapy. Also, the assessment of immune responses differs in individual laboratories, and there may be considerable variation in sensitivity and lack of concordance between tests of immunity purporting to measure the same parameter, thus reemphasizing the importance of assessing several indices of immune function in the same patient to obtain an overall impression of immune status. Even then the clinical relevance of such findings is uncertain.

IMMUNE STATUS AS A TUMOUR MARKER

Prognosis

Numerous attempts have been made to correlate immune status with prognosis. Lymphopenia per se is an unfavourable prognostic marker in Hodgkin's disease [41,42]. In our recent study of 181 consecutive untreated patients with histologically proven Hodgkin's disease, the survival in 77 patients with lymphocyte counts of less than $1.5 \times 10^9/l$ was 49.7%, significantly worse than the 74.2% recorded in those with normal counts [43]. Similar, though less well-established, observations have been made in breast carcinoma, where there seems to be an inverse correlation between pretreatment peripheral lymphocyte counts and tumour stage [44]. Likewise, impairment of cellular immunity has been associated with poor prognosis in several tumour types. In one early study, over 90% of unselected cancer patients presenting for surgery who failed to react to DNCB were either inoperable or had an early recurrence [45]. In our experience, assessment of cellular immunocompetence in malignant lymphoma is a useful pretreatment staging marker [6], advanced disease being associated with depressed immunity, but is of less value as a prognostic factor [46]. Adult acute leukaemia, however, shows a positive correlation between cellular immunocompetence and the patient's response to treatment and progress [47]. Such studies may, of course, simply reflect the fact that patients with localised tumours or good prognosis have better immunity at presentation and tolerate immunosuppressive treatment better than those who are ill and immunodepressed from the start. Comparability of these studies is also difficult in that they use different methods of immunological assessment.

Follow-up

In theory the assessment of immunity in the follow-up of patients with cancer could be an excellent marker for assessing remission, nonresponse, and relapse [7,48]. However, with the immunosuppressive effects of therapy (particularly cytotoxic chemotherapy), such follow-up findings are difficult to interpret; this has certainly been so in our studies in malignant lymphoma [34] and carcinoma of the cervix uteri [35]. The case may be different, however, in leukaemia, where deteriorating immunological function in follow-up may predict imminent relapse [47].

Immunoreactivity in the diagnosis and monitoring of tumour response

Some tests used in the assessment of immunoreactivity have been adapted for the assessment of tumour-associated antigens, the principle being to detect sensitization of peripheral blood lymphoid cells to tumour-associated antigens, thus indicating the presence of a tumour in the individual patient [49]. This depends, of course, on the availability of reasonably well characterised tumour antigen and normal tissue antigen preparations. In vivo testing involving assessing cutaneous delayed hypersensitivity reaction to tissue extracts [50] have only a limited application in the clinical situation. In vitro tests—for example, lymphocyte transformation, macrophage or leucocyte migration inhibition, macrophage electrophoretic mobility, and leukocyte adherence inhibition—have shown promise for the diagnosis and monitoring of cancer. However, in studies so far, the high degree of accuracy reported in original reports has not usually been reproduced in studies from other laboratories using the same test and the same antigens. Such tests are very sensitive to minor changes in the laboratory environment and are highly operator-dependent.

In using such investigations as a monitor of tumour response, the problems of reproducibility and sensitivity are further compounded by the surgical, radiotherapeutic, and chemotherapy procedures to which patients with cancer are exposed. In our own studies using the leucocyte migration inhibition technique, we were able to demonstrate sensitization to homogenized Hodgkin's disease spleen extract in about half of our patients with malignant lymphoma [51]. Initial sensitization responses did not correlate with presenting clinical status or with subsequent progress. However, enhancement of responses after treatment was associated with good clinical response to treatment; in patients who relapsed sensitization to spleen factor diminished [52]. Further investigations have confirmed that the factor responsible for sensitization is probably ferritin in a form different from that found in normal spleen [53].

The leucocyte adherence inhibition test [54] relies on the fact that the natural tendency of lymphoid cells to adhere to certain surfaces, such as glass, is inhibited when such cells are suspended in a medium containing an antigen to which they are sensitized. This relatively simple test, though suffering from the problems of reproducibility and sensitivity previously eluded to, may prove useful in diagnosis and in follow-up. For example, leucocyte adherence inhibition usually becomes negative several months after mastectomy; persistence or reappearance of inhibition may be associated with an increased risk of recurrence [55].

At the present time there is probably no place for the assessment of immunoreactivity on a routine basis in the preliminary assessment and follow-up of patients with cancer; the tests are expensive and fickle, and the relative yield of clinically relevant information is small. Such studies are best confined to those institutions where research groups have built up expertise in their conduct and interpretation.

CAUSES OF IMMUNOSUPPRESSION

Various immunosubversive factors have been described to account for the immunosuppression seen with cancer [56]. These include immune "blocking" factors (such as inappropriate antitumour antibodies, excess tumour antigen, and antigen/antibody complexes) and nonspecific immunosuppressive substances (such as "foetal" substances, fibrinogen degradation products, and prostaglandins). The role of the suppressor T-cell is likely to be important [57] and is being actively studied using monoclonal antibodies [58].

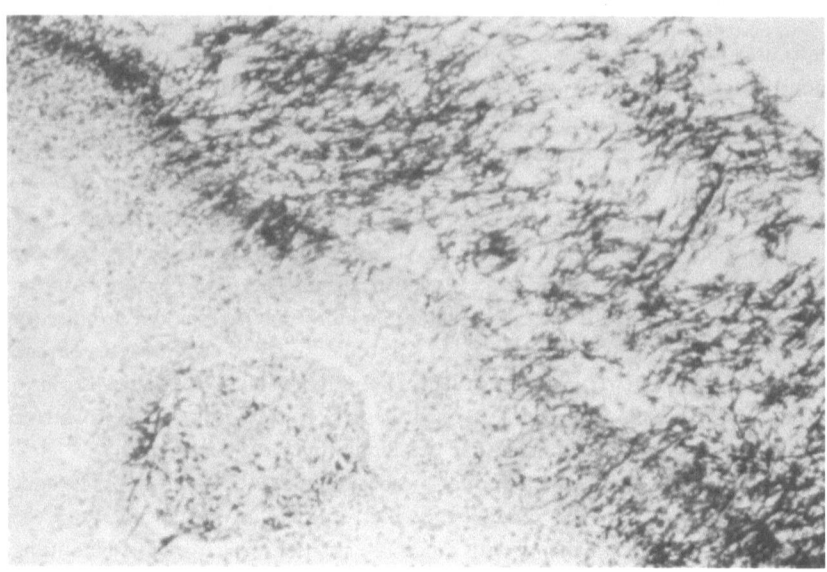

Figure 7-1. Fatal renal candidiasis.

In addition to the added immunosuppressive results of antitumour therapy numerous other factors increase the susceptibility of the patient with cancer to infection. Malnutrition, hospital pathogens, tumour necrosis, obstruction to drainage, oral and gastrointestinal ulceration, intravenous devices, urinary catheters, antibiotics, steroids, and so on—all are factors that must be taken into account before incriminating the tumour or its therapy as the underlying cause of any infection.

Surgery per se may be immunosuppressive in the short term, but splenectomy, an accepted practice in the staging of Hodgkin's disease, may lead to long-term defects (see earlier discussion on Hodgkin's disease). The possible causes of immunosuppression in cancer are also discussed in other chapters of this book.

CONSEQUENCES OF IMMUNOSUPPRESSION

Infections

A major problem encountered during the treatment of cancer is the susceptibility of the patient to infection. As we have seen, profound immunological disturbances may accompany the primary malignant condition, particularly when it is widely metastatic or primarily involves the lymphoreticular system, and these disturbances are exaggerated by the effects of therapy. Infection is a major cause of death in cancer, particularly in haematological malignancies.

The type of infection the patient will get will depend largely on the nature of the immunological deficiency. The complex interactions among lymphocytes, mononuclear phagocytes, antibody, and complement have already been stressed, and defects in any or all of these components may occur in cancer.

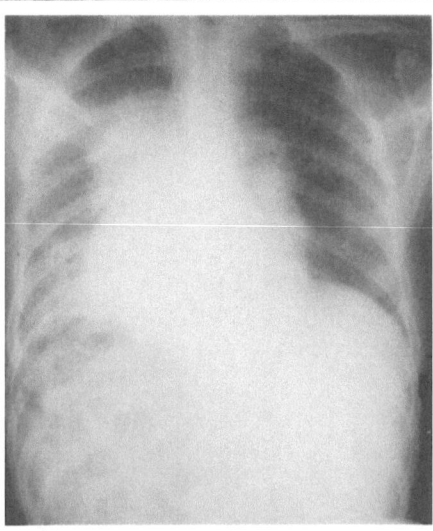

Figure 7-2. *Pneumocystis carinii* pneumonia.

When humoral (B-cell-dependent) immunity is defective (as occurs classically in myelomatosis, in chronic lymphocytic leukaemia, and after cytotoxic chemotherapy), inadequate antibody production may result in recurrent or chronic infections, particularly of the skin and respiratory tract, with organisms such as staphylococci, streptococci, pneumococcus, enterococci, and pneumocystis; such infections tend to become more severe as the disease progresses and are commonly the cause of death. Patients with defects predominantly involving mononuclear phagocytic/T-cell (cell-mediated) immunity tend to get infections with obligate or facultative intracellular parasites, for example, myobacteria, cryptococcus, candida (figure 7-1), aspergillus, pneumocystis (figure 7-2), cytomegalovirus, varicella/zoster (figure 7-3), and herpes simplex.

Quantitative and qualitative changes in neutrophil leucocytes may accompany chemotherapy or radiotherapy and are frequently a feature in the treatment of acute leukaemias. Such patients are particularly prone to recurrent bacterial infections (including normal commensal organisms), which commonly occur where membrane barriers are deficient (skin and respiratory, gastrointestinal, and genitourinary mucosa) (figure 7-4). Pus formation may be impaired and the infection not well localised. In advanced multitreated malignancies, wide-ranging immunological defects occur; opportunistic, often lethal, infections of all forms may be seen.

Second neoplasms

The fact that second malignancies may complicate certain forms of cancer treatment has been recognised for several years. The aetiology is likely to be multifactorial, relating partly to the immunological defects occuring with the primary cancer, partly to the immunosuppressive effects of intensive treatment, and partly to the direct cellular effects of radiation and chemotherapy. The possibility of an oncogenic viral aetiology has not been excluded. Much information on second malignancies has come from studies on Hodgkin's disease.

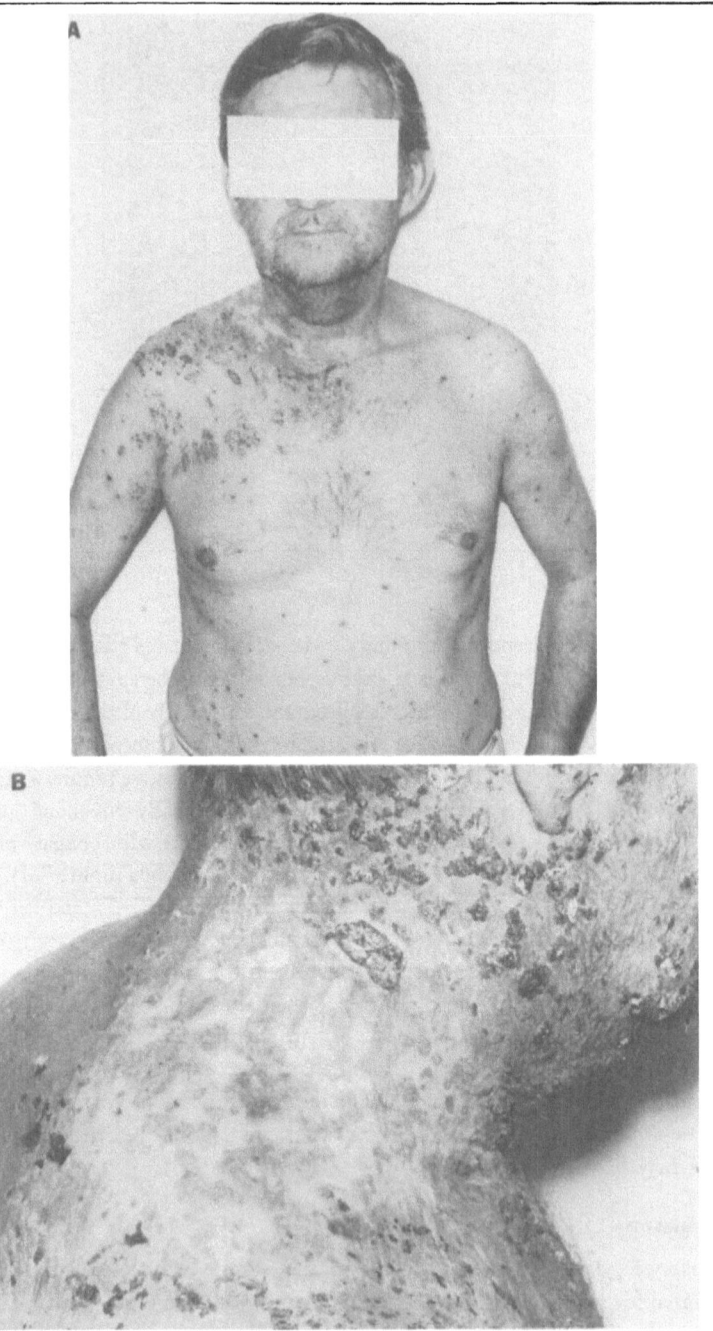

Figure 7-3. Severe herpes zoster with generalised spread.

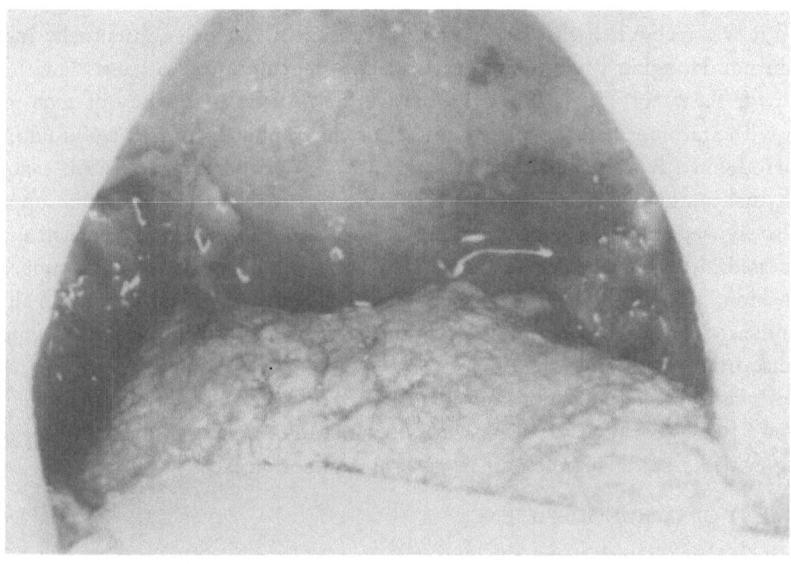

Figure 7-4. Oropharyngeal ulceration in a neutropenic patient.

There is undoubtedly an increased incidence of acute nonlymphoblastic leukaemia (ANLL) within 10 years of the initial treatment [59–62]. The risk of developing this complication may be as high as 5 to 10%, and therapy is generally accepted as the main cause. In early studies radiotherapy was assumed to be markedly leukaemagenic, analogous to the findings in atomic bomb survivors and in patients treated with irradiation for ankylosing spondylitis. More recently, it has been recognised that the role of radiotherapy is less important; in fact, high-voltage irradiation for Hodgkin's disease [62], and indeed for cervical carcinoma [63], is associated with a low risk of leukaemia. The importance of combined modality treatment (radiotherapy and chemotherapy) has been stressed by certain authorities [61], but undoubtedly chemotherapy is the major factor. An increased incidence of leukaemia has also been seen in patients with ovarian carcinoma treated with alkylating agents [64]; with non-Hodgkin's lymphoma [65], breast carcinoma [66], and polycythaemia vera [67] treated with chlorambucil; with myeloma, treated with melphalan and other agents [68]; and also in patients treated with busulphan [69]. The common denominator in these studies seems to be the alkylating agent component, often given for long periods or as maintenance.

Although leukaemia seems to be the main problem as a second malignancy, other studies have reported a high risk of solid tumours and non-Hodgkin's lymphomas [59,61]. Though the actual aetiological mechanism of these second neoplasms is still unclear, it is certain that the risk of such a neoplasm is still far exceeded by the risk of death from the primary tumour and its complications.

Cancer in patients with nonmalignant disease treated with immunosuppressive drugs

By 1970 it was recognised that renal transplant recipients were at substantially increased risk from non-Hodgkin's lymphoma (particularly "reticulum cell sarcomas" with a predilection for the brain) [70,71]. A collaborative UK/Australasian study of such patients (treated with azathioprine, cyclophosphamide, or chlorambucil) showed a 60-fold increase of non-Hodgkin's lymphoma together with an excess of squamous cell skin cancer and mesenchymal tumours [72]. Patients without transplants treated with immunosuppressive drugs also showed an excess of these tumours, though to a less extent. The mechanisms for this increased incidence of a narrow range of tumours are uncertain; immunosuppression, viral infection, graft-versus-host reaction, and chronic antigenic stimulation could all play a part. Similar factors are probably important in the increased incidence of neoplasia following cardiac transplantation [73].

Kaposi's sarcoma, recently notoriously associated with the "aquired immunodeficiency syndrome" [see 74 for review], also occurs after immunosuppressive therapy [75]; there is growing evidence for an aetiological relationship with a virus.

TREATMENT OF IMMUNODEFICIENCY

The main objectives in managing the immunosuppression seen in cancer are, first, to reduce the tumour burden and improve the patient's general clinical condition and, second, to treat any infections energetically. Therapeutic enhancement of immunity by various forms of immunotherapy has long proved attractive in theory but unfortunately has been of little practical value to date. Various forms of immunotherapy have been tried in an effort to improve cellular immunity (see chapter 9) but these have not been consistently successful, and we must await controlled studies with biologic response modifiers (for example interferons, lymphokines). One possible exception is the suggestion that transfer factor reduces the incidence of varicella/zoster infections in acute leukaemia [76], and we are at present undertaking a double blind randomised trial (transfer factor versus placebo) to see whether the same is true for Hodgkin's disease.

In cases of severe immunosuppression, for example, in the intensive therapy of acute leukaemia, the use of sterile environments may be advantageous with sterilization of the gastrointestinal tract and prophylactic use of certain antibiotics. Such patients may also require granulocyte transfusions. This is a relatively specialised area, however, and in most patients with cancer such management is not appropriate; however, the prompt recognition of infection with early and appropriate treatment may be life saving. Fever in a patient with cancer should not be assumed to be a result of the tumour or its necrosis following treatment. Infection is far more likely the cause, and the situation should be regarded as an oncological emergency. Possible bacterial infection (for example, septicaemia or chest infection) should be treated with broad-spectrum antibiotics, after taking the appropriate microbiological cultures. Viral infections such as herpes zoster/varicella and herpes simplex may be severe but fortunately not often fatal; such infections are now treatable with agents such as acyclovir and adenosine arabinoside. Other more exotic infections include pneumocystis, now potentially treatable with high-dose co-trimoxazole, and certain fungi (e.g., systemic candidiasis, aspergillosis) which may respond if given treatment early enough; amphotericin, though relatively toxic, is probably still the best agent in such cases.

In patients with antibody deficiency states where immunoglobulin levels remain depressed, immunoglobulin replacement may be required. This is often prepared from pooled blood bank plasma and its antibody activity reflects the specificities of the donor pool. It consists mainly of IgG and is usually given by intramuscular injection. Hypersensitivity reactions are unfortunately common and the injections are painful. Intravenous immunoglobulin therapy, though considerably more expensive, is now available and may be of benefit to those individuals having severe reactions to the intramuscular injections.

In immunosuppressed patients it is, of course, important to avoid immunisation with live and attenuated organisms, for example, smallpox and poliomyelitis. Killed vaccines are generally harmless and may be given if necessary, though the evoked immune response is likely to be subnormal.

REFERENCES

1. Burnet FM. Immunological surveillance in neoplasia. Transplant Rev 7: 3-20, 1971.
2. Platsoucas CD, Fernandes G, Gupta SL, Kempin S, Clarkson B, Good RA and Gupta S. Defective spontaneous and antibody dependent cytotoxicity mediated by E-rosette positive and E-rosette negative cells in untreated patients with chronic lymphocytic leukaemia: Augmentation by in vitro treatment with interferon. J Immunol 125: 1216-1223, 1980.
3. Hancock BW, Bruce L, Richmond J. Neutrophil function in lymphoreticular malignancy. Br J Cancer 33: 396-500, 1976.
4. Hersh EM, Oppenheim JJ. Impaired in vitro lymphocyte transformation in Hodgkin's disease. N Engl J Med 273: 1006-1072, 1965.
5. Young RC, Corder MP, Haynes HA, DeVita VT. Delayed hypersensitivity in Hodgkin's disease. Am J Med 52: 63-72, 1972.
6. Hancock BW, Bruce L, Sugden P, Ward AM, Richmond J. Immune status in untreated patients with lymphoreticular malignancy—A multifactorial study. Clin Oncol 3: 57-63, 1977.
7. Kaplan HS. The nature of the immunologic defect. In Hodgkin's disease, 2nd ed. Cambridge MA: Harvard, 1980, pp. 236-279.
8. Kun LE, Johnson RE. Haematological and immunologic status in Hodgkin's disease 5 years after radical radiotherapy. Cancer 36: 1912-1916, 1975.
9. Fuks Z, Strober S, Bobrove AM, Sasazuki T, McMichael A, Kaplan HS. Long-term effects of radiation on T & B lymphocytes in peripheral blood of patients with Hodgkin's disease. J Clin Invest 58: 803-814, 1976.
10. Bjorkholm M, Holm G, Mellstedt H. Persisting lymphocyte deficiencies during remission in Hodgkin's disease. Clin Exp Immunol 28: 389-393.
11. Bjorkholm M, Holm G, Mellstedt H. Immunologic profile of patients with cured Hodgkin's disease. Scand J Haematol 18: 361-368, 1977.
12. Fisher RI, DeVita VT, Bostik F, Van Haelan C, Howser DM, Hubbard SM, Young RC. Persistent immunologic abnormalities in long-term survivors of advanced Hodgkin's disease. Ann Int Med 92: 595-599, 1980.
13. Desser RK, Ultmann JE. Risk of infection in patients with Hodgkin's disease or lymphoma after diagnostic laparotomy and splenectomy. Ann Int Med 77: 143-145, 1972.
14. Hancock BW, Bruce L, Ward AM, Richmond J. Changes in immune status in patients undergoing splenectomy for the staging of Hodgkin's disease. Br Med J, 313-315, 1976.
15. Weitzman SA, Aisenberg AC, Siber GR, Smith DH. Impaired humoral immunity in treated Hodgkin's disease. N Engl J Med 297: 245-248, 1977.
16. Hancock BW, Bruce L, Whitham MD, Dunsmore IR, Ward AM, Richmond J. Immunity in Hodgkin's disease: Status after 5 years remission. Br J Cancer 46: 593-600, 1982.
17. Moroz C, Lahat N, Bianiamov M, Ramot B. Ferritin on the surface of lymphocytes in HD patients. Clin Exp Immunol 29: 30-35, 1977.
18. Bieber MM, Kaplan HS, Strober S. Polar lipid inhibitor of phytohaemagglutinin mitogenesis in the sera of untreated patients with Hodgkin's disease. In Rosenberg SA, Kaplan HS (eds.), Malignant lymphomas. Etiology, immunology, pathology, treatment. New York: Academic Press, 1982, pp. 285-294.
19. Van Haelan CPJ, Fisher RI. Increased sensitivity of lymphocytes from patients with Hodgkin's disease to concanavalin A-induced suppressor cells. J Immunol 127: 1216-1220, 1981.

20. Fisher RI, Van Haelan C, Bostik F. Increased sensitivity to normal adherent suppressor cells in untreated advanced Hodgkin's disease. Blood 57: 830-835, 1981.

21. Manifold IH, Whitman MD, Bruce L, Hancock BW. Monocyte/lymphocyte interaction in Hodgkin's disease. Br J Cancer 46: 483, 1982.

22. Hawylowicz CM, Rees RC, Hancock BW, Potter CW. Depressed natural killer cell activity in patients with malignant lymphoma, and failure of NK cells to respond to interferon treatment. Europ J Cancer 18: 1081-1088, 1982.

23. Hancock BW, Bruce L, Ward AM, Richmond J. The immediate effects of splenectomy, radiotherapy and cytotoxic chemotherapy on the immune status of patients with malignant lymphoma. Clin Oncol 3: 137-144, 1977.

24. Bruce L, Hancock BW, Richmond J. Neutrophil function in human malignant disease. J Physiol 259: 48-50, 1976.

25. Dent RG. The role of the mononuclear phagocyte system in cancer. Hospital Update 6: 469-479, 1980.

26. Kadish AS, Doyle AT, Steinhaver EH, Ghossein NA. Natural cytotoxicity and interferon production in human cancer: Deficient natural killer activity and normal interferon production in patients with advanced disease. J Immunol 127: 1817-1822, 1981.

27. Tarpley JL, Potvin C, Chretian PB. Prolonged depression of cellular immunity in cured laryngo-pharyngeal cancer patients treated with radiation therapy. Cancer 35: 638-644, 1975.

28. Stein JA, Adler A, Efraim SB, Maor M. Immunocompetence, immunosuppression and human breast cancer. Cancer 38: 1171-1187, 1976.

29. Haim N, Rudik L, Samuelly B, Mekori T, Robinson E. Immune status in patients cured of breast and gynaecological cancer. Clin Oncol 7: 141-147, 1981.

30. Bodey GP. Factors predisposing cancer patients to infection. In Spitzy KH, Karrer K (eds.) Proceedings of the 13th International Congress of Chemotherapy. 1983, pp. 3/3-3/8.

31. Aisenberg AC. Studies on delayed hypersensitivity in Hodgkin's disease. J Clin Invest 41: 1964-1970, 1962.

32. Gross L, Manfredi DL, Protos AA. The effect of cobalt-60 irradiation upon cell-mediated immunity. Radiology 106, 653-655, 1973.

33. Hancock BW, Bruce L, Heath J, Sugden P, Ward AM. The effect of radiotherapy on immunity in patients with localised carcinoma of the cervix uteri. Cancer 43: 118-123, 1979.

34. Hancock BW, Bruce L, Dunsmore IR, Ward AM, Richmond J. Follow-up studies on the immune status of patients with Hodgkin's disease after splenectomy and treatment in relapse and remission. Br J Cancer 36: 347-354, 1977.

35. Hancock BW, Bruce L, Whitham MD, Ward AM. The effects of radiotherapy on immunity in patients with cured localised carcinoma of the cervix uteri. Cancer 53: 884-887, 1984.

36. Halili M, Bosworth T, Romney S, Moukhtar M, Gossein NA. The long-term effect of radiotherapy on the immune status of patients cured of gynaecological cancer. Cancer 37: 2875-2878, 1976.

37. Harris J, Sengar D, Stewart T, Hyslop D. The effect of immunosuppressive chemotherapy on immune function in patients with malignant disease. Cancer 37: 1058-1069, 1976.

38. Serrou B, Dubois JB, Silva R. Immunological overshoot phenomenon chemotherapy of solid tumours. Proc Am Assoc Cancer Res 15: 125, 1974.

39. Borella L, Green AA, Webster RG. Immunologic rebound after cessation of long-term chemotherapy in acute leukaemia. Blood 40: 42-51, 1972.

40. Chang TC, Stutzman L, Sokal JE. Correlation of delayed hypersensitivity responses with chemotherapy results in advanced Hodgkin's disease. Cancer 36: 950-955, 1975.

41. Swan HT, Knowelden J. Prognosis in Hodgkin's disease related to lymphocyte count. Br J Haematol 21: 343-349, 1971.

42. MacLennan KA, Vaughan Hudson B, Jelliffe AM, Haybittle JL, Vaughan Hudson G. The pre-treatment peripheral blood lymphocyte count in 1100 patients with Hodgkin's disease: The prognostic significance and relationship to the presence of systemic symptoms. Clin Oncol 7: 333-339, 1981.

43. Hancock BW, Dunsmore IR, Swan HT. Lymphopenia a bad prognostic factor in Hodgkin's disease. Scand J Haematol 28: 193-199, 1982.

44. Papatestas AE, Lesnick GJ, Genkins G. Aufses AH. The prognostic significance of peripheral lymphocyte counts in patients with breast carcinoma. Cancer 37: 164-168.

45. Eilber FR, Morton DL. Impaired immunologic reactivity and recurrence following cancer surgery. Cancer 25: 362-367, 1970.

46. Hancock BW, May K, Bruce L, Dunsmore IR, Clark A, Ward AM. Haematological and immunological markers in malignant lymphoma. Tum Diagn 3: 140-144, 1980.

47. Hersh E, Gutterman JU, Mavligit GM, McCredie KB, Burgers MA, Matthews A, Freireich EJ. Serial

studies of immunocompetence of patients undergoing chemotherapy for acute leukaemia. J Clin Invest 54: 401-408, 1974.

48. Eilber FR, Nizze JA, Morton DL. Sequential evaluation of general immune competence in cancer patients: Correlations with clinical course. Cancer 35: 660-665, 1975.

49. Herbermann RB. Immunologic approaches to the diagnosis of cancer. Cancer 37: 548-561, 1976.

50. Herbermann RB. Delayed hypersensitivity skin reactions to antigens on human tumours. Cancer 34: 1469-1473, 1974.

51. Hancock BW, Bruce L, Richmond J. Cellular immunity to Hodgkin's disease splenic tissue as measured by leucocyte migration inhibition. Br J Med 1: 556-557, 1976.

52. Hancock BW, Bruce L, Richmond J. Sensitisation to Hodgkin's disease spleen tissue in patients with malignant lymphoma—A follow-up study. Br Med J 2: 35-352, 1976.

53. Hancock BW, May K, Bruce L, Richmond J. Ferritin, a sensitising factor in the leucocyte migration inhibition test in malignant lymphoma. Br J Haematol 43: 223-233, 1979.

54. Halliday WS, Maluish AE, Isbister WH. Detection of anti-tumour cell mediated immunity and serum blocking factors in cancer patients by the leucocyte adherence inhibition test. Br J Cancer 29: 31-35, 1974.

55. Flores M, Maiti JH, Grosser N, MacFarlance JK, Thompson DMP. An overview: Anti-tumour immunity in breast cancer assayed by the tube leukocyte adherence inhibition. Cancer 39: 84-505, 1977.

56. Kamo I, Friedman H. Immunosuppression and the role of immunosuppressive factors in cancer. Adv Cancer Res 25: 271-321, 1977.

57. Noar D. Suppressor cells: Permitters or promotors of malignancy. Adv Cancer Res 29: 45-125, 1976.

58. Robbins DS, Fudenberg HH. Human lymphocyte subpopulations in metastatic neoplasia—Six years later. N Engl J Med 308: 1595-1597, 1983.

59. Arsenau JC, Canellos GP, Johnson R, DeVita VT. Risk of new cancers in patients with Hodgkin's disease. Cancer 40: 1912-1916, 1977.

60. Coleman CN, Williams CJ, Flint A, Glatstein EJ, Rosenberg SA, Kaplan HS. Haematologic neoplasia in patients treated for Hodgkin's disease. N Engl J Med 297: 1249-1252, 1977.

61. Valagussa P, Santoro A, Kenda R, Fossati Bellani F, Franchi F, Banfi A, Rilke F, Bonadonna G. Second malignancies in Hodgkin's disease: A complication of certain forms of treatment. Br Med J 280: 216-219, 1980.

62. Pederson-Bjergaard J, Larsen SO. Incidence of acute nonlymphocytic leukaemia, preleukaemia and acute myeloproliferative syndrome up to ten years after treatment of Hodgkin's disease. N Engl J Med 307: 965-971, 1982.

63. Boice JD, Hutchison GB. Leukaemia in women following radiotherapy for cervical cancer: Ten-year follow-up of an international study. J Natl Cancer Inst 65: 115-129, 1980.

64. Reimer RR, Hoover R, Fraumeni JF, Young RC. Acute leukaemia after alkylating-agent therapy of ovarian cancer. N Engl J Med 297: 177-181, 1977.

65. Steigbigel RT, Kim H, Potolsky A, Schrier SL. Acute myeloproliferative disorders following long-term chlorambucil therapy. Arch Intern Med 134: 728-731, 1974.

66. Lerner HJ. Acute myelogenous leukaemia in patients receiving chlorambucil as long-term adjuvant chemotherapy for stage II breast cancer. Cancer Treat Rep 62: 1135-1138, 1978.

67. Berk PD, Goldberg JD, Silverstein MN, Weinfeld A, Donovan PB, Ellis JT, Landaw SA, Laszlo J, Najean Y, Pisciotta AV, Wasserman R. Increased incidence of acute leukaemia in polycythaemia associated with chlorambucil therapy. N Engl J Med 304: 441-447, 1981.

68. Bersagel DE, Bailey AJ, Langley GR, MacDonald RN, White DF, Miller AB. The chemotherapy of plasma-cell myeloma and the incidence of acute leukaemia. N Engl J Med 30: 743-748, 1979.

69. Strott H, Fox W, Girling DJ, Stephens RJ, Galton DAG. Acute leukaemia after busulphan. Br Med J 2: 1513-1517, 1977.

70. Penn I, Hammond W, Brettschneider L, Starzel TE. Malignant lymphomas in transplantation patients. Transplant Proc 1: 106-111, 1969.

71. Doll R, Kinlen L. Immunosurveillance and Cancer: Epidemiological evidence. Br Med J 4: 420-422, 1970.

72. Kinlen LJ, Sheil AGR, Peto J, Doll R. Collaborative United Kingdom/Australasia study of cancer in patients treated with immunosuppressive drugs. Br Med J 2: 1461-1466, 1979.

73. Krikorian JG, Anderson JL, Bieber CP, Penn I, Stinson EB. Malignant neoplasms following cardiac transplantation. J Am Med Assoc 240: 639-643, 1978.

74. Waterson AP. Aquired immune deficiency syndrome. Br Med J 286: 743-746, 1983.

75. Gange RW, Jones EW. Kaposi's sarcoma and immunosuppressive therapy: An appraisal. Clin Exp Dermatol 3: 135-146, 1978.

76. Steele RW, Myers MG, Vincent MM. Transfer factor for the prevention of varicella/zoster infection in childhood leukaemia. N Engl J Med 303: 355-359, 1980.

8. MONOCLONAL ANTIBODIES

K. SIKORA

H. SMEDLEY

INTRODUCTION

Molecular biology has made many advances over the last ten years. One of its most important achievements has been the development of monoclonal antibodies (MCAs). Similar to
conventional polyclonal antibodies in their structure and function, the significance of
MCAs lies in their specificity and immortality. A virtually endless supply of a MCA can be
made available in a completely purified form. We will outline the essential steps in the
manufacture of MCAs and discuss their potential uses in the fields of biology and clinical
medicine related to cancer. In particular we shall stress how these sophisticated immunological agents can be used as tools to unravel complicated immunological problems
such as the body's response to malignant disease and the antigenic structure of certain common solid tumours, as well as having immense potential in the management of patients
with cancer (table 8–1).

WHAT IS A MONOCLONAL ANTIBODY?

When a foreign antigen is introduced into an animal its immunological response is
polyclonal; many different clones of B-lymphocytes are stimulated to produce antibodies.
Each of these clones produces an antibody of unique sructure that in turn will recognise
unique components of the antigen. Each discrete region of an antigen so recognised is
known as an antigenic determinant or epitope. Complex antigenic molecules may contain
several epitopes, although more simple molecules may contain just one. Such complexity in
the immune response creates problems in understanding the individual components of the

B.W. Hancock and A.M. Ward (eds.), Immunological Aspects of Cancer. Copyright © 1985, Martinus Nijhoff Publishing, Boston/Dordrecht/Lancaster.

Table 8-1. Potential uses of monoclonal antibodies in oncology

DIAGNOSIS

Circulating Tumour Markers:

  Screening
  Diagnosis
  Monitoring
  Prognosis
  Treatment Decisions

Histology

  Prognosis
  Treatment Decisions

Cytology

  Sputum, Urine, Vaginal Smears, Effusions and Bone Marrow

Immunoscintigraphs

  Detection
  Localisation

THERAPY

Bone Marrow Clearance

Systemic Therapy

  Antibody alone
  Coupled with drugs, toxins, radionucleides

---

system. Although each B-lymphocyte produces one and only one antibody, no method was available for selecting out particular lymphocytes and propagating them in cell culture until the advent of MCAs. Much ingenious work had been performed in attempting to establish stable lines of cloned B-lymphocytes but no method was found to be reliable. It therefore was a tremendous advance when Kohler and Milstein [1] first made a monoclonal antibody to sheep red cells.

In making a MCA a lymphocyte is immortalised by fusing it to a myeloma cell. First of all the antigen against which it is required is selected, purified, and used to immunise experimental animals, usually mice or rats. The antigen is introduced into the animal on several occasions following an immunisation schedule. After a suitable period the animal will mount a response to the antigen and produce antibodies against it. In the case of a complex immunogen such as a tumour cell membrane preparation, literally thousands of antibodies may be produced. At this point the animal is sacrificed and the spleen dissected out. From this organ many lymphocytes can be recovered and a single cell suspension prepared. It is possible to hybridise these cells with a myeloma line from the same species as the experimental animal. The essential feature of this line is that as in all other malignant cells it is clonogenic: it is capable of infinite division from a single cell as long as adequate nutritional support is available. After cell fusion a hybridoma cell is constructed that in ideal circumstances will contain the DNA and therefore the characteristics of both parent cells. What is looked for is the ability to manufacture the desired antibody from a B-lymphocyte and the ability to undergo infinite cell division conferred by the myeloma genes (figure 8-1). Such a hybridoma cell can readily be cultured in the laboratory. It is therefore possible to have available a culture of hybridoma cells producing a single antibody in endless quantity. It should

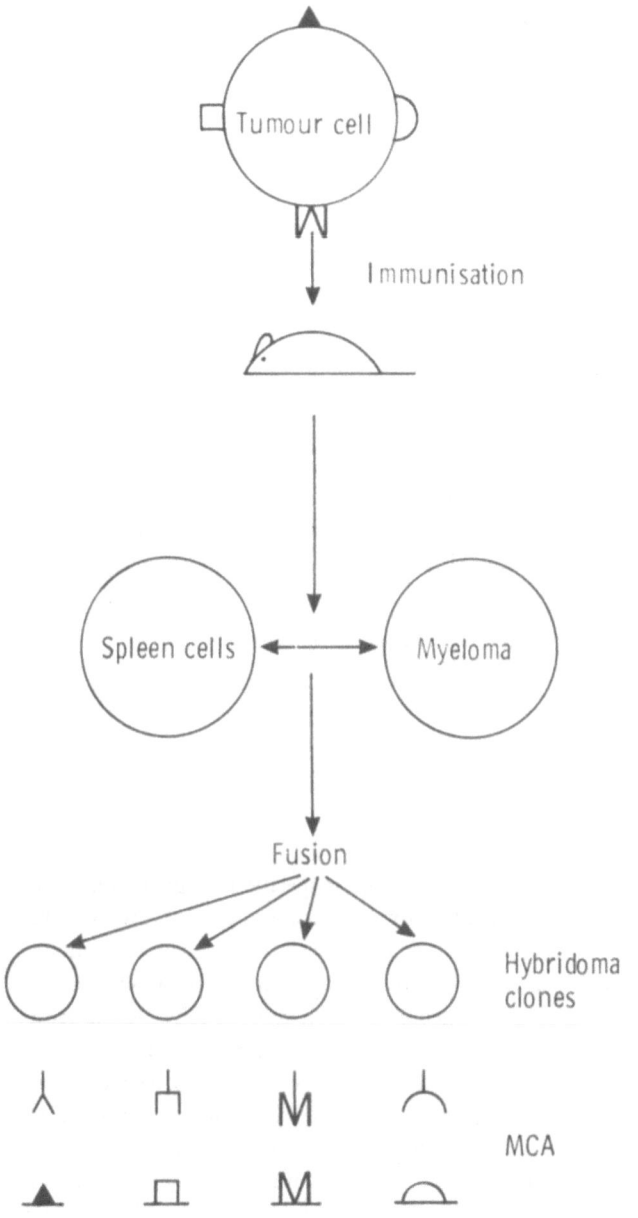

Figure 8-1. The production of MCAs to a complex antigen such as the molecular pattern on a cancer cell surface.

be stressed that although an immortal antibody-producing cell is the ideal result of such a fusion, many imperfect and uninteresting hybridisations will occur. Many of these will not have the necessary gene structure for immortality and will rapidly die out. Other cells may be viable, but will not produce the antibody required. These may be selected out at the cloning stage by the use of specific assays for antibody activity. The construction of useful antibody-producing hybridoma cells is not yet routine, and great effort is required in the screening and selection of hybridomas in order to make useful clones after even the simplest of immunisation schedules.

HUMAN TUMOUR ANTIGENS

There is considerable evidence that the immune system is able to recognize tumour cells, but almost nothing is known about the molecular nature and genetic specificity of the components on the cancer cell surface involved in this recognition. A variety of immunological assays have been used to examine components present on the cell surface (chapters 3 and 4). Several groups of antigens can be detected on tumour cells, some of which are shared with normal cells (table 8–2). Normal transplantation antigens can be detected serologically and by cell-mediated lympholysis in vitro. These histocompatibility antigens are important in studying immune response to cancer for two reasons. The first is that unless syngeneic systems are used there will be confusion in the detection of antigens specific for transformed cells and not on normal counterparts [2]. Second, some tumour-specific transplantation antigens may in fact be modified forms of histocompatibility antigens [3].

Table 8–2. Human tumour antigens

Histocompatibility antigens
Tumour-specific transplantation antigens
Embryonic antigens
Viral antigens
Differentiation antigens

In a variety of animal systems, tumour-specific transplantation antigens (TSTA) have been detected. These are defined by a rejection assay that involves the immunization of groups of syngeneic animals, either by excision of the growing tumour or by repeated injections of tumour cells made inactive by irradiation or by other means [4]. After a suitable interval the animals are challenged with viable tumour cells and the growth of the resultant tumours is compared with that of a group of unimmunized animals. Several observations have been made from rejection assays. There appears to be a considerable range of immunogenicities amongst different experimental tumours. Chemically induced tumours often possess specific rejection antigens; that is, immunization with one tumour confers immunity only to itself and not to others, even if induced by the same carcinogen in another location in the same animal. Clearly, such assays are not possible with human tumours and so we do not know if human TSTAs exist. In virally induced experimental tumours, the surface antigen characteristic of the transforming virus can, under certain circumstances, act as a transplantation antigen. Embryonic antigens are defined by antisera and cytotoxic lymphocytes prepared in syngeneic animals by injection of preparations of embryonic tissue. Such sera detect antigens on a wide variety of tumour cells that may well represent products expressed during the rapid growth of cells, both in embryogenesis and tumourigenesis [5]. Normal tissue antigens that appear during differentiation can also be expressed in neoplastic cells (chapter 11). Under certain circumstances such antigens may appear tumour specific. An example is the idiotype of the immunoglobulin expressed on neoplastic B-lymphocytes in certain lymphomas.

MONOCLONAL ANTIBODY PRODUCTION STRATEGIES

The requirements of the antibody

Before embarking on the production of an MCA, it is necessary to consider the purpose for which it is to be used. The inherent properties of different classes of antibody naturally confer different physical and chemical properties, and therefore different strategies may be more relevant to a particular purpose (figure 8–2). When considering the preparation of antibodies for cancer therapy, for example, it may be that the production of human MCAs using human lymphocytes and myeloma cells would have advantages. Human MCAs do not elicit strong immune responses when administered to a patient, thus eliminating the danger of anaphylactic reactions always present when mouse or rat monoclonal antibodies are used. When prepared for use in immunohistology, however, no such considerations apply. If the antibody is to be used to destroy a human solid tumour in patients, then the stringency of its required specificity will depend on the tissue distribution of the antigen concerned. In breast cancer, an MCA that causes the destruction of all breast cells as well as the malignant cells may be useful for the breast but is not necessary for the survival of the patient. However, in a tumour of colorectal tissue, clearly the destruction of all the normal colon would be catastrophic. If, however, the antibody is to be used for localisation and detection of tumour, then true tumour specificity is less important, as the consequences of binding a small amount of antibody to normal tissues are insignificant to the patient. The class of the antibody is also important. IgG antibodies have relatively low molecular weights and can diffuse easily within the extracellular space compared with the relatively massive IgM molecule. On the practical front, the antibody should be secreted in high concentration by a hybridoma line that is capable of growth in a serum-free medium to allow for easy purification.

Immunisation

Immunisation schedules relating to different biological systems vary widely. We will concentrate here on schedules of proven value in the study of human solid tumours. First, clearly, immunisation with tumour antigens from humans is possible only with experimental animals. The injection of tumour antigens into normal human subjects would be unethical and impractical. The antigenic material used for xenogeneic immunisation has included cell lines grown in vitro, homogenised fresh tumour tissue, membrane preparations, or fractionated, solubilised components from fresh tumour cell membranes [6]. The timing of administration of the immunogens appears to be critical. Most schedules involve weekly administration of antigen for at least three weeks. This is followed by an intravenous injection of antigen three days prior to sacrifice of the animal. This final boost stimulates the splenic lymphocytes concerned with antibody production into division—the optimal state for hybridisation.

Many of the antibodies raised in xenogeneic immunisation are against blood group and histocompatibility antigens. Human hybridomas allow the analysis of the immune response

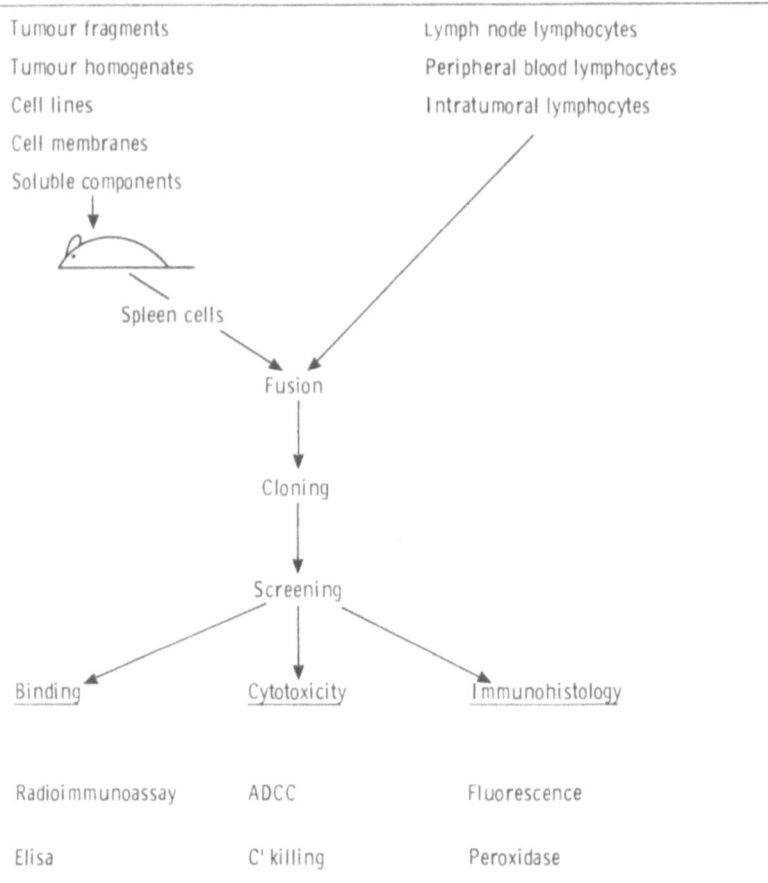

Figure 8-2. Strategies in the production of MCAs to human tumour cells.

of an individual to his own tumour. The best results reported so far for human hybridomas have involved the fusion of B-lymphocytes taken from the regional lymph node draining tumour sites obtained from patients undergoing surgery. In patients with carcinoma of the lung the hilar lymph nodes are often enlarged and of course contain many lymphocytes [7]. Similarly in patients with glioma, a malignant brain tumour, up to 30% of the cells found within the tumour have been shown to be lymphocytes [8]. As lymphocytes are not normal components of the brain, it is likely that their presence fulfills a biological function: the mounting of a response to the tumour. Fusion of such cells with a human myeloma line can be performed and human monoclonal antibodies produced [9].

Myeloma cells

A large number of myeloma cells that are suitable for fusion are now available. These cells have been selected for rapid growth. After fusion, however, it is important that a mechanism exists to destroy those myeloma cells that have failed to hybridise. The most commonly used self-destruct system involves the selection of myelomas that lack the enzyme hypoxanthine phosphoribosyl transferase (HPRT). Cells lacking a functional gene for this protein can be selected by growth in 8-azaguanine (8AG). This synthetic nucleoside analogue is incorporated into DNA by HPRT, so that cells that lack HPRT (HPRT$^-$)will grow in high concentrations of 8AG. when HPRT$^-$ cells are placed in a medium containing hypoxanthine, aminopterin, and thymidine (HAT medium), they will die. Aminopterin blocks the synthesis of new nucleosides by the cell, and thymidine and hypoxanthine provide the necessary nucleotide precursors. Normal cells can utilize the hypoxanthine whereas HPRT$^-$ cells cannot and so die in HAT. After fusion with immune lymphocytes the hybrid cells will survive by possessing the immortality of the myeloma and the HPRT gene of the lymphocyte (figure 8–3) [10]. The use of myelomas that do not secrete immunoglobulin simplifies the analysis of the antibody products of the hybrid cells.

Fusion

The fusion procedure used to manufacture hybridomas is now standardised. Originally, myeloma and immune lymphocytes were mixed in the presence of *Sendai* virus. Polyethylene glycol is now used to destroy the surface tension forces that keep cells apart. Myeloma and splenocytes are mixed and washed in a serum-free medium. Polyethylene glycol at a concentration of 35 to 45% w/v is added to the medium and the cells gently contrifuged at forces of up to 400/g. The cells are washed, added to selective HAT medium, and dispensed into plastic microwell dishes for culture. After 14 days, hybrids will appear in most wells. The supernatants are removed and assayed for activity and the relevant wells are cloned by limiting dilution [11].

Screening

Whichever immunisation schedule and fusion system are used, the eventual spectrum of MCAs produced will depend on the methods used for screening to find suitable immunoglobulins. Three main screening methods are used: radioimmunoassay, by binding to membranes or whole cell lines; immunohistology, using either fluorescence or peroxidase techniques; and cytotoxicity, either by the addition of complement or by antibody-dependent cell-mediated cytotoxicity (figure 8–2). In searching for antihuman tumour MCAs, there are advantages in the use of immunohistology in a primary screen [12]. As well as providing a rapid screening technique, this method also allows the acquisition of information about the exact location of an antigen and its distribution within a tumour. Binding radioimmunoassays provide the most rapid way of screening large numbers of supernatants for antibody activity but may not pick up all antibodies that have clinical use, such as those that activate cell-mediated cytotoxicity. Successive rounds of screening and cloning are often required to produce the required MCA. At each stage it is possible to lose the hybrid cells by infection or by growth problems. It is therefore important to freeze-down cells in liquid nitrogen after each successive round of cloning.

Although it is relatively easy to construct sets of MCAs that have activity against a particular tumour, it is much more difficult to characterize specificity and produce antibodies reacting with defined target antigens. The most common method to characterize MCAs is to study binding to a panel of different cell lines. In a particularly elegant study, MCAs were raised by immunizing mice with human melanoma cell line and tested for binding to

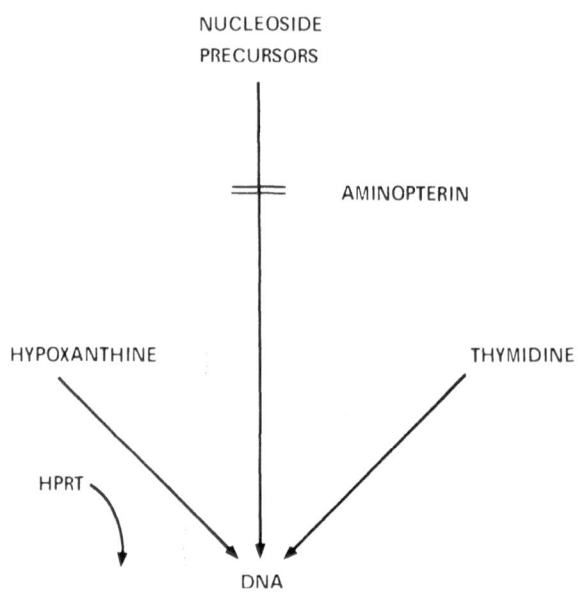

NUCLEOSIDE
PRECURSORS

AMINOPTERIN

HYPOXANTHINE   THYMIDINE

HPRT

DNA

Figure 8-3. The HAT selection system used to destroy unfused myeloma cells.

a large panel of different tumour lines [13]. By increasing the sensitivity of these binding assays, apparent specificity often disappears. A good example of this is the work of Brown et al. [14]. The binding to cells and tissues of an apparently specific antimelanoma antibody was investigated in a highly sensitive assay system using a second MCA (double determinant immunoassay). Its target antigen was shown to be present, although in small quantities, on normal tissue as well as on tumour cells. The search for MCAs with well-defined specificity is clearly essential if antibodies are to be of use for targeting drugs or toxic agents. For tumour localisation, or in vitro removal of tumour cells from bone marrow during autologous marrow transplantation, fine specificity may not be so essential for clinical usefulness.

DIAGNOSIS

Histology

The diagnosis and classification of human malignancy is made by the histopathologist from biopsy material provided by the clinician. Although the light microscopic appearance of tissue sections may be sufficient in most cases to provide an unequivocal diagnosis, this is not always the case. It is well recognised, for example, that undifferentiated carcinoma and lymphoma may have very similar appearances, but the choice of therapy and prognosis for the two diseases is radically different. In addition, the recognition of variants of major diseases is also vital if our understanding of tumour biology and approaches to treatment is to improve. In the case of non-Hodgkin's lymphoma, for example, at least 15 different varieties are recognised with a wide spectrum of clinical outcome. Highly purified conventional polyclonal antibodies reacting against certain tumour types can be labeled with specific reagents in order to make the identification of certain subpopulations within the tumour more readily visible (chapter 9). The techniques most widely employed are immuno-peroxidase staining and immunofluorescence. Monoclonal antibodies add to the usefulness of immunohistology by increasing the specificity of the antibodies available. In addition to identifying certain cell types, it is also possible to recognise certain subpopulations. There are series of MCAs capable of recognising different lymphocyte subsets. These can be used to distinguish different types of lymphoma and leukaemia [16].

Tumour markers

By its very nature cancer is a disease that has a propensity to spread throughout the body. The development of such distant disease is what leads to treatment failure. The accurate detection of metastatic disease in patients with common solid tumours would be a great advance in their management. First, metastases could be detected at a point when the total number of cells present is relatively small. Thus, chemotherapy would have a greater chance of success, and the patient's general health might still be sufficiently good to allow the use of aggressive and possibly debilitating therapy. The detection of occult micrometastases would also have a role in determining the choice of primary management in many patients. It is known, for example, that up to 40% of women with breast cancer have micrometa-static disease at the time of presentation. The majority of treatment failures arise from this group of patients. If these patients could be identified at presentation, then the choice of treatment to the primary lesion may be modified and these patients selected for immediate adjuvant systemic therapy [17].

Although certain rare tumours do shed products that may be detected in the blood, they tend to be in the minority. In patients with testicular teratoma, for example, alphafeto-protein and human choriogonadotrophin may be detected in the blood. The concentration of these proteins reflects the size of the tumour tissue present. MCAs can be used in assays to detect small quantities of these compounds and so detect the presence of extremely small quantities of malignant tissue. The search is underway for new tumour markers for other tumours, using MCAs raised against surface components [18].

Immunoscintigraphy

Antibodies to tumour-associated antigens may be useful in the localisation of malignant disease. In principle, if an antigen is expressed in high quantity on a tumour cell surface, it should be possible to manufacture an antibody that binds to the tumour cell better than any other tissue present in the body. When injected into a patient with cancer, such an antibody will ultimately bind to tumour cell membranes. If prior to injection that antibody is labeled with a radioisotope such as [131]iodine, then conventional nuclear medicine techniques can be used to scan the patient externally and locate areas of relative high uptake of the labeled antibody. Such areas of high uptake will correspond to areas of tumour deposits.

Several groups have now shown that MCAs can localise colorectal cancer [19,20], ovarian cancer [21], and melanoma [22]. The techniques used were identical. To provide an insight into this approach, we will describe our studies in producing localising MCAs for colorectal cancer. From fresh surgical specimens of colorectal tumour, membranes were

prepared and injected into rats on three separate occasions. After a final booster immunisation the rats were sacrificed and spleen lymphocytes fused with a rat myeloma line. The
resulting hybrids were cloned and screened for activity using a radioimmunoassay against a
human colorectal cell line available in culture. Those hybrids exhibiting binding to the cell
line were selected for further investigation using a series of in vitro and in vivo testing including immunohistology and human tumour xenograft localisation in immunosuppressed
mice. One of these antibodies was selected for clinical use. The antibody was iodinated
with ^{131}I using a modification of the chloramine T-method. In vitro experiments demonstrated that radioiodination resulted in no appreciable loss of immunoreactivity. Using this
purified radiolabeled antibody, a series of patients with known colorectal carcinoma were
studied. First, the patients received potassium iodide 120/mg daily by mouth for two days
prior to injection in order to saturate the thyroid uptake of iodine. After obtaining consent
and ensuring no clinical history of allergy to rodents, the patients received a slow intravenous infusion containing 1/mg of antibody labeled with 1 mCi of ^{131}iodine. Forty-eight
hours later the patients received a second injection of 99-technetium labeled human serum
albumin and technetium pertechnetate. The purpose of the second injection was to
delineate the normal blood pool. A computer is used to subtract the image obtained on the
technetium (blood pool) channel from the image obtained on the iodine channel. In this
way the presence of circulating-labeled antibody does not interfere with the image of
tumour-bound antibody. Using this subtraction method, accurate tumour localisation has
been observed in 24 out of 27 patients studied (figure 8–4). Although many problems still
exist with the radiolocalisation of tumour deposits, they are gradually being overcome.
Such work has clearly demonstrated that the use of labeled MCAs to detect the presence of
cancer is entirely feasible and may have important practical use in the near future.

THERAPY

Serotherapy for cancer using conventional antibodies has been attempted for more than 50
years, so far with no success. Most of such sera have poor specificity and also a low titre
against putative tumour antigens. MCAs may overcome both these problems; in addition,
the development of human monoclonal antibodies may prevent the immunological reactions against the administered antibodies with the associated adverse side effects. There
are several mechanisms by which the administration of a suitable monoclonal antibody can
result in tumour cell death (table 8–3). Most of these mechanisms are unlikely to destroy
large numbers of tumour cells. Table 8–4 lists some of the clinical trials on the use of MCAs
for therapy. However, drugs, toxins, and radionucleides can be coupled to MCAs in such a
way that their immunological activity remains unaltered. The antibody, therefore, provides
a targeting mechanism, whilst the coupled agent acts as a warhead.

Targeting

The development of antitumour MCAs to carry diagnostic agents, as previously described,
is a necessary first step in developing MCAs for targeting. If an antibody could be manu-
factured that recognised a tumour with a high degree of specificity and had no cross-reaction
with normal tissues, then it is conceivable that such an antibody could be conjugated to a

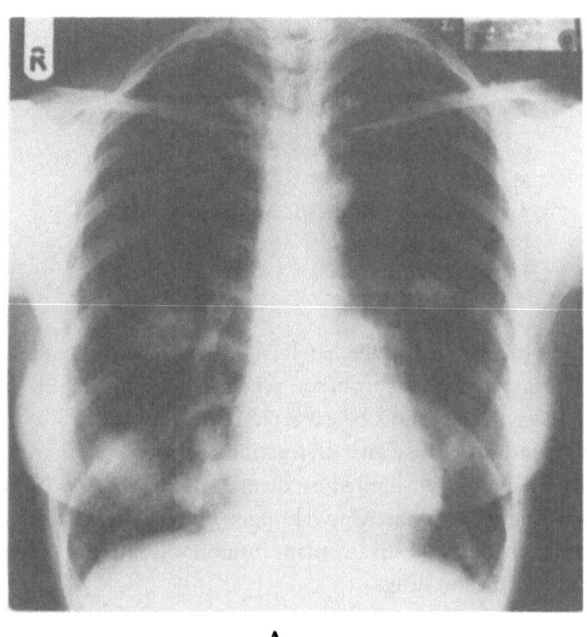

A

B

Figure 8–4. The detection of lung metastases in a patient with colorectal cancer by the administration of monoclonal antibody.

Table 8–3. Killing mechanisms of MCAs

Complement cytotoxicity
Macrophage activation
Antibody-directed cell-mediated cytotoxicity
Natural killer cell activation
Immunoregulation

therapeutic agent. As can be seen immediately, however, the technique of subtraction as used in immunoscintigraphy is inappropriate when considering highly toxic agents. An agent suitable for cancer therapy must be expected to destroy any cell with which it comes into contact and therefore the unselective destruction of normal tissue would be dangerous. At present this type of approach is limited by the lack of antibodies with sufficient tumour specificity. Another limitation is the relatively poor blood supply of many tumours. The presence of a necrotic, hypoxic centre in many tumours limits the usefulness of existing agents such as radiotherapy and drugs.

Drugs

Many drugs are currently available that interfere with malignant cell growth by a variety of mechanisms. Unfortunately, their therapeutic ratio is often low, causing profound effects on normal cells. Patients undergoing cancer chemotherapy develop bone marrow suppression and other side effects that limit the dose of chemotherapy. Targeting such drugs with MCAs may achieve high concentrations of drug around the tumour without an unacceptable high level of systemic toxicity. Although several animal models exist for this sort of approach using drugs such as chlorambucil, adriamycin, and methotrexate, clinical studies are only just beginning.

Toxins

Toxins are naturally occurring bacterial or plant products that cause the death of any cell they enter at very low concentrations. The targeting of such agents by MCAs could result in tumour destruction. Particularly attractive is the use of a group of plant toxins that consist of two parts (figure 8–5). The A-chain, or active chain, enters the cell to inhibit protein synthesis whilst the B-chain, or binding chain, is necessary for binding the cell sur-

Table 8–4. MCA therapy and cancer

Antibody	Antigen	Disease studied	Response	Ref
L17F12	α-T-cell	mycosis fungoides	yes	[23]
J5-CALLA	α-leukaemia	ALL	transient	[24]
T65	α-CLL cells	CLL	transient	[25]
17-1A	α-colon cell	colon ca	no	[26]
MoAB225	α-melanoma	melanoma	no	[27]
4D6	α-idiotype	lymphoma	yes	[28]
ID6	α-glioma	glioma	no	[29]

BINDING   ENTRY   KILLING

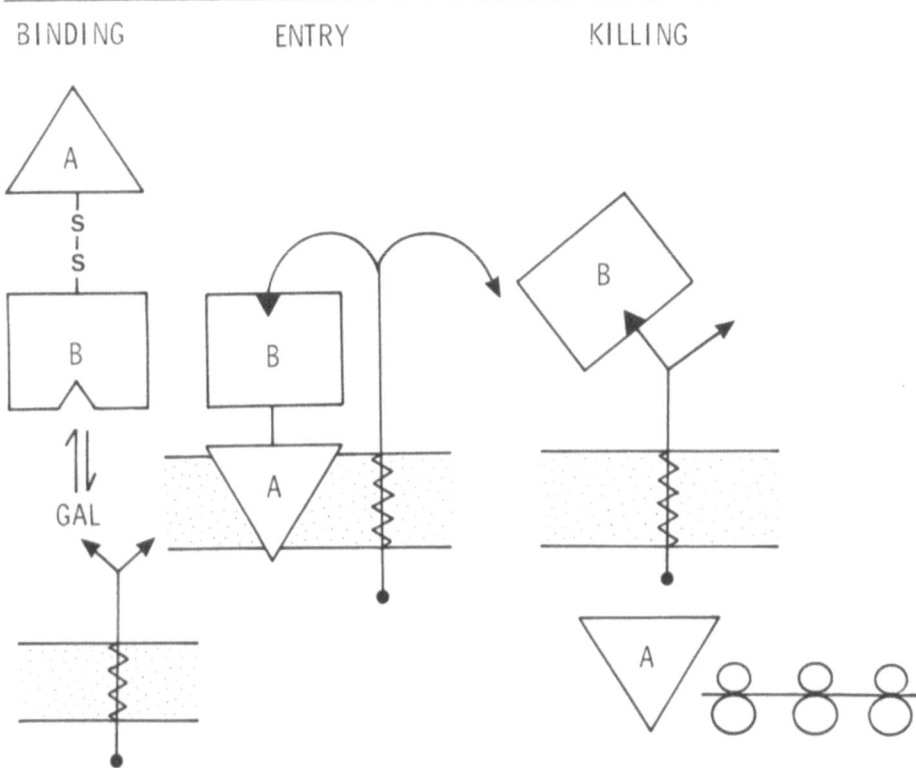

Figure 8-5. The killing mechanism of ricin.

face. Isolated A-chains are not toxic because no binding can occur. If, however, A-chains are coupled chemically to a suitable MCA, then an ideal magic bullet can be constructed, with the MCA providing specific binding to the tumour cell surface. Experimental work in rodents has already shown that such systems are capable of causing tumour regression [30].

Isotopes

Although isotopes such as ^{131}I that emit high-energy gamma rays may be used to detect the presence of malignant cells, isotopes with other physical properties may be used for cell destruction. Ideally, an isotope so employed would be of short half-life, have stable non-toxic decay products, and emit alpha particles that have limited penetration into adjacent tissue. Isotopes such as [211]astatine when conjugated to a MCA can achieve relatively high concentrations within a tumour. Sufficient radiation damage then occurs to a localised volume of tumour so as to cause destruction of that tumour but with little or no damage to adjacent normal tissue. Again, encouraging results are available from animal models.

Bone marrow clearance

The bone marrow is important for patients with common solid tumours for two reasons. First, it is a common site for metastatic disease to develop, where relatively large amounts of tumour may be present. Second, the response of normal bone marrow to many conventionally available cytotoxic agents is often critical in determining the amount of chemotherapy that may be employed in one particular patient. One therapeutic tactic to overcome these problems is to remove a quantity of a patient's bone marrow prior to giving very high-dose cytotoxic therapy. The patient then receives therapy at a supralethal dose in the hope of destroying all tumour cells present. After this, the patient's own bone marrow containing stem cells is reinjected. Following appropriate support measures, the reconstituted bone marrow will repopulate the patient's own marrow and provide haematological stability. Such a system is, however, useless if the bone marrow harvested prior to cytotoxic therapy itself contains malignant cells that can be reintroduced into the patient. MCAs are now available that can recognise leukaemia cells and breast cancer cells in bone marrow samples [31]. By using complement fixation cytotoxicity, MCAs can destroy malignant cells when present in bone marrow in small quantities. In this way the patient's bone marrow may be "laundered" while the patient is receiving high-dose cytotoxic therapy.

REFERENCES

1. Kohler G, and Milstein C. Continuous cultures of fused cells secreting antibody of predefined specificity. Nature 256: 495–497, 1975.
2. Sikora K, Lennox ES. Tumour antigens. In Lachmann PJ, Peters DK (eds.), Clinical aspects of immunology. Oxford: Blackwell, 1982.
3. Invernizzi G, and Parmiami G. TSTA's of chemically induced sarcomas cross-react with allogeneic histocompatibility antigens. Nature 254: 713–716, 1975.
4. Sikora K, Koch G, Brenner S, Lennox ES. Partial purification of TSTA from methyl cholanthrene induced murine sarcomas. Br J Cancer 40: 831, 1979.
5. Chism SE, Wallis S, Burton RC, Warner NL. Analysis of immune oncofoetal antigens as tumour associated transplantation antigens. J Immunol 117: 1870–1877, 1976.
6. Lennox ES, Sikora K. Definition of human tumour antigens. In McMichael AJ, Fabre JW (eds.), Monoclonal antibodies in clinical medicine. London: Academic Press, 1982.
7. Sikora K, Wright R. Human monoclonal antibodies to lung cancer antigens. Br J Cancer 43: 696–702, 1981.
8. Yasuda K, Alderson T, Phillips J, Sikora K. The characterisation of infiltrating lymphocytes in malignant glioma. J. Neurol Neurosurg Psychiatry: 46: 734–740, 1983.
9. Sikora K, Neville M. Human monoclonal antibodies. Nature: 316: 300, 1982.
10. Kennett E. Plasmocytoma cell lines. In Kennett, McKearn, Bechtol (eds.), Monoclonal antibodies, New York: Plenum, 1980, p. 364.
11. Gerhard W. Fusion of cells in suspension and outgrowth of hybrids in conditioned medium. Kennett, McKearn, Bechtol (eds.), Monoclonal antibodies. New York: Plenum, 1980, p. 370.
12. Finan PJ, Grant RM, Mattos CD, Takei F, Berry PJ, Lennox E, Bleehen NM. The use of immunohistochemical techniques as an aid in the early screening of monoclonal antibodies. Br J Cancer: 46: 9–17, 1982.
13. Dippold WG, Lloyd KO, Lucy TC, Ikeda H, Oettgen HF, Old LJ. Cell surface antigens of human malignant melanoma: Definition of six antigenic systems with mouse monoclonal antibodies. Proc Natl Acad Sci 77: 6114–6118, 1980.
14. Brown, JP, Woodbury RG, Hart CE, Hellstrom I, Hellstrom KE. Quantitative analysis of melanoma associated antigen p97 in normal and neoplastic tissues. Proc Natl Acad Sci 78: 539–543, 1981.
15. Blom J. Malignant lymphoma. In Bergevin, Blom, and Tormey (eds.), Guide to therapeutic oncology. Baltimore: Williams & Wilkins, 1979, p. 290.
16. Janossy G, Thomas JA, Pizzolo G, Granger SM, McLaughlin J, Habeshaw JA, Stansfeld AG, Sloane J. Immunohistological diagnosis of lymphoproliferative diseases by selected combinations of antisera and monoclonal antibodies. Br J Cancer 42: 224–242, 1980.
17. Tormey DC, Cohen P. Breast cancer. In Bergevin, Blom, and Tormey (eds.), Guide to neoplastic oncology. Baltimore: Williams & Wilkins, 1979, p. 43.

18. Koprowski H, Herlyn M, Steplewski Z, Sears HF. Specific antigen in serum of patients with colon carcinoma. Science 212: 53–54, 1980.
19. Mach JP, Buchegger F, Forni M. Use of radiolabelled monoclonal anti-CEA antibodies for the detection of human carcinomas. Immunol Today 2: 239–249, 1981.
20. Smedley HM, Finan P, Lennox E, Ritson A, Wraight P, Sikora K. Localisation of metastatic carcinoma by a radiolabelled monoclonal antibody. Br J Cancer 286: 262–264, 1983.
21. Epenetos AA, Britton KE, Mather S. Targeting of ^{123}I labelled tumour associated monoclonal antibodies to ovarian, breast and gastrointestinal tumours. Lancet 2: 999–1006, 1982.
22. Larson SM, Brown JP, Wraight PW, Carnosquillo JA, Hellstrom I, Hellstrom KE. Imaging of melanoma with ^{131}I labelled monoclonal antibodies. J Nucl Med 24: 123–129, 1983.
23. Miller RA, Levy R. Response of cutaneous T cell lymphoma to therapy with hybridoma monoclonal antibody. Lancet 2: 226–230, 1981.
24. Ritz J, Pesando JM, Sallan SE, Clavell LA, Notis-McConarty J, Rosenthal P, Schlossman SF. Serotherapy of acute lymphoblastic leukaemia with monoclonal antibody. Blood 58: 361–372, 1981.
25. Dilman RO, Sobol RE, Collins H, Beauregard J, Royston I. T101 monoclonal antibody therapy in chronic lymphocytic leukaemia. In Mitchell MS, Oettgen HF (eds.), Hybridomas in cancer diagnosis and treatment. New York: Raven Press, 1982, pp. 151–1971.
26. Sears HF, Atkinson B, Mattis J, Ernst C, Herlyn D, Steplewski Z, Hayry R, Koprowski H. Phase-I clinical trial of monoclonal antibody in treatment of gastrointestinal tumours. Lancet 1: 762–765, 1982.
27. Sobol RE, Dillman RO, Smith JD, Imai K, Ferrone S, Shawler D, Glassy MC, Royston I. Phase I evaluation of immune monoclonal anti melanoma antibody in man. In Mitchell MS; Oettgen HF (eds.), Hybridoma in cancer diagnosis and treatment. New York: Raven Press, 1982.
28. Miller RA, Maloney DG, Warnke R, Levy R. Treatment of B cell lymphoma with monoclonal anti idiotype antibody. N Eng J Med 306: 517–522, 1982.
29. Watson JV, Alderson T, Sikora K, Phillips J. Subcutaneous culture chamber for continuous infusion of monoclonal antibodies. Lancet 1: 99–100, 1983.
30. Thorpe PE, Edwards DC, Davies AJS, Ross WCJ. Monoclonal antibody—Toxin conjugates: Aiming the magic bullet. In McMichael AJ, Fabre JW (eds.), Monoclonal antibodies in clinical medicine. London: Academic Press, 1982.
31. Buckman R, McIlhinney RA, Sheperd V, Patel S, Coombes RC, Neville AM. Elimination of carcinoma cells from human bone marrow. Lancet 2: 428, 1982.

9. IMMUNOPATHOLOGY OF TUMOURS

J.C.E. UNDERWOOD

N. ROONEY

INTRODUCTION AND HISTORICAL ASPECTS

The cells that participate in immunological and inflammatory reactions are commonly found infiltrating human tumours [1]. This observation has excited much interest because many studies have shown that it has prognostic significance; it has been suggested that the presence of these cells in tumours may therefore reflect some sort of host defense.

Virchow [2] was the first to draw any conclusions from the presence of lymphocytes in tumours: he considered that they indicated previous chronic inflammation at that site, thus reinforcing the popular contemporary hypothesis that chronic inflammation was an important cause of cancer.

The first clue that infiltrates of lymphocytes and related cells might have some functional importance came from the histology of regressing human and animal tumours. Handley [3] concluded that lymphocytic infiltration in malignant melanomas indicated a "regressive process," and Wade [4] poetically described a regressing canine sarcoma being "borne away on a lymphocyte tide." Animal experiments, admittedly not performed with syngeneic strains, seemed to emphasise the importance of lymphocytes in tumour defense; Da Fano's meticulous histological study of tumour grafts in resistant mice led to the conclusion that peritumoural lymphocytes and plasma cells were a hallmark of defensive reaction [5]. At that time, however, the function of lymphocytes was not clearly understood, but it was not long before the immunological significance of these cells was appreciated.

These early experiments in tumour immunology using animal models were largely discredited by Woglom's influential review published in 1929 [6]. Until then all the work had been done with outbred animals; rejection of a tumour transplanted from one animal

B.W. Hancock and A.M. Ward (eds.), Immunological Aspects of Cancer. Copyright © 1985, Martinus Nijhoff Publishing, Boston/Dordrecht/Lancaster.

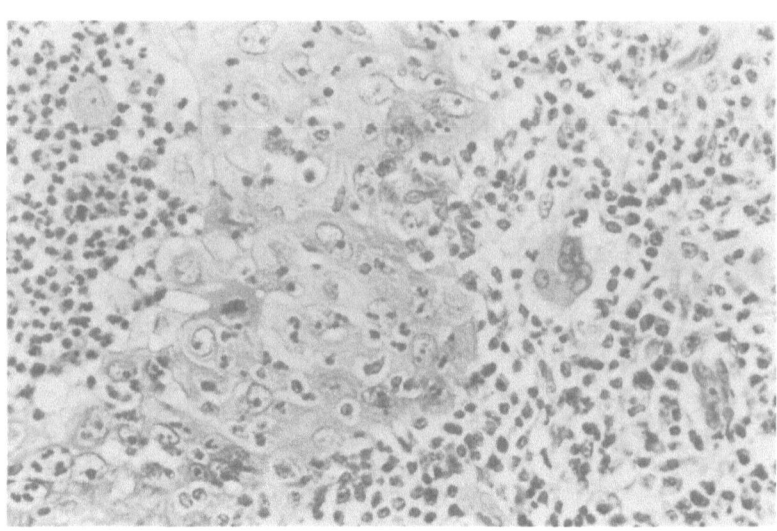

Figure 9-1. Stromal infiltration in a squamous cell carcinoma of cervix. Lymphocytes and plasma cells with a solitary multinucleate giant cell infiltrate the stroma (right); neutrophil polymorphs have infiltrated between tumour cells to reach necrotic area (left). Haematoxylin and eosin × 460.

to another was therefore attributable to individual-specific antigens resident on all cells rather than to tumour-specific antigens peculiar to the cancer cells. Also, with regard to human tumours, several investigators considered that lymphoid cells accumulated in tumours merely in response to necrosis [7]. Interest in tumour immunology waned.

The prognostic advantage allied to lymphocytic infiltration in human tumours, first reported by MacCarty and his collaborators [8,9,10] in carcinomas of breast, stomach, colon, and rectum, remained unarguable however. When Gross [11] and others, using syngeneic mice, unequivocally established the existence of tumour-associated transplantation antigens, interest in the biological significance of the lymphoid cell infiltration in tumours was renewed.

Electron microscopy and other sophisticated techniques had been used to study the immune cells infiltrating rejected grafts of normal tissues, such as kidney, and it seemed wholly appropriate to use these same techniques to examine the infiltrating cells in tumours to see what morphological analogies, if any, could be drawn. More recently, the precise nature of the infiltrating cells has been determined by immunostaining with antibodies to surface markers of lymphocyte subpopulations. Understanding the true nature of the local cellular response to tumours may enable us to modify it to the patient's advantage.

GENERAL FEATURES

The stroma of most nonlymphoid tumours comprises variable proportions of three components: vascular network, fibroblast or myofibroblast framework, and infiltrating lymphoid cells (figure 9-1). The lymphoid infiltrate is seen in several locations: around the periphery of the tumours, either diffusely or around vessels; infiltrating the fibrovascular septa within the tumour; and infiltrating actually among the tumour cells.

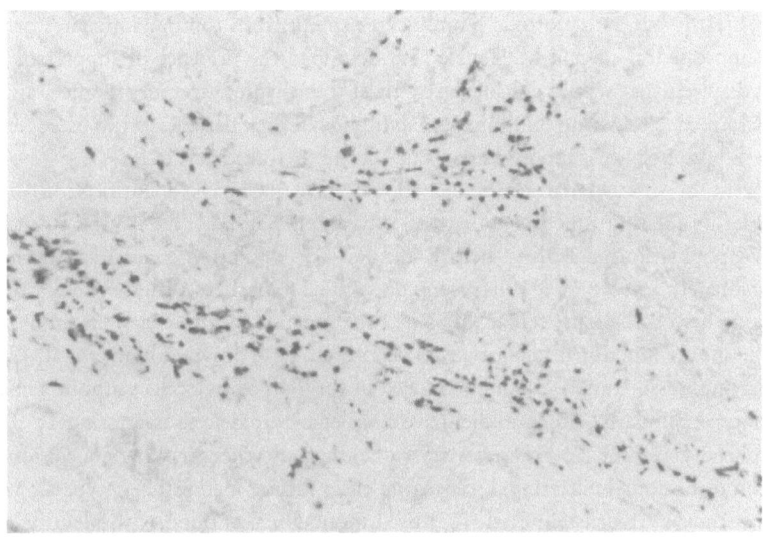

Figure 9-2. T$_{11}$-positive (Pan T) lymphocytes infiltrating the stroma of an invasive ductal adenocarcinoma of the breast. (Positive cells appear black.) Frozen section/immunoperoxidase × 140.

Infiltrates of lymphocytes at the edge of malignant neoplasms often contain venules lined by tall endothelial cells similar to those in the paracortical T-zone of lymph nodes [12]. In lymph nodes much lymphocytic traffic takes place across these venules—lymphocytes enter the node from the blood in this way—and these venules may similarly act as an avenue for lymphocytes to enter tumours.

Ultrastructural studies reveal that some of the infiltrating cells, notably lymphocytes and macrophages, are in intimate contact with tumour cells [13]. The ultrastructural evidence does not, however, point to any cytotoxic consequences of these interactions.

COMPOSITION OF TUMOUR INFILTRATES

Before considering the cellular infiltrate in terms of the different cell types involved, it must be emphasised at the outset that no consistent features have been identified: the composition of the infiltrate varies from one tumour to another even within the same histogenetic type and sometimes within different regions of a single tumour. In some tumours, lymphocytes predominate, in others plasma cells, and so forth. Within this variation there may be an element of consistency, but it has yet to be determined. We shall concentrate on observations made on human tumours.

Lymphocytes

Lymphocytic infiltration of tumours is a common phenomenon and has been associated with improved prognosis (figure 9-2). Numerous studies on peripheral blood lymphocytes from tumour-bearing animals and humans have revealed circulating lymphocytes with specific cytotoxicity toward autologous tumour cells [14,15]. Are specific cytotoxic lymphocytes present in the local cellular reaction to a tumour? Most investigators agree that the cytotoxic activity of lymphocytes extracted from tumours is lower than that in the peripheral blood [16,17,18]; but are cytotoxic lymphocytes absent from tumour infiltrates or is their function suppressed? Lala and McKenzie [19] described the presence of suppressor cells in thymus and spleen that would enhance growth of transplanted tumours in mice, and Yu et al. [20] described circulating inhibitory T-lymphocytes in patients with osteogenic sarcoma; these lymphocytes suppressed tumour-specific cytotoxicity.

The advent of monoclonal antibodies should have made the identification of T-cell subsets easier by relating function to surface-antigen phenotype. This is valid to the extent that the T4 population generally "helps" and the T8 population generally "suppresses," but, unfortunately, cytotoxic T-cells also express the T8 marker. Whether these two functions go together on the same cell at the same time remains controversial. As more research is done, the simple functional-phenotype relationship breaks down. Thomas et al. [21] have shown that suppressor function can be induced in the T4 positive cells without a change in their phenotype. Similarly, clonal studies have revealed cytotoxic cells expressing T_8^+ T_4^- and T_8^- T_4^+ phenotypes [22]. So it is necessary to be cautious when drawing conclusions about the function of tumour-infiltrating T-cells from their surface marker phenotype alone.

A recent study by Kornstein et al. [23] used monoclonal antibodies to identify, in situ, T-cell subsets infiltrating melanocytic lesions. They found a mixed population of T4 and T8 positive cells in both naevi and malignant melanoma with no obvious difference between them. We have obtained similar results from a wide range of human epithelial malignant neoplasms [24]. Interpretation of the results must be done with caution, since although monoclonal antibodies are raised against specific T-cell components, the same epitope may be expressed on another cell, particularly in malignancy. Kornstein et al. [23] found staining of melanoma cells with T4 antibody in two cases and B1 antibody in one case. In general, T4-positive cells exceed T8-positive cells in tumour infiltrates.

In recent years most work has concentrated on the T-lymphocyte and its subclasses. B-lymphocytes are also found in tumours but tend to occur in aggregates at the edge of the lesion, unlike T-cells, which can often be found penetrating between the tumour cells [24,25].

Monoclonal antibodies have been available for only a relatively short time. As the original clones are replaced by new ones, new specificities will emerge, and it may yet be possible to identify functionally important lymphocyte subgroups infiltrating tumours.

Macrophages

Macrophages may be abundant in tumours; in animal tumours up to 40% of the cells may be infiltrating macrophages [26]. They are relatively inconspicuous on light microscopy unless they are detected histochemically or by immunostaining for markers of mononuclear phagocytes such as lysozyme or α_1-antitrypsin. The macrophages in tumours are often mature cells, large and rich in primary lysosomes, with undulating plasma membranes. Electron microscopy of animal and human tumours has disclosed frequent apposition between macrophages and tumour cells, but rarely is evidence seen that might be interpreted as indicating cytotoxic consequences except in animal models where tumour growth is retarded or reversed by immunological manipulation [27].

Macrophage-derived epithelioid cells or polykaryons (giant cells) are a very occasional feature in human tumours, and in the latter instance may be simply a phagocytic reaction, for example, to dead cells or keratin. Stromal granulomas are uncommon except in seminomas; granulomas in regional nodes are similarly rare [28]. This may be a sarcoid tissue reaction to the presence of tumour.

Interest in the macrophages infiltrating tumours may be rekindled by the recognition that these cells may have natural cytotoxic activity similar to that of natural killer cells.

Natural killer cells

Cells capable of killing tumour cells without prior antigenic stimulation are now attracting much attention [29]. The discovery of these "natural killer" (NK) cells aroused interest because of their possible role in surveillance against neoplasia. However, the precise lineage of NK-cells remains uncertain, largely because the surface markers on which many cell lines are defined are variable. A recent study by Abo et al. [30] highlighted this problem by identifying in humans phenotypic, morphological, and functional changes in NK-cells in all lymphoid compartments from the fetus to the adult. Functionally mature NK-cells were found in largest numbers in adult peripheral blood and spleen and morphologically corresponded to the large granular lymphocyte described in previous studies. Cells from other compartments (lymph node and bone marrow) in the adult had lower NK activity. Furthermore, cells that are obviously macrophages also have "natural killer" activity. At a recent workshop [31] the following definition was agreed: "NK cells are effector cells with spontaneous cytotoxicity against various target cells; these cells lack the properties of classical macrophages granulocytes and cytotoxic T-lymphocytes and the observed cytotoxicity does not show restriction mediated by the major histocompatibility complex."

What is the role of the NK-cells in vivo? By injecting a cloned cell line with NK activity into mice deficient in NK-cells, Warner and Dennert [32] have shown that NK-cells can reject allogeneic bone marrow grafts, reduce the incidence of lung metastases from implanted tumour, and reduce the incidence of radiation-induced thymomas.

In humans the role of the NK-cells has not been investigated as thoroughly for obvious reasons. Most work has been done on the NK activity of peripheral blood lymphocytes and lymphocytes extracted from tumours. There are major differences between the two sources. Whereas peripheral blood cells may have detectable and enhanceable NK activity, tumour-infiltrating cells have low levels of activity unaffected by interferon [33,34,35]. The mixing of tumour-infiltrating cells with peripheral blood cells does not affect the NK activity of the latter; this suggests that low NK function is not due to the presence of suppressor lymphocytes but to either suppression of function by tumour products or failure of infiltration by NK-cells. The latter possibility was explored by Intona et al. [36], who found low numbers of morphologically and phenotypically (HNK1 +) defined NK-cells. It does not, of course, exclude the possibility that morphology and phenotype may change along with the suppression of function. In contrast to this, Gremin et al. found that tumour-infiltrating cells did suppress the NK activity of peripheral blood cells [33]. Obviously the situation is not resolved. It seems likely that once a primary tumour has become established, the NK-cell has ceased to have significant local effects; but it may well be important in the control of metastasis.

Polymorphonuclear leukocytes

The presence of neutrophil polymorphs in malignant neoplasms is assumed, with some justification, to be of little consequence because these cells quite probably appear simply in in response to the necrosis commonly seen in tumours. In any cytotoxic immunological reaction against a tumour, they probably scavenge dead or dying cells killed by other effector cells.

Eosinophil polymorph infiltration in tumours is less frequently encountered but is generally acknowledged to have prognostic significance. Paradoxically, eosinophilia in the blood of cancer patients is an ominous sign [37], whereas stromal eosinophilia denotes a favorable prognosis for most tumour types [38]—though there are exceptions, such as has been found in some studies on cervical carcinoma [39].

Recruitment of eosinophils into the stroma of tumours may accompany mast cell degranulation; mast cells produce an eosinophil chemotactic factor. Mast cell infiltration is, however, often negligible; in a few instances it has been shown that the tumour cells themselves directly recruit eosinophils by producing a similar chemotactic factor [40]. Alternatively, eosinophil infiltration may accompany a T-cell-mediated immune reaction.

Mast cells

Mast cells are infrequently mentioned in descriptions of the cellular infiltrate in tumours, probably because they are inconspicuous in sections conventionally stained with haematoxylin and eosin. Special staining methods are usually required to see the characteristic cytoplasmic granules that enable their identification. Mast cells are, however, commonly present in human tumours, though rarely in large numbers. They tend to be more numerous at the tumour edge than within the stroma, and the overall mast cell content is, with few exceptions, less than that of the normal parent tissue [41].

Their presence in cervical carcinomas has been found to be correlated positively with prognosis [42]; these authors speculated that heparin from the mast cells might retard the growth of the tumour cells.

Langerhans' cells

The monocyte-macrophage system is widely distributed around the body and has been ascribed many functions—from phagocytosis of particulate matter to inducing B- and T-lymphocyte proliferation. In the epidermis there is a population of macrophagelike cells—Langerhans' cells (LC)—characterised by the presence of intracytoplasmic Birbeck granules. They are present in all layers of the epidermis and send out dendritic processes between the keratinocytes. Langerhans' cells can also be detected in dermal lymphatics and in the sinuses of regional lymph nodes. Evidence that they have a central role in immunological reactions involving the skin is well documented [43]. LC pick up antigenic material in the epidermis and convey it to local nodes by migrating along the dermal lymphatics. Whether LC act as antigen-presenting cells or pass the material on to other nodal dendritic cells is debatable. The fate of LC once they reach the local node is similarly not known.

LC are not found only in cutaneous squamous epithelium but also in the mouth and in the oesophagus. They have also been reported in experimentally induced squamous metaplasia. It has been shown in animals that LC are derived from monocytes, and it seems likely that contact with squamous epithelium is the stimulus to differentiation. It is not surprising, therefore, to find LC in the neoplasms derived from squamous epithelium [44,45] (figure 9–3), in a pleomorphic salivary adenoma with squamous metaplasia, and in a tera-

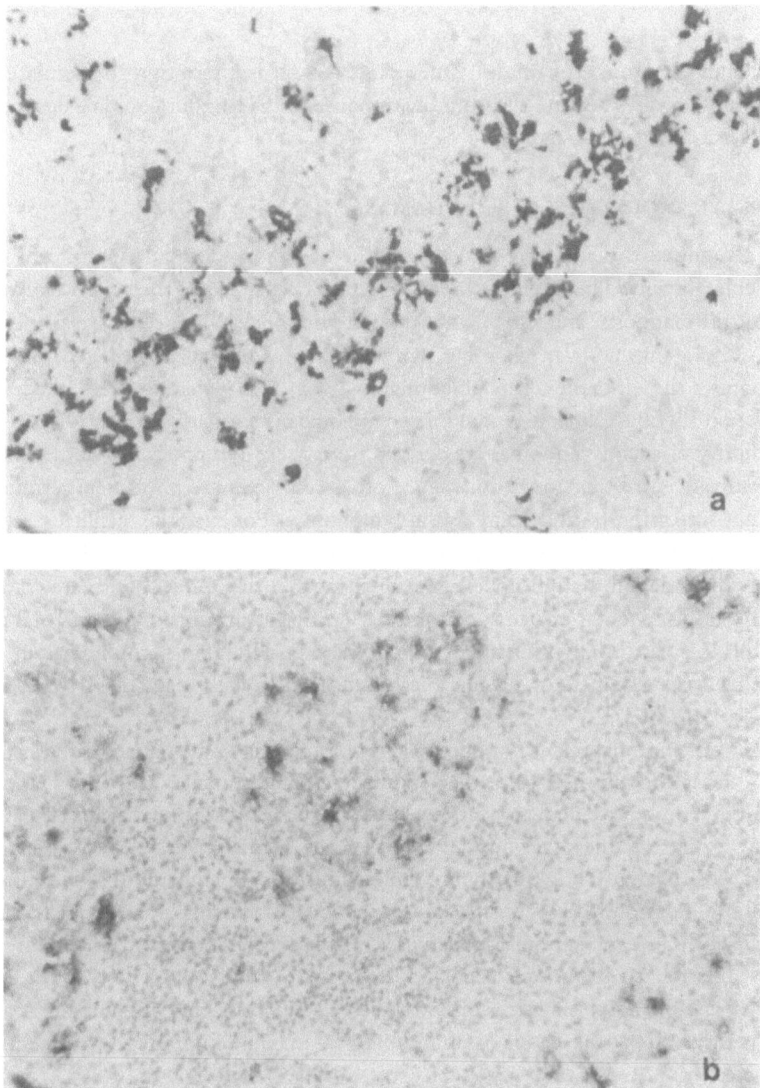

Figure 9–3. T_6-positive (Langerhans' cells) in squamous cell carcinomas:

(**A**) invasive squamous cell carcinoma of cervix;

(**B**) lymph node metastasis in which T_6-positive cells are typically restricted to the islands of carcinoma. Frozen sections/immunoperoxidase. (**A**) × 360 (**B**) × 288.

toma containing stratified squamous tissue [24,46,47]. It is interesting to speculate on the role of LC in such cases because the immune response to the tumour could be dependent on the presence of intratumoural LC.

REACTIVE LYMPHOID CELLS IN LYMPHOMAS

It is well recognised that in Hodgkin's disease there is a mixed population of cells causing the nodal enlargement. These cells include the Reed-Sternberg cell, the presence of which is essential for the diagnosis, and variable numbers of lymphocytes. Indeed the classification of Hodgkin's disease into nodular sclerosing, lymphocyte predominant or depleted, and mixed-types recognises the different cell populations involved. It is generally overlooked that the cell population involved in non-Hodgkin's lymphomas is similarly mixed.

The majority of such lymphomas are derived from the B-lymphocyte at some stage during its germinal-centre transformation. Since other cell types are present in germinal centres, it is not surprising to find them also in lymphomas. For example, dendritic reticulum cells are found surrounding the B-cells in normal germinal centres; they are also found in follicular lymphomas, in lymph nodes, and in extranodal sites [48]. T-cells are commonly found in B-cell lymphomas and may comprise a significant proportion of the total cellular content [49]. It is particularly interesting to note that non-Hodgkin's lymphomas are unique in containing large numbers of phenotypically and functionally defined NK-cells [50,51] (figure 9–4).

The role of the nonmalignant lymphoid cell in lymphoma tissue remains subject to speculation. In Hodgkin's disease, since the lymphocyte-predominant form has a better prognosis than the lymphocyte-depleted variety, it would be heuristically attractive to attribute a protective role of the lymphocytes against the "malignant" Reed-Sternberg or Hodgkin's cells. In non-Hodgkin's lymphoma it must be remembered that T-cells can induce B-cell proliferation, so we must be cautious about attributing a protective function or a neoplastic label. The presence of natural killer cells in lymphomas is extremely interesting and needs to be related to tumour type and prognosis.

Functional and phenotypic analysis of lymphoid-cell subgroups in lymphoma is at an early stage but perhaps offers some hope of immunological manipulation in the treatment of this form of cancer.

PROGNOSTIC SIGNIFICANCE

The positive correlation between cellular infiltrates in tumours and good prognosis stimulated much of the research into the significance of the phenomenon. MacCarty and his colleagues first noted the association in a study of breast and gastric carcinomas [8,9,10]. The correlation between infiltration and prognosis has been variously confirmed or refuted for these tumours and others [1,52]. Medullary breast carcinomas and seminomas of the testis are both characterised by dense stromal infiltrates, sometimes granulomatous in the latter instance, and a remarkably good prognosis. Precisely how this prognostic benefit is mediated remains uncertain, and a direct causal relationship remains unestablished.

In some of these studies, which particular cell type is being assessed is not always clear and the rather nondescript "round cell" or "mononuclear cell" features all too frequently

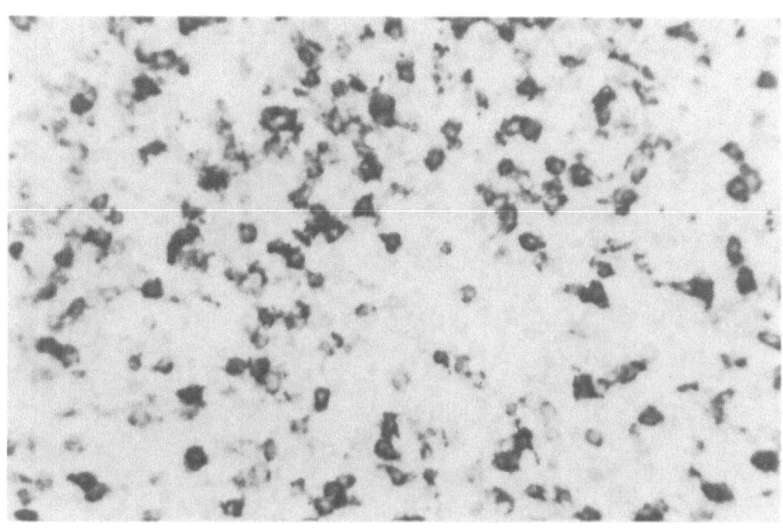

Figure 9-4. Leu-7 positive (NK) cells in a follicle centre cell lymphoma. Many cells in B-cell lymphomas are not B-lymphocytes. Frozen section/immunoperoxidase × 460.

in early reports. Lymphocytes are certainly the most prominent cell on routine light microscopy; plasma cells [53] and eosinophils [54] are also variously recorded as prognostically significant. Mast cells and macrophages will be revealed only by special techniques, so these cells are rarely mentioned except when they have been deliberately sought out [42,55]. Now that lymphocyte subpopulations can be identified by monoclonal antibodies (subject to certain caveats described earlier) it is likely that attempts will be made to link their presence in tumour infiltrates to the clinical behaviour of the lesions.

The favorable prognostic association is not absolutely consistent, however, and the published data may be biased toward a positive correlation because of the reluctance of authors and editors to publish negative results. Particularly interesting in this regard is a simultaneous study from Britain, Japan, and the United States in which an inconsistent correlation between infiltration and prognosis was found in breast carcinomas from the three centres [56].

NODAL REACTIONS

Reactive changes in regional lymph nodes (e.g., follicular hyperplasia, sinus histiocytosis, paracortical expansion) may be either an immunologically specific response to tumour antigens, a reaction to secondary infection, or a consequence of tumour necrosis (figure 9-5).

Black et al. [57] studied Halsted's observation that reactive changes in the axillary lymph nodes of women with breast cancer correlated with prolonged survival after mastectomy: sinus histiocytosis was the most significant feature. Since then many investigations on this theme have been published and the consensus has been reviewed recently by Brynes et

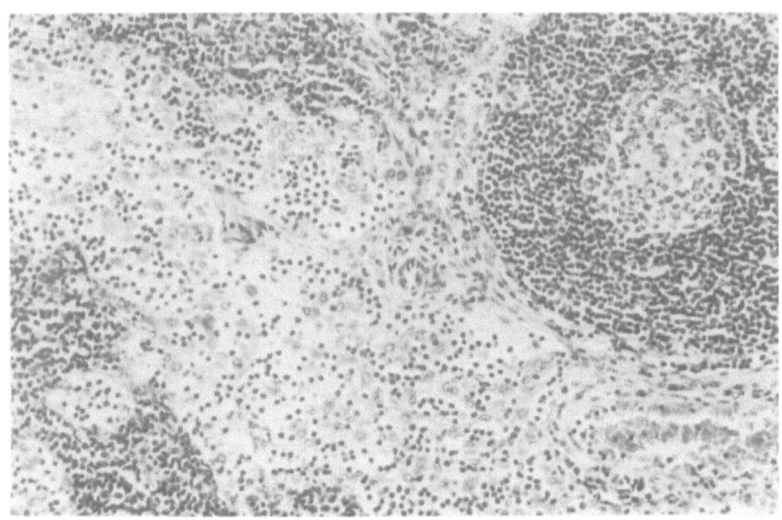

Figure 9-5. Sinus histiocytosis in lymph node draining a carcinoma of breast. In addition to histiocytes, the sinus contains numerous lymphocytes. A lymphoid follicle (top right) contains a small germinal centre. Haematoxylin and eosin × 288.

al. [58]; they commend the classification system of Tsakraklides et al. [59]—lymphocyte predominance (sometimes with sinus histiocytosis), germinal-centre predominance, lymphocyte-depletion, and unstimulated. With most tumour types, lymphocyte predominance in regional nodes is associated with a better prognosis; lymphocyte depletion or an unstimulated pattern often heralds a poor prognosis.

The phenomenon of sinus histiocytosis in nodes-draining breast cancers has been reexamined recently by Fisher et al. [60], who conclude that the observation has no significant association with survival. On the other hand, there seems to be a correlation between the morphology of lymph-nodes-draining breast cancers and the in vitro cytotoxicity of the nodal lymphoid cells to breast cancer target cells [61]: high cytotoxicity levels were exhibited by cells from lymph nodes showing sinus histiocytosis; low levels of cytotoxicity were associated with germinal-centre hyperplasia. A similar study, done with lymph-nodes-draining colorectal carcinomas, found a correlation between sinus histiocytosis and cytotoxicity [62]. Lymph nodes bearing metastatic breast cancer contain a higher proportion of B-lymphocytes than uninvolved nodes [63].

The combination of perivascular lymphocyte cuffing near the primary tumour and paracortical hyperplasia in regional lymph nodes appears to be prognostically advantageous in patients with Dukes's B colorectal carcinomas [64].

Very occasionally sarcoidlike lesions are seen in nodes draining cancers [28]. Insufficient cases have been studied for any significant prognostic conclusions to be drawn.

CONCLUSIONS

Patients whose tumours are densely infiltrated by lymphocytes and related cells tend to survive longer than patients whose tumours lack infiltrates or bear sparse infiltrates. The composition of the infiltrates is variable and includes a wide range of cell types—helper and suppressor/cytotoxic T-lymphocytes, B-lymphocytes, NK-cells, monocytes/macrophages, mast cells, and, in some squamous epithelial tumours, Langerhans' cells. Although close contact often occurs between these defensive cells and tumour cells, there is as yet no clear evidence of direct cytotoxicity.

Reactive changes are often seen in lymph-nodes-draining tumours, and there is a slight positive correlation between certain features and prognosis. Assessment of the lymphoid cell infiltrate in tumours enables histopathologists to obtain prognostically useful information even though how the effect on survival is mediated is not yet known precisely.

Despite the frequency and density of lymphoid cell infiltration in a wide variety of tumours and the repeatedly confirmed prognostic advantage, we are only beginning to understand the real signifiance of the phenomenon. Now that monoclonal antibodies are being used to identify precisely the infiltrating cells, we may be able to draw more coherent conclusions about their immunological role. Advances in our understanding of tumour munology in general may enable us to augment the cellular reaction in the stroma of tumours to the patient's advantage.

REFERENCES

1. Underwood JCE. Lymphoreticular infiltration in human tumours: Prognostic and biological implications: A review. Brit J Cancer 30: 538–548, 1974.
2. Virchow R. Krankhaften Geschwülste. Berlin, 1863.
3. Handley WS. The pathology of melanotic growths in relation to their operative treatment. Lancet 1: 927–933, 1907.
4. Wade H. An experimental investigation of infective sarcoma in the dog, with a consideration of its relationship to cancer. J Pathol Bact 12: 384–425, 1908.
5. Da Fano C. A cytological analysis of the reaction in animals resistant to implanted carcinomata. Fifth Sci Rep Imp Cancer Res Fund, 57–78, 1912.
6. Woglom WH. Immunity to transplantable tumours. Cancer Rev 4: 129–214, 1929.
7. Dawson EK, Tod MC. Prognosis in mammary carcinoma in relation to grading and treatment. Edin Med J 41: 61–98, 1934.
8. MacCarty WC. Factors which influence longevity in cancer. Ann Surg 76: 9–12, 1922.
9. MacCarty WC, Mahle AE. Relation of differentiation and lymphocytic infiltration to postoperative longevity in gastric carcinoma. J Lab Clin Med 6: 473–480, 1921.
10. Sistrunk WE, MacCarty WC. Life expectancy following radical amputation for carcinoma of the breast: A clinical and pathologic study of 218 cases. Ann Surg 75: 61–69, 1922.
11. Gross L. Intradermal immunization of C3H mice against a sarcoma that originated in an animal of the same line. Cancer Res 13: 835–837, 1943.
12. Freemont AJ. The small blood vessels in areas of lymphocytic infiltration around malignant neoplasms. Brit J Cancer 46: 283–288, 1982.
13. Underwood JCE, Carr I. The ultrastructure of the lymphoreticular cells in nonlymphoid human neoplasms. Virchows Arch Abt B Zellpath 12: 39–50, 1972.
14. Hellstrom KE, Hellstrom I. Cellular immunity against tumour antigens. Adv Cancer Res 12: 167–223, 1969.
15. Fossati G, Canevari S, Della Parta G. Cellular immunity to human breast carcinoma. Int J Cancer 10: 391–396, 1972.

16. Kaszubowski PA, Husby G, Tung KSK, Williams RC Jr. T-lymphocyte subpopulations in peripheral blood and tissues of cancer patients. Cancer Res 40: 4643–4657, 1980.
17. Vose BM, Gallagher P, Moore M, Schofield PF. Specific and non-specific lymphocyte cytotoxicity in colon carcinoma. Brit J Cancer 44: 846–855, 1981.
18. Hutchinson GH, Heinemann D, Symes MO, Williamson RCN. Differential immune reactivity of tumour intrinsic and peripheral-blood lymphocytes against autoplastic colorectal carcinoma cells. Brit J Cancer 44: 396–402, 1981.
19. Lala PK, McKenzie IFC. An analysis of T lymphocyte subsets in tumour-transplanted mice on the basis of Lyt antigenic markers and functions. Immunol 47: 663–667, 1982.
20. Yu A, Watts H, Jaffe N, Parkman R. Concomitant presence of tumour-specific cytotoxic and inhibitor lymphocytes in patients with osteogenic sarcoma. N Engl J Med 297: 122–127, 1977.
21. Thomas Y, Rogogwiki L, Irgojen OH. Functional analysis of T cell subsets defined by monoclonal antibodies. IV. Induction of suppressor cells within the OKT$_4$ population. J Exp Med 154: 459–467, 1981.
22. Moretta L, Mirigani MC, Sekaly PR, Moretta A, Chapuis B, Ceroltine JC. Surface markers of cloned human T cells with various cytolytic activities. J Exp Med 154: 569–574, 1981.
23. Kornstein MJ, Brooks JSJ, Elder DE. Immunoperoxidase localisation of lymphocyte subsets in the host response to melanoma and nevi. Cancer Res 43: 2749–2753, 1983.
24. Rooney N, Day CA, Underwood JCE. Identification of the cells infiltrating human tumours using monoclonal antibodies. J Pathol 141: 525, 1983.
25. Shimokawara I, Imanwa M, Yamanaka N, Ishii Y, Kckuchi K. Identification of lymphocyte subpopulations in human breast cancer tissue and its significance. Cancer 49: 1456–1464, 1982.
26. Alexander P, Eccles SA, Gauci CL. The significance of macrophages in human and experimental tumours. Ann NY Acad Sci 276: 124–133, 1976.
27. Carr I, Underwood JCE, McGinty F, Wood P. The ultrastructure of the local lymphoreticular response to an experimental neoplasm. J Pathol 113: 175–182, 1974.
28. Gresham GA, Ackerley AG: Giant cell granulomata in regional lymph nodes of carcinoma. J Clin Pathol 11: 244–250, 1958.
29. Herberman RB (ed.). NK and other effector cells. New York: Academic Press, 1982.
30. Abo T, Miller CA, Gartland L, Balch CM. Differentiation stages of human natural killer cells in lymphoid tissue from fetal to adult life. J Exp Med 157: 273–284, 1983.
31. Koren HS, Herberman RB. Natural killing—Present and future. J Natl Cancer Inst 70: 785–786, 1983.
32. Warner JF, Dennert G. Effect of a clonal cell line with NK activity on bone marrow transplants, tumour development and metastasis in vivo. Nature 300: 31–34, 1982.
33. Gremin O, Coombs RRA, Ashby J. Lymphocytes infiltrating human breast cancer lack K activity and have low levels of NK cell activity. Br J Cancer 44: 166–176, 1981.
34. Moore M, Vose BM. Extravascular natural cytotoxicity in man: Anti K562 activity of lymph node and tumour infiltrating lymphocytes. Int J Cancer 27: 265–272, 1981.
35. Dehandazuri MO, Lopez-Botet M, Timonen T, Ortaldo JR, Herberman RB. Human large granular lymphocytes: Spontaneous and interferon boosted NK activity against adherent and nonadherent tumour cell lines. J Immunol 127: 1380–1383, 1981.
36. Introna M, Allavena P, Biardi A, Colombo N, Villa A, Montovani A. Defective natural killer activity within human ovarian tumours: Low numbers of morphologically defined effectors in situ. J Natl Cancer Inst 70: 21–27, 1983.
37. Lowe D, Jorizzo J, Hutt MSR. Tumour-associated eosinophilia: A review. J Clin Pathol 34: 1343–1348, 1981.
38. Yoon IL. The eosinophil and gastrointestinal carcinoma. Am J Surg 97: 195–200, 1959.
39. Bostrom SG, Hart WR. Carcinomas of the cervix with intense stromal eosinophilia. Cancer 47: 2887–2893, 1981.
40. Wasserman SI, Goetzl EJ, Ellman L, Austen FK. Tumour-associated eosinophilotactic factor. N Engl J Med 290: 420–424, 1974.
41. Lascano EF. Mast cells in human tumours. Cancer 11: 1110–1114, 1958.
42. Graham RM, Graham JB. Mast cells and cancer of the cervix. Surg Gynec Obstet 123: 3–9, 1966.
43. Balfour BM, Drexhage HA, Kamperdijke EWA, Hoefsmit ELM. Antigen presenting cells, including Langerhans' cells, veiled cells and interdigitating cells cells. In Microenvironments in haemopoietic and lymphoid differentiation. Ciba Foundation Symposium No. 84, p. 281–301, Pitman Medical, 1981.
44. Schenk P. Langerhans' cells in invasive laryngeal carcinoma. Laryngo Rhinol Otol 59: 232–237, 1980.
45. Löning T, Caselitz J, Seifert G, Weber K, Osborn M. Identification of Langerhans' cells: Simultaneous use of sera to intermediate filaments, T6 and HLA-DR antigens on oral mucosa, human epidermis and their tumours. Virchows Arch (Pathol Anat) 398: 119–128, 1982.

46. Raffade D, Buchner A. Langerhans' cells in a pleomorphic adenoma of submandibular salivary gland. J Pathol 131: 127–135, 1980.
47. Flotte TJ, Bell DA. Langerhans' cells in ovarian benign cystic teratomas. Lab Invest 42: 117, 1980.
48. Naiem M, Gerdes J, Abdulaziz Z, Stein H, Mason DY. Production of a monoclonal antibody reactive with human dendritic reticulum cells and its use in the immunohistological analysis of lymphoid tissue. J Clin Pathol 36: 167–175, 1983.
49. Habeshaw JA, Bailey D, Stansfeld AG, Greaves MF. The cellular content on non-Hodgkin lymphomas: A comprehensive analysis using monoclonal antibodies and other surface marker techniques. Brit J Cancer 47: 327–351, 1983.
50. Banerjee D, and Thibert RF. Natural killer-like cells found in B-cell compartments of human lymphoid tissues. Nature 304: 270–272, 1983.
51. Mari S, Mohri N, Movita H, Yamagashi K, Shimenwie T. The distribution of cells expressing a natural killer cell marker (HNK1) in normal human lymphoid organs and malignant lymphomas. Virchows Arch B (Cell Pathol) 43: 253–263, 1983.
52. Haskill S. Some historical perspectives on the relationship between survival and mononuclear cell infiltration. In Haskill S (ed.), Tumour immunity in prognosis: The role of mononuclear cell infiltration. New York and Basel: Dekker, 1982, pp. 1–10.
53. Berg JW. Inflammation and prognosis in breast cancer: A search for host resistance. Cancer 12: 714–720, 1959.
54. Pretlow TP, Keith EF, Cryar AK, Bartolucci AA, Pitts AM, Pretlow TG, Kimball PM, Boohaker EA. Eosinophil infiltration of human colonic carcinomas as a prognostic indicator. Cancer Res 43: 2997–3000, 1983.
55. Lauder I, Aherne W, Stewart J, Gainsbury R. Macrophage infiltration of breast tumours: A prospective study. J Clin Pathol 30: 563–568, 1977.
56. Morrison AS, Black MM, Lowe CR, MacMahon B, Yuasa S. Some international differences in histology and survival in breast cancer. Int J Cancer 11: 261–267, 1973.
57. Black MM, Kerpe S, Speer FD. Lymph node structure in patients with cancer of the breast. Am J Pathol 29: 505–521, 1953.
58. Brynes RK, Hunter RL, Vellios E. Immunomorphologic changes in regional lymph nodes associated with cancer. Arch Pathol Lab Med 107: 217–221, 1983.
59. Tsakraklides V, Anastassiades OT, Kersey JH. Prognostic significance of regional lymph node histology in uterine cervical cancer. Cancer 31: 860–868, 1973.
60. Fisher ER, Kotwal N, Hermann C, Fisher B. Types of tumour lymphoid response and sinus histiocytosis: Relationship to five-year, disease-free survival in patients with breast cancer. Arch Pathol Lab Med 107: 222–227, 1983.
61. Check IJ, Cobb M, Hunter RL. The relationship between cytotoxicity and prognostically significant histologic changes in lymph nodes from patients with cancer of the breast. Am J Pathol 98: 325–338, 1980.
62. Pihl E, Nairn RC, Nind AP, Muller K, Hughes ESR, Cuthbertson AM, Rollo AJ. Correlation of regional lymph node in vitro antitumour immunoreactivity histology with colorectal carcinoma. Cancer Res 36: 3665–3671, 1976.
63. Eremin O, Roberts P, Plumb D, Stephens JP. Human regional tumour lymph nodes: Alterations of microarchitecture and lymphocyte subpopulations. Brit J Cancer 41: 62–72, 1980.
64. Pihl E, Malahy MA, Khankhanian N, Hersh EM, Marligit GM. Immunomorphologic features of prognostic significance in Dukes' class B colorectal carcinoma. Cancer Res 37: 4145–4149, 1977.

10. IMMUNOLOGICAL LYMPHOCYTE MARKERS IN LYMPHOID NEOPLASIA

J.S. LILLEYMAN
R.F. HINCHLIFFE

INTRODUCTION

Over the last decade or so the classification of the lymphocyte-related leukaemias and lymphomas has been expanded from being an essentially clinical and morphological exercise to one for which more sophisticated cell recognition systems are employed. Such systems involve the identification of so-called immunological "markers," which are chemical structures found on or in normal lymphocytes reflecting their stage of maturation or differentiation. These structures are not, as was initially thought in some cases, indicative of malignancy as such and do not represent tumour-specific phenomena, but may only be present in very few normal cells.

Markers are identified in three basic ways: by their capability of attaching themselves to a miscellany of specific structures (such as sheep or mouse erythrocytes or the Fc portion of human immunoglobulin); by their antigenicity, which is recognised by an appropriate antibody; or if they happen to be enzymes, by their bioactivity. Antibodies used to identify marker antigens are either oligoclonal absorbed heterologous antisera, usually from rabbits [1] or, more commonly in recent years, murine and other monoclonal antibodies made by the hybridoma technique. As the number of monoclonal antibodies is rapidly increasing and potentially limitless, not surprisingly, an already bewildering variety from both academic and commercial sources have become available. Some show similar and well-documented specificity, others less so. Nomenclature has also been confusing, as coded names for antibodies have not done more than hint at what their specificity might be. The nonexpert might be forgiven, for instance, for failing to realise immediately that OKT1 (OKT series: Ortho Diagnostic Systems Limited); Leu – 1 (Leu series: Becton Dickinson & Co. Labora-

B.W. Hancock and A.M. Ward (eds.), Immunological Aspects of Cancer. Copyright © 1985, Martinus Nijhoff Publishing, Boston/Dordrecht/Lancaster.

tory Systems); 17F12, T101 (Hybridtech Inc.); 10.2 (Lyt − 2) (Lyt series: New England Nuclear); SC1, and A50 all recognise the same antigen found on T-lymphocytes and thymocytes [2].

There are two approaches to the use of markers in oncology: first, the classification of new or untried markers and the definition of their distribution in known tumours, and second, the use of established markers to classify unrecognisable lymphocyte neoplasia. Importantly, these two approaches must not be confused, otherwise both missile and target become unknowns and sensible conclusions become impossible. Most service laboratories will be interested only in the second, the use of established techniques to aid classification of undefined lymphoproliferative diseases. For this reason, this chapter will not dwell further on exhaustive lists of marker techniques that are either not widely available, have not had their specificity determined, or do not yet provide relevant information to the clinician. It will instead concentrate on the more tried and trusted techniques that are relatively easy to use and can be undertaken in most laboratories without great expense or sophisticated equipment.

The first section will deal with the actual techniques involved, and the second will examine the patterns of results found in the lymphoid leukaemias and lymphomas, their frequencies, and their clinical significance.

LYMPHOCYTE MARKER METHODOLOGY

The theory and practice of marker technology has recently been reviewed in detail [3]. The techniques involved have been described in the literature with an often bewildering range of variations, and so precise details of methodology are not given here. Those interested in introducing such techniques are advised to try several and use those that best fit their purpose; our experience has been that complex modifications are unnecessary, providing care is taken with such simple, but important, procedures as thorough washing and gentle resuspension of cells.

At present the most important piece of equipment in this type of work is the fluorescence microscope. A number of very good models are available incorporating incident light excitation, which has several advantages [3]. Although scoring of fluorescence-labeled material can be tedious, it has the great advantage, when combined with phase contrast, of allowing the experienced observer to detect contaminating nonlymphoid cells and concentrate on the cells of interest. With increasing use of immunoenzyme techniques, however, a fluorescence microscope may become less essential. Monoclonal antibody methodologies usually recommend that cells are washed at 4°C in a refrigerated centrifuge, but this also may not be essential.

A problem in smaller laboratories is that some time may pass in which no patients present for investigation, during which time reagent deterioration can occur. We have found it useful to study cells from normal persons on a regular basis, a practice that largely overcomes this problem and simultaneously allows the laboratory to build up its own normal range.

Sample requirements

In the acute leukaemias, bone marrow is the sample of choice. Most cases show gross infiltration (i.e., a "pure" population), whereas peripheral blood may have relatively few blast cells and contamination with circulating normal lymphocytes will occur. In chronic lymphoid leukaemias, on the other hand, with a high peripheral count, the great majority of cells will belong to the malignant clone and blood samples are acceptable. When the lymphocyte count is low and normal cells are likely to be present, double staining techniques can be used to identify, for example, B-cells by their HLA-DR positivity combined with specific antikappa and antilambda reagents to search for monoclonality. Alternatively, antikappa and antilambda reagents, labeled with different fluorochromes, can be used in the same tube.

Separation of mononuclear cells

Mononuclear cells are usually separated on Ficoll-Isopaque following the method devised by Boyum [4]. A number of commercial preparations are available, but the reagent is easily prepared [3]. Small volumes of marrow collected into a culture medium need no further dilution; blood with a normal leucocyte count is diluted 1 in 3, and samples with high counts should be diluted to bring the count down to $<20 \times 10^9/l$. Occasional samples contain a proportion of light density red cells; a reagent containing a red cell aggregant such as Lympho-paque (Nyegaard) may overcome this problem. Other technical problems, including the identification of monocytes in the mononuclear preparation, are discussed by Aiuti et al. [5]. It is important at some point after the separation step to determine the viability (e.g., with trypan blue) and the purity (by cytocentrifugation) of the test population; viability of blood and marrow cells should be $>90\%$ but is likely to be lower in suspensions produced from lymph nodes.

Sheep erythrocyte rosette technique

The ability of a large proportion of peripheral blood lymphocytes to form rosettes with sheep erythrocytes was reported by two groups of workers in 1970 [6,7]. Proof of the T-cell nature of those cells soon followed, and the technique has become the most widely used method for enumerating T-cells. A variety of technical modifications have been reported. Pretreatment of red cells with neuraminidase, papain, or 2-aminoethyl-isothiouronium bromide hydrobromide enhances rosetting, although this effect may also be achieved by incubation for 2 to 24 hours at 4°C with untreated cells. Metabolic inhibitors, useful in immunofluorescence, should be avoided, as rosette formation is energy-dependent. Gentle resuspension prior to counting is important, as rosettes (conventionally only those cells clearly binding three or more red cells) are easily disrupted. Cells may be counterstained with, for example, methylene blue or fluorescein diacetate. Here fluorescence microscopy is used and gives two advantages: (1) avidly rosetting cells completely surrounded by RBC can be distinguished from RBC clumps, and (2) dead cells do not fluoresce and can thus be ignored. Further technical details are considered by Aiuti et al. [5].

In health the T-cell population comprises about 50 to 80% of circulating lymphocytes. A proportion of peripheral "active" T-cells form rosettes at room temperature or 37°C and appear to comprise those cells that rapidly form rosettes. Thymocytes form such rosettes, as do the blast cells in most cases of T-cell acute lymphoblastic leukaemia (T-ALL) [8,9].

The E-rosette technique has been reliable in the detection of T-cell variants of chronic lymphoproliferative disorders [2], but has a lower detection rate in T-ALL when compared with results obtained with heterologous anti-T-cell sera [9] and monoclonal antibodies [2]. These T-antigen positive, E-rosette negative cells form the pre-T or minor-T subgroup of ALL.

Recent work indicates that the culture of chronic lymphocytic leukaemia B-cells (B-CLL) and hairy cell leukaemia B-cells (B-HCL) in the presence of mitogens and T-cells results in the development of the E-receptor on these cells [10,11], a finding that may help to explain some of the rare cases of "mixed" lymphoproliferative disorders.

Several monoclonal antibodies have been developed to the E-receptor. The antibody OKT 11 blocks E-rosette formation when preincubated with lymphocytes, and the percentage of OKT 11+ cells correlates closely with that of E-rosetting cells [12]. There is also a close correlation between E-rosetting cells and those positive with the pan-T-cell monoclonal antibody OKT 3 [13].

Mouse erythrocyte rosette technique

Lymphocytes forming rosettes with mouse erythrocytes have been shown to be increased in patients with CLL [14], and the test has proved to be of considerable value in differentiating CLL from other lymphoproliferative disorders [15,16], especially as surface immunoglobulin staining is often weak or undetectable in CLL. The technique is similar to that used for sheep E-rosettes, being performed at room temperature or 4°C for periods of up to 24 hours. Erythrocytes from CBA, Balb/c, and C57BL strains of mice have all proved suitable.

Prior incubation of lymphocytes with neuraminidase results in a selective increase of mouse rosetting cells in CLL, but not in normal subjects or patients with other lymphoproliferative disorders [15].

CLL cells obtained from marrow, nodes, and spleen have been reported to show much reduced rosetting abilities [17], and it has been suggested that the ability to form rosettes may reflect a property determining whether a cell enters the blood or remains in the tissues. In view of this, blood cells should be used when investigating patients with this technique.

Detection of surface membrane-bound immunoglobulin

Surface membrane-bound immunoglobulin (SMIg) is the classical marker of mature B-cells but is not present on more primitive cells that can be identified by other methods (e.g., the demonstration of cytoplasmic immunoglobulin) to be committed to the B-cell line. SMIg is the cell's receptor for antigen and confers on a cell its specificity for certain antigens.

SMIg is usually detected by direct immunofluorescence, using antiimmunoglobulin sera conjugated to a fluorochrome, either fluorescein (fluorescein isothyocyanate) or rhodamine (tetramethyl-rhodamine-isothyocyanate). Early results were sometimes conflicting due to lack of understanding of the problems of this technique. The most important problems are as follows:

1. Use of nonspecific reagents contaminated with antibodies to other immunoglobulin classes or other cell surface antigens.
2. Use of antisera containing Ig aggregates that may bind to Fc receptors.
3. Binding of antisera to extrinsic SMIg, which may be of two types: either SMIg bound to Fc receptors or antibody bound to another membrane component.

The first two problems can be largely overcome by the use of high-quality monospecific reagents from which the Fc fragments have been removed by pepsin digestion (F[ab']$_2$ reagents), and the third by prior incubation of the test cells in a culture medium or by using an acetate wash.

Care and some experience are needed when scoring immunofluorescence, as a variety of reactions may be observed, some artifactual [3]. When a number of samples or reagents are being tested, "capping" (the movement of antigen-antibody complex to a pole of the cell and its ultimate shedding or internalization) may occur, which should be kept to a minimum by keeping cells on ice in the presence of azide; alternatively, cells may be fixed with formalin.

Direct immunofluorescence gives weaker staining than the indirect method, and SMIg staining may be weak or undetectable in CLL. Catovsky et al. [18] reported 21% of 120 cases of CLL as SMIg negative, and of 93 SMIg positive cases only 6 showed a strong staining reaction. In our department we have usually failed to detect SMIg on CLL cells by this method; and direct immunofluorescence is by no means the best method of detecting SMIg in CLL. Dhaliwal et al. [19] have stated that the technique is "working at the very limit of sensitivity in studies on CLL cells." Johnstone and Millard [20], using a sensitive radioimmunoassay, showed that CLL cells express only 20% of the surface IgM of normal B-cells but carry more cytoplasmic IgM (see the following section). Most cases of CLL express both μ and δ heavy chains on the cell surface [21], and the majority of cases of HCL show multiple heavy chain determinants [22]. In order to demonstrate monoclonality it is therefore important to determine the ratio of kappa-positive to lambda-positive cells. The criteria for monoclonality are kappa-lambda ratios of $> 10:1$ or $< 1:5$ [3].

Detection of cytoplasmic immunoglobulin

Cytoplasmic immunoglobulin (CIg) may be demonstrated in B-lymphoid cells (including early precursors) using the same fluorochrome-labeled antibodies used to detect SMIg. Fixed smears or cytospin preparations are used and may be stored unfixed at $-20°C$ for several months at least, allowing batches of positive and negative controls to be kept. Once fixed, staining should be carried out immediately, and it is important not to allow the area of cells to dry out. We have found the method of Worman [23] acceptable.

Plasma cells show intense activity and mature B-cells are also positive, but the point in B-cell maturation at which CIg becomes detectable is a matter of debate. B-CLL cells have generally been reported as CIg-negative, but Han et al. [24] have reported moderate to strong positivity in each of a series of 20 cases. They suggest CIg staining may be better than SMIg staining as a way of determining monoclonality, since it is not affected by problems of binding of extrinsic Ig. Johnstone and Millard's report [20] of a 1.6-fold increase in cytoplasmic IgM in CLL supports the report of Han et al. [24] as do our own findings.

The presence of μ-chain alone in a proportion of cases of childhood ALL [25] indicates the presence of a pre-B subgroup of this disease.

Antibodies to cell membrane components

Antibodies to cell membrane components have been widely used in immunology, and several have proved of value in the diagnosis and classification of lymphoid malignancy.

An important milestone was the detection of the so-called common ALL antigen by Greaves [1] and Greaves et al. [26] using a highly absorbed rabbit antiserum. A number of workers raised similar heterologous antisera to other lymphoid antigens, such as T-cell antigens and the P28, 33 (HLA DR) antigens. The rationale and methodology of production are outlined by Janossy [3]. Nowadays monoclonal antibodies are available and have largely taken the place of heterologous sera; most laboratories have neither the facilities nor the workload to warrant production of their own heteroantisera but have the modest financial resources needed to purchase selected monoclonal antibodies. Their advantage lies in the fact that they are uniform and highly specific and supply is no problem, enabling greater diagnostic consistency.

Both types of antibody have been used with a similar range of techniques, of which indirect immunofluorescence, with or without a cell sorter, (e.g., Fluorescence Activated Cell Sorter, FACS, Becton Dickinson) has been the most common. Some monoclonal reagents (Ortho Diagnostic Reagents) are available directly coupled to a fluorochrome, but other methods, including immunoenzyme and rosette techniques [27,28], have been described.

The monoclonal reagents we have used have given satisfactory results by indirect immunofluorescence with high intensity of staining of positive cells in most cases. Commercial companies give details of recommended methodology that are easy to follow. These reagents are not cheap, however, and may be sold only in large-pack sizes, making their stability after reconstitution an important factor. This factor should be discussed with the seller prior to purchase. A useful panel of antibodies would include pan-T and pan-B reagents, anticommon ALL, and anti-HLA-DR. Antimonocytic and antimyeloid reagents are available. Those detecting antigens produced early in myeloid differentiation (e.g., MY7) may be helpful in the classification of poorly differentiated leukaemias.

The common ALL antigen

This 100,000 MW membrane glycoprotein is found on a very small number of lymphoid percursors in normal bone marrow. It is present on the blasts of a large proportion of cases of childhood ALL but in significantly fewer cases of adult ALL. Of the commercial monoclonal reagents, J5 (Coulter) has been widely used and has given satisfactory results in our hands.

T-Cell antigens

Heterologous antisera have been historically valuable in the detection of T-cell malignancies that fail to form sheep E-rosettes [9,29], but normal T-cells have now been studied in some detail using panels of monoclonal reagents [30], mainly the OKT (Ortho) and Leu (Becton-Dickinson) series. Tentative attempts have been made to match the detailed phenotypes of T-cell malignancies to their normal counterparts [2], but this has sometimes proved difficult in T-cell acute leukaemia [31].

The main value of T-cell antibodies lies in detecting sheep E-rosette-negative T-cell diseases. The pan-T-cell reagent Leu-1 appears to be very useful in this respect in detecting pre-T-ALL [2], although both this and OKT-3, another pan-T reagent, also react with B-CLL and B-cell prolymphocytic leukaemia (B-PLL) cells.

B-cell antigens

The monoclonal antibodies BA-1 (Hybridtech) and B1 (Coulter) are commercially available. These pan-B-cell reagents have been reported to stain normal B-cells and cells of chronic and acute B-lymphoid malignancies. We have not found B1 to stain common ALL blasts, although the antigen defined is present in relatively low density [R. Jarvis, personal communication].

HLA-DR antigens

The gene products of the HLA-DR locus (previously known as Ia and p28, 33 antigens) are found on B-lymphoid cells, primitive myeloid cells, monocytes, activated T-cells, and a subpopulation of peripheral T-cells. They are also found on some nonhaemic cells. Their widespread presence detracts from their value in the classification of lymphoid neoplasia, although T-cell forms are usually HLA-DR negative.

Terminal deoxynucleotidyl transferase

This deoxynucleotide polymerase was shown to be abundant in cells from patients with ALL and in some cases of CML blast crisis ("Lymphoid blast crisis") by McCaffrey et al. [32]. Terminal deoxynucleotidyl transferase (TdT) determination has become a cornerstone of the laboratory investigation of acute leukaemia. High levels are found in almost all cases of ALL, with lower levels in the pre-B form. The rare B-cell form is usually TdT negative. Lymphoblastic lymphoma cells are usually strongly positive as are cells in lymphoid blast crisis of CML, but only very few blast cells in a small proportion of AML patients.

The enzyme may be estimated quantitatively by biochemical assay [33] or qualitatively by indirect immunofluorescence [34]. Here the degree of fluorescence allows a semiquantitative estimate of activity to be made. A commercial kit is available (Bethesda Research Laboratories). We have found this to give reliable results in close accordance with those obtained by a reference laboratory (Membrane Immunology Labs., ICRF London). TdT activity is soon lost (it is not detectable immunologically after storage of slides for seven days at $-20^{\circ}C$),and the test should be performed as soon as possible.

The biochemical assay is complex and requires a large number of cells, whereas the immunological test is simple and can be performed using two blood or marrow smears (one used as a negative control). Individual cells can be observed, and this may be important, for example, when searching for small numbers of infiltrating leukaemic cells in cerebrospinal fluid or a testicular biopsy.

Bethesda Research Laboratories has recently introduced an immunoperoxidase kit for estimation of TdT. It offers the advantages of allowing the test to be performed with ordinary light microscopy, with the production of a permanent preparation.

CLINICAL APPLICATION OF IMMUNOLOGICAL LYMPHOCYTE MARKERS IN THE LYMPHOPROLIFERATIVE DISEASES

The various immunological markers just described can be used in the identification and classification of the lymphoproliferative disorders by helping to answer one or more of three questions:

1. *Does a clonal neoplastic disease exist?* Uncertainty can arise where an excess of morphologically normal lymphocytes circulates or infiltrates the bone marrow. The differentiation is usually between a reactive lymphocytosis or some variety of CLL without bone marrow failure or physical signs (Rai Stage 0) [35]. Most cases of CLL are B-cell derived [36], and the cells have low density surface immunoglobulin on them with usually a single light chain determinant indicative of clonality. Occasionally, they are T-cell derived. While they may react with antibodies against T-cell-specific antigens, this does not demonstrate clonality as such, and some cases of T-CLL cannot be reliably distinguished from a reactive T-lymphocytosis.

2. *Is a leukaemia lymphocyte related or derived?* Where there is no doubt that a leukaemia exists, if it is undifferentiated, conventional morphology and cytochemistry may fail to indicate unequivocally whether it is granulocyte/monocyte or lymphocyte related. Presently such a distinction is clinically important, as the treatments and response rates of the two groups are different. In such cases some immunological markers have greatly helped to categorise what is an otherwise unrecognisable ALL. As mentioned above, particularly useful in this respect is the DNA polymerase TdT, which is found in nearly all varieties of ALL cells but not to any significant degree in granulocytic leukaemias.

3. *To what place in the lymphocyte lineage does the malignant cell correspond?* It is perhaps in this area that, historically, immunological markers have played a unique role. With the recognition of the different lymphocyte subsets came the realisation that they could have their malignant counterparts in the lymphoproliferative disorders. The parallel tracks of defining different normal lymphocytes and examining the phenotypes of malignant cells have merged, and most lymphocyte related sarcomas have now been at least tentatively placed at a developmental stage in lymphocyte ontogeny. The reader is referred elsewhere to recent excellent detailed reviews of this topic [2,37]. What follows here is an essentially clinically orientated approach to the use of the commonly available markers described above in the classification of three groups of lymphoid cancer: ALL, CLL, and non-Hodgkin's lymphoma.

Acute lymphoblastic leukaemia

This heterogeneous group of disorders has been the most extensively studied using immunological lymphocyte markers. The first subtype to be recognised was T-ALL [38] and, following the definition of the CALL antigen, so-called "common" ALL [1]. This led to three definable types for comparison: "T," "common," and "null." It was apparent that patients so defined could be distinguished by other criteria, the most important of which was their response to treatment [39]. The advent of more markers, chiefly monoclonal antibodies and enzymes, further modified the immunological classification of ALL, and these, plus the recognition of the rare, SMIg-bearing, B-ALL has led to the general current acceptance of six immunological phenotypes: "common" ALL, pre-B ALL, T-ALL (major group), T-ALL (minor group), B-ALL, and "null" ALL [40]. These six can be recognised by seven of the markers described above; their relative frequencies in a large unselected series of patients with ALL are shown in table 10-1. The pattern of marker results found in the six phenotypes is given in table 10-2.

Table 10-1. Frequency of immunological markers in childhood ALL

	CALLA	ER	T*	SMIg	TdT	HLADR	CIg
Proportion of cases	73%	12%	14%	<1%	99%	87%	18%

*T-cell antibody positive.
Source: Data from Greaves et al. [1981].

Table 10-2. Pattern of markers found in immunologically defined subtypes of ALL

	Proportion of cases	CALLA	ER	T*	SMIg	TdT	HLADR	CIg
Common ALL	73%	+	−	−	−	+	+	−
Pre B-ALL	18%	+	−	−	−	+	+	+
T-ALL Major Group	12%	−	+	+	−	+	−	−
T-ALL Minor Group	2%	±	−	+	−	+	−	−
Null ALL	13%	−	−	−	−	+	+	−
B-ALL	<1%	−	−	−	+	−	+	−

*T-cell antibody positive.
Source: Data from Greaves et al. [1981].

Despite the initial impression that the immunologically defined features of ALL were independent indicators of prognosis [39], larger numbers and multivariate statistical analyses have shown that this is not always so and that while, for example, T-ALL usually has a poor outlook, this is because it usually relates to a high circulating white cell count, a poor prognostic feature whatever the cell phenotype. T-ness as such, if associated with a low count, does not carry the same sinister significance [40]. Nonetheless, T-cell and B-cell ALL are both distinct biological syndromes with clinical and cytogenetic features different to common ALL [38,41,42,43]. At present, however, such clinically significant differences are recognised only between four of the six described immunological subtypes of ALL. They are listed in table 10-3 alongside their major distinctive features. Pre-B and minor-T disease are clinically indistinguishable from "common" and "T" ALL, respectively.

All markers, on the other hand, have done more than enable clinicians to catalogue the different varieties of the disease. They have given insight into the biology of the condition and suggested stages of differentiation at which normal cell development is arrested. Furthermore, they have given rise to a hypothesis about the curability of the condition from the suggestion that within a tumour cell population are the clonogenic proliferating cells and the nonproliferating end-stage variety. The latter make up the majority and determine the disease phenotype, whereas the former, although infrequent, determine the curability of the disease by their successful eradication [41].

Chronic lymphocytic leukaemia

Clinically the most benign lymphoid leukaemias, the CLLs nonetheless encompass a spectrum of severity from an incidentally discovered accumulative clonal lymphocytosis that

Table 10-3. Clinical correlates to immunologically defined ALL subtypes

	High (>20.0) WBCC %	Mediastinal mass %	Males %	CNS infil- tration %	Specific chromosome abnormality %
"Common" ALL	28[*]	0[*]	56[*]	5§	<10§§
T-ALL	63[*]	52[*]	82[*]	45§	<10§§
Null ALL	35[*][**]	0[*]	60[*][**]	<10'	<10§§
B-ALL	(25)	0	(50)	–	90§§

Sources: [*]Greaves et al. [1981].
            §Lilleyman and Sugden [1982].
            §§Lawler [1982].
            [**]Numbers too small for accuracy.

Table 10-4. Immunological phenotypes found in nonacute lymphocytic leukaemias

	SMIg	MR	ER	TdT	OKT8	OKT4	OKT3	B1
B-CLL	±	+	–	–	–	–	–	+
T-CLL	–	–	+	–	+	–	+	–
B-PLL	+	±	–	–	–	–	–	+
T-PLL	–	–	+	–	some	most	+	–
HCL	+	±	–	–	–	–	–	?
Waldenström's macroglobulinaemia	+	–	–	–	–	–	–	+

Source: Data from Catovsky et al. [1982], Galton and MacLennan [1982], and Foon et al. [1982].
P-Prolymphocytic HC-Hairy cell.

does not shorten life to a more progressive condition with intractable bone marrow failure. Immunological markers show that over 95% are B-cell derived and less than 5% T-cell derived [36]. They are essentially adult diseases and occur rarely, if at all, in children. Since the majority of the tumour cells are more differentiated than those of the acute lymphoid leukaemias, it is not surprising that early developmental markers, such as the CALL antigen, are absent. The B-CLLs show low density SMIg (which can be hard to demonstrate) but usually avid receptors for an unidentified structure on mouse erythrocytes [15], which are thought to be a feature of "early" B-cells. T-CLL, on the other hand, shows a mature T-cell phenotype with, usually, the pattern found in the T-suppressor cell population [36]. Table 10-4 shows the pattern of markers found in T-CLL and B-CLL compared, together with that found in four other clinically distinct conditions conveniently tabulated here, B-PLL, T-PLL, HCL [21] and Waldenstrom's macroglobulinaemia. These four are all rare and usually identified on morphological criteria or the presence of abnormal plasma proteins.

The main practical use of immunological markers in the CLLs lies not so much in determining disease subtype and prognosis—this relies more on clinical criteria [35]—but more in helping to determine whether a clonal neoplasm exists at all. Light chain specificity of SMIg in the B-cell diseases will determine this, but in the T-cell diseases (fortunately more rare), no markers exist that are not found in a reactive lymphocytosis. Cytogenetics may help in this group. Marker analysis may also be useful, however, in distinguishing an "ordinary" CLL from a PLL (where doubts exist) or from a non-Hodgkin's lymphoma.

Non-Hodgkin's lymphoma

The non-Hodgkin's lymphomas form a miscellany of lymphocytic tumours, all of which, at least in their early stage, do not involve the blood and bone marrow. Such a distinction breaks down in many cases as the disease evolves, and, indeed, at times the difference between lymphocytic lymphomas and leukaemias can be somewhat subtle. The situation is further confused by the long-running debate on the histological classification of these cancers (whether or not they involve the haemic system), and in the United Kingdom at least three major classification systems favoured by different pathologists have led to the present "semantic quagmire" [44].

Immunologically, most NHLs are B-cell tumours, a few are T-cell derived, and the small remainder so-called null lymphomas. They can be broadly grouped into two types: the low-grade (more benign) variety, which does not occur in children to any significant extent, and the high-grade, which, apart from the immunoblastic variety, occurs more often in younger patients. It must be said that cell marker studies have not greatly helped to clear the confusion surrounding NHLs, partly because they have been studied less for technical reasons and partly because the cell marker phenotypes have been pegged on to the various morphologically defined groups rather than vice versa. Nonetheless, information is accumulating, and it is apparent that, purely from the marker analysis angle, NHL can again be divided into two categories: tumours of immature immunologically incompetent cells with features similar to the various types of ALL, and tumours of differentiated lymphocytes expressing the phenotypic features of B-cells arrested at one of several stages of an antigen-dependent immune response [45]. These types broadly correspond to the high- and low-grade tumours mentioned above. Table 10-5 indicates the pattern of markers that may

Table 10-5. Immunological markers in non-Hodgkin's lymphomas

	CALLA	ER	SMIg	B1	HLADR	MR	Leukaemic counterpart
HIGH GRADE							
*Diffuse undifferentiated							
¥(Lymphoblastic)							
Unclassified type	+	−	−	−	+	−	CALL
T-cell type	±	+	−	−	−	−	**T-ALL
B-cell type (Burkitt)	−	−	+	+	+	−	B-ALL
*Diffuse histiocytic	−	±	+	+	+	−	(NHL with overspill)
¥(Immunoblastic)							
LOW GRADE							
*Diffuse poorly differentiated							
¥(Centroblastic/centrocytic)	−	−	+	+	+	−	(NHL with overspill)
*Nodular poorly differentiated							
¥(Centroblastic/centrocytic follicular)	±	−	+	+	+	−	(NHL with overspill)
*Diffuse well-differentiated							
¥(Centrocytic, lymphocytic)	−	−	+	+	+	±	B-CLL
Mycosis fungoides	−	+	−	−	−	−	Sézary
Myeloma	−	−	±	−	±	−	Plasma cell leukaemia

*Rappaport classification system.
¥ Kiel classification system (Lennert 1981).
**T-ALL may have differing, less mature, phenotype to MLDU(T).

be encountered in NHLs defined according to the Rappaport and Kiel classification systems [46]. Only tumours that do not usually present as leukaemias are included, but for comparison the approximate leukaemic counterpart is indicated for each. Where there is none, the term NHL with overspill is used. Perhaps the most practical current application of markers to NHLs is in distinguishing between one of the B-follicular centre cell tumours and large-cell CLL when the former is exfoliating into the circulation. The density of SMIg is greater in the lymphoma, and the CLL cell will show mouse rosette formation to a discriminating degree [16].

REFERENCES

1.   Greaves MF. Clinical application of cell surface markers. Prog Haematol 9: 255–303, 1975.
2.   Foon KA, Schroff RW, Gale RP. Surface markers on leukaemia and lymphoma cells: Recent advances. Blood 60: 1–19, 1982.
3.   Janossy G. Membrane markers in leukaemia. In Catovsky D (ed.), The leukaemic cell. Edinburgh: Churchill Livingstone, 1981, pp. 129–183.
4.   Boyum A. Isolation of mononuclear cells and granulocytes from human blood. Scand J Clin Lab Invest 21: Supplement 97: 77–89, 1968.
5.   Aiuti F, Cerottini JC, Coombs RRA, Cooper M, Dickler HB, Froland S, Fudenberg HH, Greaves MF, Grey HM, Kunkel HG, Natvig J, Preud'homme J-L, Rabellino E, Ritts RE, Rowe DS, Seligmann M, Siegal FP, Stjernsward J, Terry WD, Wybran J. International Union of Immunological Societies (IUIS) Report. July 1974. Identification, enumeration and isolation of B and T lymphocytes from human peripheral blood. Clin Immunol Immunopathol 3: 584–597, 1975.
6.   Brain P, Gordon J, Willets WA. Rosette formation by peripheral lymphocytes. Clin Exp Immunol 6: 681–688, 1970.
7.   Coombs RRA, Gurner BW, Wilson AB, Holm F, Lindgren B. Rosette formation between human lymphocytes and sheep red cells not involving immunoglobulin receptors. Int Arch Allergy Appl Imunol 39: 658–663, 1970.
8.   Borella L, Sen L. E-receptors on blasts from untreated acute lymphoblastic leukaemia (ALL): Comparison of temperature dependence of E-rosettes formed by normal and leukaemic lymphoid cells. J Immunol 114: 187–190, 1975.
9.   Melvin SL. Comparison of techniques for detecting T-cell acute lymphocytic leukaemia. Blood 54: 210–215, 1979.
10. Worman CP, Beverley PCL, Cawley JC. Alterations in the phenotype of hairy cells during culture in the presence of PHA: Requirement for T cells. Blood 59: 895–899, 1982.
11. Worman CP, Cawley, JC. B-chronic lymphocytic leukaemia cells express true endogenous E receptor after culture with T-cells and mitogens. Br J Haematol 52: 205–210, 1982.
12. Ip SH, Rittershaus CW, Struzziero CL, Hoxie JA, Hoffman RA, Healey KW, Lifter J. Evaluation of E-rosetting human lymphocytes with OKT11 and other monoclonal antibodies. Blood 60: 795–799, 1982.
13. Cock W, Cree J, Verhaegen H. Enumeration of human peripheral T lymphocytes with E-rosettes and OKT3 PAN monoclonal antibody: A close correlation. Thymus 2: 133–137, 1980.
14. Stathopoulos G, Elliott EV. Formation of mouse or sheep red-blood-cell rosettes by lymphocytes from normal and leukaemic individuals. Lancet 1: 600–601, 1974.
15. Catovsky D, Cherchi M, Okos A, Hegde U, Galton DAG. Mouse red-cell rosettes in B lymphoproliferative disorders. Br J Haematol 33: 173–177, 1976.
16. Sugden PJ, Lilleyman JS. Mouse red cell rosette formation and colchicine sensitivity test: Relative usefulness in the differential diagnosis of chronic lymphocytic leukaemia and B lymphocytic lymphoma. J Clin Pathol 35: 376–379, 1982.
17. Cherchi M, Catovsky D. Mouse red blood cell rosettes in chronic lymphocytic leukaemia: Different expression in blood and tissues. Clin Exp Immunol 39: 411–415, 1980.
18. Catovsky D, Pittman S, O'Brien M, Cherchi M, Costello C, Foa R, Pearce E, Hoffbrand AV, Janossy G, Ganeshaguru K, Greaves MF. Multiparameter studies in lymphoid leukaemias. Am J Clin Pathol 72: 736–745, 1979.
19. Dhaliwal HS, Ling NR, Bishop S, Chapel H. Expression of immunoglobulin G on blood lymphocytes in chronic lymphocytic leukaemia. Clin Exp Immunol 31: 226–236, 1978.

20. Johnstone AP, Millard RE. The type and subcellular distribution of immunoglobulin in normal adult, neonatal and chronic lymphocytic leukaemic cells. Br J Haematol 53: 346, 1983.
21. Galton DAG, MacLennan ICM. Clinical patterns in B lymphoid malignancy. Clin Haematol II: 561–587, 1982.
22. Jansen J, Schuit HRE, Meijer CJLM, van Nieuwkoop JA, Hijmans W. Cell markers in hairy cell leukaemia studied in cells from 51 patients. Blood 59: 52–60, 1982.
23. Worman C. Cytoplasmic immunofluorescent staining: A micro method with counterstain. J Immunol Methods 23: 193–194, 1978.
24. Han T, Ozer H, Bloom M, Sagawa K, Minowada J. The presence of monoclonal cytoplasmic immunoglobulins in leukaemic B cells from patients with chronic lymphocytic leukaemia. Blood 59: 435–438, 1982.
25. Vogler LB, Crist WM, Lawton AR, Bockman DE, Pearl ER, Cooper MD. Pre-B-cell leukaemia. New Engl J Med 298: 872–878, 1978.
26. Greaves MF, Brown G, Rapson NT, Lister TA. Antisera to acute lymphoblastic leukaemia cells. Clin Immunol Immunopathol 4: 67–84, 1975.
27. McMillan EM, Wasik R, Everett MA. OKT-6 positive cells: Their demonstration in human thymus and the effect of fixation on the immunoperoxidase reaction. Arch Pathol Lab Med 106: 9–12, 1982.
28. Bernard J, Ternynck T, Zagury D. A general method for the cytochemical and ultrastructural studies of human lymphocyte subsets defined by monoclonal antibodies. Immunol Lett 4: 65–73, 1982.
29. Thiel E, Rodt H, Huhn D, Netzel B, Gross-Wilde H, Ganeshaguru K, Thierfelder S. Multimarker classification of acute lymphoblastic leukaemia: Evidence for further T subgroups and evaluation of their clinical significance. Blood 56: 759–772, 1980.
30. Reinherz EL, Scholssman SF. Regulation of the immune response—Inducer and suppressor T-lymphocyte subsets in human beings. New Engl J Med 303: 370–373, 1980.
31. Koziner B, Gebhard D, Denny T, McKenzie S, Clarkson BD, Miller DA, Evans RL. Analysis of T-cell differentiation antigens in acute lymphatic leukaemia using monoclonal antibodies. Blood 60: 752–757, 1982.
32. McCaffrey R, Harrison TA, Parkman R, Baltimore D. Terminal deoxynucleotidyl transferase activity in human leukaemic cells and normal thymocytes. New Engl J Med 292: 775–780, 1975.
33. Coleman MS, Hutton JJ. Terminal transferase. In Catovsky D (ed.), The leukaemic cell. Edinburgh: Churchill Livingstone, 1981, pp. 203–219.
34. Goldschneider I, Gregoire K, Barton RW, Bollum FJ. Demonstration of terminal deoxynucleotidyl transferase in thymocytes by immunofluorescence. Proc Natl Acad Sci, USA, 74: 3993–3996, 1977.
35. Rai KR, Sawitsky A, Cronkite EP, Channa AD, Levy RN, Pasternack BS. Clinical staging of chronic lymphocytic leukaemia. Blood 46: 219–234, 1975.
36. Catovsky D, Linch DC, Beverley PCL. T cell disorders in haematological diseases. Clin Haematol II: 661–695, 1982.
37. Moretta L, Mingari MC, Moretta A, Fauci AS. Human lymphocyte surface markers. Sem Haematol 19: 273–284, 1982.
38. Catovsky D, Goldman JM, Okos A, Frisch B, Galton DAG. T-lymphoblastic leukaemia: A distinct variety of acute leukaemia. Br Med J 2: 643–646, 1974.
39. Chessels JM, Hardisty RM, Rapson NT, Greaves MF. Acute lymphoblastic leukaemia in children: Classification and prognosis. Lancet 2: 1307–1309, 1977.
40. Greaves MF, Janossy G, Peto J, Kay H. Immunologically defined subclasses of acute lymphoblastic leukaemia in children: Their relationship to presentation features and prognosis. Br J Haematol 48: 179–197, 1981.
41. Greaves MF. Biology of acute lymphoblastic leukaemia. London: Leukaemia Research Fund, 1981.
42. Lilleyman JS, Sugden PJ. T lymphoblastic leukaemia and the CNS. Br J Cancer 43: 320–323, 1981.
43. Lawler SD. Significance of chromosome abnormalities in leukaemia. Sem Haematol 19: 257–272, 1982.
44. Wright DH. The identification and classification of non-Hodgkin's lymphoma: A review. Diagn Histopathol 5: 73–111, 1982.
45. Habeshaw JA, Catley PF, Stansfeld AG, Brearley RL. Surface phenotyping histology and the nature of non-Hodgkin lymphoma in 157 patients. Br J Cancer 40: 11–34, 1979.
46. Lennert K. Histopathology of non-Hodgkin's lymphomas. Berlin: Springer Verlag, 1981.

11. VIRUSES, IMMUNITY, AND CANCER

C.W. POTTER
R.C. REES

INTRODUCTION

Reading the scientific and medical literature is difficult without feeling swamped by suggested causes of human cancer: genetic factors have been implicated; epidemiological studies based on geographic variations in cancer incidence have suggested a variety of environmental factors [1]; multiple elements in our food and diet have been indicted at various times; and many fashions of western and eastern society have been held to contain factors that increase the incidence of malignant diseases [2]. With this in mind, it is not surprising that virus infection has been associated with the aetiology of cancer; however, this theory deserves attention, since it is supported by a large body of circumstantial evidence, and under strictly controlled conditions, viruses can be shown to induce many forms of cancer in a variety of animal species. These observations have led many authorities to suggest that viruses are aetiological agents of malignant disease in man, but the inability to carry out the experiments that proved the association of viruses and cancer in animals has meant that direct proof of association cannot be made for human cancers.

The theory that viruses can cause human malignant diseases has emotional attractions; many virus infections can be controlled by vaccines, and the possibility that some cancers may be controlled in a similar way is a hope of many. In addition, the study of virus-induced tumours of animals has yielded much information on the mechanism of tumour induction, the genotypic and phenotypic changes associated with cell transformation, the antigenicity of tumour cells, and the immune responses to these cells. Thus, the study of virus-induced

B.W. Hancock and A.M. Ward (eds.), Immunological Aspects of Cancer. Copyright © 1985, Martinus Nijhoff Publishing, Boston/Dordrecht/Lancaster.

tumours produced in laboratory animals may be relevant to the aetiology of natural human cancer, providing information on the immune response of the host and on methods of immunotherapy that may help in the understanding of the immunology and treatment of human cancer.

As might be expected, therefore, the subject of virus-induced tumours has been studied by a large number of researchers during the past 20 years, and the results of these studies have been published in tens of thousands of papers. The value of this work rests on two premises: first, that viruses do cause human cancer, and second, that the immune response to virus-induced cancers of laboratory animals has parallels in naturally arising tumours of man. These two theories are examined in this chapter.

VIRUS-INDUCED TUMOURS OF ANIMALS

Oncogenic viruses

Evidence that viruses may be a cause of malignant diseases was first put forward by Ellerman and Bang [3], who described a filterable and transmittable agent able to induce erythro-myeloblastic leukaemia in chickens. Three years later, similar agents were demonstrated for a chicken sarcoma and a rabbit tumour [4,5]. These findings remained items of curiosity and speculation for some 20 years after their discovery; however, infective agents for rabbit fibroma and papilloma were next reported [6,7], and the infective agent of lymphomatosis in chickens was described at approximately the same time [8]. Bittner [9] subsequently identified an agent capable of producing mammary tumours in mice, and a filterable agent of frog kidney sarcoma was also found [10].

The identification of viruses as a cause of cancer was established in the above studies, and in subsequent years the data were extended; however, all the results were for cancers of animals, and the relevance of the findings to naturally occurring human cancers remained suspect. Attention was focused on viruses and cancer in man, when early batches of inactivated poliovirus vaccines given to tens of thousands of subjects were found to contain a live virus from the monkey kidney cells used for vaccine virus growth [11]; this virus, termed simian virus type-40 (SV40), induced tumours when inoculated into a range of rodents [12]. Later, Trenton and his colleagues [13] reported that human adenovirus type-12 caused tumours when inoculated into newborn hamsters; subsequent studies showed that 8 of 31 human adenoviruses could induce tumours in hamsters [14] and that many of these viruses were common infective agents of man [15]. These findings initiated major enquiries into the role of viruses as causes of tumours in animals—studies that would hopefully identify tumour-inducing viruses of man, establish the mechanism(s) of tumour induction, provide models for investigative work, lead to the development of methods of prevention by the use of vaccines, and identify therapeutic agents for immunotherapy. As a result of this work carried out during the last two decades by numerous researchers, over 150 viruses have been identified either as infective agents causing naturally occurring malignant diseases or capable of inducing tumours when inoculated into experimental animals. A variety of both RNA and DNA viruses were found to cause tumours. The malignancies arising as a result of virus infection include leukaemia, lymphomas, carcinomas, and sarcomas; and animals in which virus-induced tumours occur include frogs and other cold-blooded species, mice, rats, birds, chickens, hamsters, dogs, cats,

Table 11-1. Some oncogenic DNA viruses of animals

Family	Virus	Natural host	Occurrence of tumour		Histology
			Species		
Papovaviridae	Papilloma	Various	Natural host		Papilloma to carcinoma
	Polyoma	Mouse	Natural host		Adenoma, adenocarcinoma
			Hamster, etc.		Fibroma, fibrocarcinoma
	SV40	Monkey	Hamster/mouse		Fibrosarcoma, ependyoma
Adenoviridae	Human (8 types)	Man	Hamster		Sarcoma
	CELO (1 type)	Fowl	Hamster		Sarcoma
	Monkeys (6 types)	Monkey	Hamster		Sarcoma
	Others	Cow, dog, etc.	Hamster		Sarcoma
	Human (other types)	Man	Rat		Sarcoma
Herpesviridae	Lucké agent	Frog	Natural host		Adenoma, adenocarcinoma
	Marek's agent	Fowl	Natural host		Neurolymphomatosis
	H. Ateles	Spider monkey	Natural host		Lymphoma, leukaemia
	H. Saimiri	Spider monkey	Natural host		Lymphoma, leukaemia
	H. Hominis	Man	Hamster/rat/mouse		Fibrosarcoma
Poxviridae	Yaba virus	Rhesus monkey	Natural host		Fibroma
	Shope fibroma	Rabbit	Natural host		Fibroma
	Kilham virus	Squirrel	Natural host		Fibroma

Table 11-2. Some oncogenic RNA viruses of animals

Group	Virus	Host	Tumours
Type C	Rous sarcoma	Fowl	Fibrosarcoma, sarcoma
	Gross leukaemia	Mouse	Lymphosarcoma, leukaemias
	Moloney sarcoma	Mouse	Rhabdosarcoma
	Feline leukaemia	Cat	Lymphosarcoma
	Simian sarcoma	Monkey	Fibrosarcoma
	Bovine lymphosarcoma	Cow	Lymphosarcoma, leukaemia
	Gibbon leukaemia	Gibbon	Lymphosarcoma, leukaemia
Type B	Mammary tumour	Mouse	Adenocarcinoma

deer, monkeys, and many other species. A list of some of the viruses associated with animal cancers is given in tables 11-1 and 11-2. From this weight of circumstantial evidence, many authorities concluded that viruses were a cause of cancer in man but that the direct experimentation that would give proof to this hypothesis was denied for ethical considerations; to show that human cancer was also caused by viruses would require experimental approaches distinct from those that had been so successfully applied to animal cancers.

Tumours induced by viruses

The oncogenic viruses and the tumours induced by these agents (shown in tables 11-1 and 11-2) represent only a fraction of the total number of oncogenic viruses described in the literature; however, the examples selected illustrate the diversity of the viruses involved, the number of species affected, and the range of malignancies induced by these agents. Two broad groupings may be further considered: those viruses that induce malignancies in the species that are the natural virus host, and those that induce tumours in heterologous species and only under experimental conditions. For these latter viruses, such as the adenovirus, proof that they can induce naturally occurring tumours under natural conditions is absent.

The family of viruses termed the *Papovaviridae* are divided into two genera: the Papillomaviruses and the Polyomaviruses. The Papillomaviruses include the agents of papillomas in a wide variety of species, including man, rabbits, cows, and cats; these viruses cause papillomas under natural conditions and in the natural host [16]. Although by definition papillomas are tumours, these growths are not a malignant disease; occasionally, however, they can progress to metastasising carcinomas [17]. The Polyomaviruses include Polyomavirus, which is a widespread agent infecting mice, and SV40, which has been isolated from a number of species of monkeys, including Rhesus and Cymologus monkeys. Investigations of natural malignant diseases arising in these species have never shown association with infection by these viruses; however, their inoculation into other animals, particularly newborn hamsters, has been shown to induce rapidly growing tumours [11,18]. The tumours produced by these viruses originate and remain localised to the site of virus inoculation, are encapsulated with extensive central necrosis, and do not metastasise. Metastasis, probably as a result of tumour pressure, can be found in the popliteal and inguinal lymph nodes following foot-pad inoculation of transplanted SV40-induced tumour cells, but this is a highly contrived system [19]. Despite these observations, the tumours grow rapidly and once palpable can increase rapidly in size to over 50 mms diameter in two to three weeks: histologically, they are classed as fibrosarcomas or adenocarcinomas and show the cellular properties of highly malignant cancers (figure 11-1).

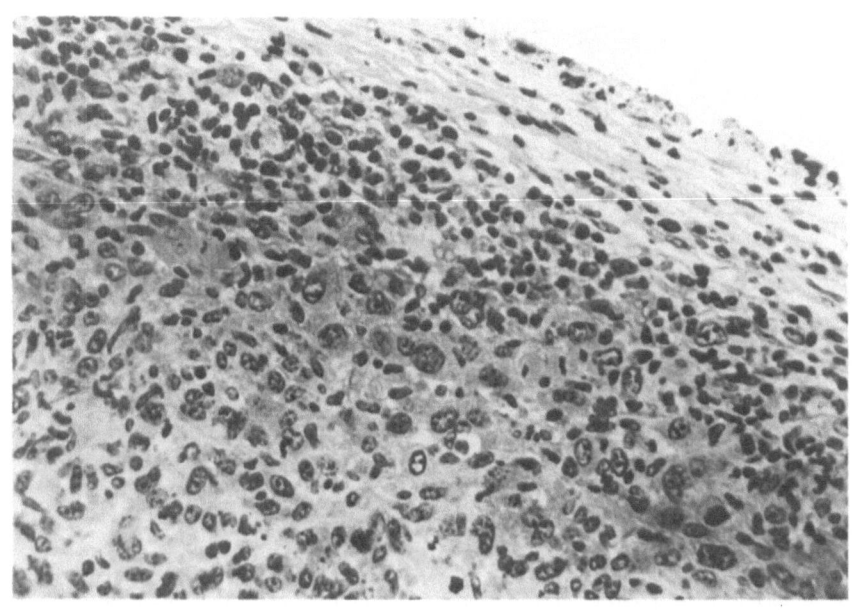

Figure 11–1. Histological appearance of SV40-induced tumour in hamster (X500).

The family *Adenoviridae* includes a large number of viruses that are common infective agents of a variety of species. Eight of 31 species that infect man produce sarcomas when inoculated into newborn hamsters [20]; and the same property is shown by an avian adenovirus termed CELO virus [21], six serotypes of which naturally infect monkeys [22] and other types of which infect cows and dogs [23]. Human adenoviruses can be divided into three groups on the basis of their oncogenicity: the highly oncogenic types 12, 18, and 31; the weakly oncogenic types 3, 7, 14, 16, and 21; and the nononcogenic types 1, 2, 5, 6, and 11 [2]. All these viruses are common infective agents of man: many infections are subclinical, but the weakly oncogenic serotypes are common causes of severe and epidemic respiratory infections in children and adults [24], and more than 50% of children have acquired antibody to two or more of these strains by the age of 10 years [25]. In addition, antibody to the highly oncogenic adenovirus type-12 and type-18 is detectable in over 50% of sera from adults over 30 years of age [26]. The tumours induced in hamsters by these viruses are all similar and have been histologically classed as sarcomas: the tumours in hamsters have properties very similar to those described for Polyomavirus-induced tumours in vivo, and the cells show the same highly malignant microscopic appearance (figure 11–2). None of these viruses appears to induce tumours in their natural hosts, and extensive studies have failed to produce evidence that adenoviruses are involved in human cancer [27].

The family *Herpesviridae* include a number of agents causal of various types of cancer in the natural or related host. Thus, the Lucké agent is a natural infection of leopard frogs and is the aetiological agent of adenoma and adenocarcinoma of the kidney in this species [28, 29]. Marek's disease is an infection of fowls characterised by neurofibromatosis [30]. Many

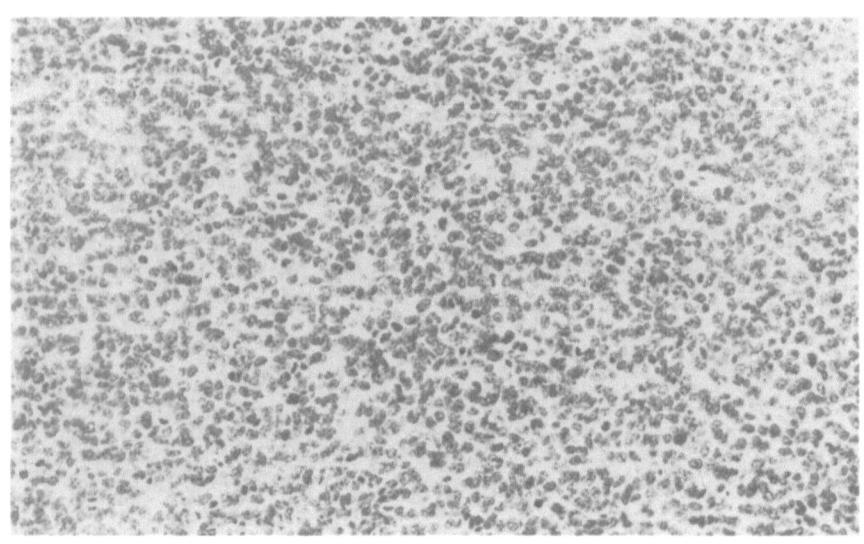

Figure 11-2. Histological appearance of adenovirus 12-induced tumour in CBA mouse (X500).

pathologists would not classify this disease as truly malignant; however, it is an active proliferative disease of T-lymphocytes that infiltrate the nerves and distal organs in a manner similar to true lymphoma. The disease is spread among fowl flocks and first affects young birds aged two to eight months; the fowls develop paralysis and die within three to four weeks of the first appearance of symptoms [31]. *Herpesvirus saimiri* and *Herpesvirus atelis* are widely distributed, natural infective agents of spider monkeys but do not cause clinical disease in this species; however, both viruses can cause a T-lymphocyte lymphoma and leukaemia in marmosets [32]. The family *Poxviridae* includes several viruses that induce fibromas in the natural host [33]; three examples are given in table 11-1.

The oncogenic RNA viruses belong to the single large famly termed *Retroviridae*, and are divided into three genera of type A, type B and type C on the basis of their appearance under the electron microscope. The type B mammary tumour virus is associated with adenocarcinoma in mice, but the incidence of this malignancy varies greatly for different strains of mice [34]: the agent is transferred from mother to litter as a milk-borne factor, but the virus can be transmitted horizontally among susceptible newborn mice [9]. It is now known that there are several strains of mammary tumour virus, some of which can be transmitted only vertically, whilst others have a hormone dependency for the expression of the oncogenic property [35]. The type C oncogenic RNA viruses are a very large group of agents capable of producing leukaemia and sarcoma in a variety of animal species including fish, reptiles, birds, and mammals; the examples shown in table 11–2 represent only a few of the viruses of this group. Type C viruses are widely distributed in their natural host and do not usually cause diseases other than the malignancy that gives the virus its name; however, glomerulonephritis due to virus-antibody-complex deposition has been described in some species [36]. A clustering of type C–induced malignancies has been described in some species [36], and this suggests horizontal spread of the transmissible agent; thus, the spread of feline leukaemia among space-related cats has been documented [37]. Some of the type C viruses have been shown to cross species barriers to produce malignancies [38], and the possibility that these or similar animal viruses may infect man, with all the implications involved, is a subject of intense enquiry at the present time; however, there is no evidence at present to associate these viruses with human cancers.

Table 11-1 lists two virus groups that can transform animal cells in vitro, and these cells can then replicate to form tumours in vivo; these are the nononcogenic adenoviruses and *Herpesvirus hominis* types 1 (HSV-1) and 2 (HSV-2). Thus, infection of rat or hamster embryo cells in vitro with a nononcogenic adenovirus induces cell transformation, and the inoculation of these cells into homologous animals produces tumours [39]. Attempts to produce tumours in animals by direct virus inoculation have been largely unsuccessful, but have been reported [40]. In addition, although the induction of tumours by HSV-2 by direct virus inoculation of mice has been described [41,42], the production of tumours with cells transformed in vitro is better recognised. Thus, virus infection of cells in vitro, using HSV-2 partially inactivated by exposure to UV-light or under conditions in which the cytolytic effects of virus are limited by incubation of infected cells at nonoptimum temperatures, can result in transformation of cells; and these cells produce tumours when inoculated into homologous animals [43]. The results of some of these studies are shown in table 11-3. The histogenesis of tumours induced in hamsters by the inoculation of cells transformed in vitro by HSV-2 is variable, depending on the nature of the original transformed cells, but fibrosarcomas are most commonly seen [44,45]. The tumours grow rapidly, are encapsulated with much central necrosis, and metastasise to the lung and later to other organs; in this respect the tumours resemble more closely naturally occurring human tumours [45].

Mechanism of virus oncogenesis

The mechanism by which viruses induce cell transformation in vitro and cancers in vivo has been a major concern in recent years of many virologists, biochemists, geneticists, and molecular biologists. Much of the earlier work was inhibited by a lack of suitable materials and techniques and was limited in many cases to studies on tumour induction in live, heterogeneic animals. The more recent development and use of highly inbred strains of many laboratory animals, the application of new tissue culture techniques for studying in vitro cell transformation, and the use of methods of molecular virology have combined to give a broad understanding of the mechanism of cell transformation by some viruses; however, the process is far from fully understood. Some workers assume that the mechanisms established by these laboratory studies are paralleled by natural in vivo events, but this assumption may not be justified. Many of the viruses capable of inducing tumours in laboratory animals can also transform cells grown in vitro from a normal to a cancerous state [51,52]; these transformed animal cells can be shown to be tumourigenic by inoculating the cells into syngeneic animals and producing tumours [53]. These techniques provide a method for studying the transformation of human cells; however, these cells cannot be proven to be tumourigenic. Data from animal studies indicate that the in vitro prop-

Table 11-3. Transformation of cells in vitro with Herpesvirus hominis type 2

Treatment	Cell transformed	Criteria of transformation			
		Altered cell morphology/growth	Virus-specific antigens	Cell growth in soft agar	Tumours in animals
UV-irradiated virus	Mouse	+	+	–	+
	Rat	+	+	NT	+
	Hamster	+	±	+	+
Growth at 20°C	Rat	+	NT	+	+
Growth at 40°C	Hamster	+	±	+	+
Growth at 42°C	Rat	+	NT	+	+
	Human	+	+	NT	NT

NT = Not tested.
± = conflicting results.

erty of transformed cells that correlates best with tumourigenicity is the loss of contact inhibition. Thus, transformed cells grown in vitro produce densely packed, multilayered colonies easily recognised by the naked eye; and the observation of this feature in transformed human cells can be taken as the best indication of tumourigenicity in vivo.

The interaction of virus with a cell may have several outcomes. First, infection and subsequent replication of virus in the cell and the subsequent release of newly formed infective virus particles can lead to cell destruction either by exhaustion of the cell's resources or by active cytolysis. Second, the cell may be nonpermissive for virus replication due to the absence of specific receptors on the cell surface or to the lack of enzymes and metabolic pathways necessary for virus replication. Third, virus infection of a cell may lead to abortive replication and the production of either no or very few infectious virus particles. It is from this result of virus-cell interaction that transformed cells may arise, since transformation is dependent on virus-induced changes and on the survival and further replication of the cells in which these changes occur. Thus, SV40 virus replicates and destroys monkey cells but can transform human or hamster cells in which only abortive infection takes place [46,47]. HSV is cytolytic for a variety of animal cells but virus partially inactivated by UV light can transform cells, since only abortive replication occurs [48,49]. The mechanism of cell transformation or tumour induction by viruses is distinct for DNA and RNA viruses and the phenomena are best considered separately.

DNA viruses

For the oncogenic DNA viruses the portion of the virus that initiates cell transformation is the virus nucleic acid [50]; however, only a fraction of the total virus genome is necessary. Thus, studies have shown that fragments of virus nucleic acid produced by restrictive enzyme treatment can cause cell transformation in vitro; for adenovirus type-12 a fragment of 4 to 20% of the total virus DNA, and for HSV-2 a fragment of approximately 10% of the total DNA can induce cell transformation [51–57].

The consequences of virus infection are many and include chromosome breakage, an increase in DNA synthesis, and the transcription into RNA of that part of the DNA coding for early functions [58]; however, the development and persistence of the properties of cell transformation are probably dependent in many cases on chromosome repair and ''accidental'' integration of the transforming fragment of the virus DNA into the host-cell chromosome [59]. Following this the virus DNA will persist in the cell and by parallel replication also in the cells of all subsequent generations; the activity of this DNA, or more probably the action of products coded for by this DNA, produces and maintains the transformed cell. Although only a fraction of the virus DNA is required to integrate, induce, and maintain transformation, most or all the virus DNA may persist. In this latter case small quantities of infective virus can be produced, and this has been described for some lines of SV40-transformed cells [59].

The identification of a specific fragment of virus DNA that can induce transformation indicates that the change in cell behaviour is probably induced by a limited number of gene products; and since the DNA fraction responsible for transformation is relatively small, transformation may be due to the action of a single product [60]. The size of the fragment of SV40 or Polyomavirus DNA that can induce transformation has been determined, and this is compatible with the translation of a protein with a molecular weight of approximately 90,000 daltons [56]. A protein of this size has been identified in the nucleus of virus-transformed cells, and is termed the tumour or T-antigen. This antigen may be found in a number of different forms [61], and genetic studies have shown that its presence is essential to the initiation and/or maintenance of the transformation property [60]. For SV40-virus-transformed cells there are two species of T-antigen. Large T-antigen (MW 94,000) is found mostly in the nucleus of infected cells, is essential for cell transformation, binds to DNA, and probably functions as an initiator of viral DNA synthesis; the role of small t-antigen (MW 17,000), which is largely found in the cytoplasm, is not known, although a role in cell transformation has been proposed [62].

For Polyomavirus the T-antigen also has two forms. Middle T-antigen is found in the nucleus of transformed cells and has properties similar to those of SV40 large T-antigen except that, although it is essential for the initiation of transformation, it is not necessary for the maintenance of this property: little t-antigen is probably equivalent to SV40 t-antigen. Both large T-antigen for SV40 and middle T-antigen for Polyomavirus may be present on the surface of transformed cells and here they function as specific virus-induced antigens. Since the presence of large T-antigen is essential for SV40-induced cell transformation, the nature and function of this protein is of particular interest. The results of preliminary studies have suggested that these proteins are phosphoproteins with kinase activity, particularly in the phosphorylation of tyrosine; this finding is particularly interesting in view of similar results obtained with RNA tumour viruses. Also, the large T-antigen is complexed with a protein, p53; this is a cellular protein found in normal cells and in increased concentrations in all tested transformed cells and is suggested to be important in transcriptional regulation [58]. If this latter suggestion can be confirmed, the virus-induced T-antigen, which can regulate p53 concentrations, could enhance p53 production in the cell, which in turn could increase and alter the transcriptional properties of the cell to express the transformed state. The subject is of great interest but many problems remain; confirmation of the results is needed. Whether the T-antigen is the kinase or is associated with the enzyme is not known, and the exact nature and function of T-antigen in transformation remains to be determined.

RNA viruses

The replication of oncogenic RNA viruses has been studied in numerous laboratories, and although the viruses vary in many respects, the essential mechanisms of cell transformation may be broadly common. The Rous sarcoma virus (RSV) is nondefective and can replicate in infected cells, a factor that has facilitated studies of transformation by this agent. The RNA of RSV is made up of four genes, each coding for a discrete function, and these functions have been identified by using mutant forms of virus [64]. Thus, the *pol* gene codes for the enzyme reverse transcriptase, the *env* gene specifies the surface glycoproteins of the virus particle, the *gag* gene specifies core protein, and the *sarc* gene codes for a phosphoprotein; genetic studies have shown that the *sarc* gene specifies the product essential for the initiation and maintenance of cell transformation [64,65] but has no other known properties. The *sarc*-encoded protein, termed pp60 v-sarc, has been identified as phosphoprotein of MW approximately 60,000 daltons; it is localised in the cell cytoplasm, probably at the cell membrane, and exhibits protein kinase activity, particularly phosphorylating tyrosine [66,67]. It now remains for researchers to extend these findings to establish the exact biochemical sequence of reactions that determine cell transformation by this virus. The continued presence of the *sarc* gene is essential for the maintenance of the transformed cell state, and the gene must be present in subsequent generations of cells to maintain this property. The perpetuation of the *sarc* gene in cells is due to the activity of the reverse transcriptase encoded by the *pol* gene; this enzyme reverse transcribes a DNA copy from the RNA *sarc* gene, which is then integrated into the host cell genome to persist by parallel replication with the host DNA [64]. A similar *sarc* gene product has been identified for avian sarcoma virus [68].

Many other C-type viruses, such as mouse, rat, and feline sarcoma viruses, can transform cells in vitro: all these viruses are defective for one of the genes required for replication and require a "helper" virus to supply missing genetic material for virus replication. In addition, these viruses all contain gene sequences comparable to the *sarc* gene of RSV and termed the *onc* gene, which is not located at a specific point but can be inserted in any part of the virus RNA. This is the gene conferring oncogenic properties and presumably encodes for the transforming product similar to the *sarc* encoded product of the RSV [69]. Considerable interest surrounds the nature and properties of the protein encoded by the *onc* gene though no clear indication of the nature of this protein has been reported [69]. It has been suggested that the *onc* gene product is a phosphoprotein [70], mimics a normal cell product—which would account for the specificity of cells which can be transformed by these viruses [71]—or mimics growth factors [72–74]. One product of Abelson leukaemia virus is a protein with protein kinase activity and since the T-antigens of some DNA tumour viruses are essential for virus transformation and are probably kinases, confirmation of the results with Abelson leukaemia virus and association of this protein with the *onc* gene would tend to suggest a unified mechanism for transformation by different viruses [75,76].

A third group of C-type viruses are agents such as some avian and murine leukaemia viruses, which are nondefective and induce leukosis in vivo but do not transform cells in vitro. The mechanisms of tumourigenesis for these agents is not known [58]. It is suggested that the induction of tumours is by virus induction of host cell genes, by integration of reverse transcribed DNA from viral genes in the host cell chromosomes—which disturbs growth regulation [73]—or by recombination between these viruses and endogenous host cell viruses to produce strains with altered properties and oncogenic potential [75]. The above theories are purely speculative, and much work remains to be done to determine the mechanism of tumourigenesis by these agents.

ANTIGENS OF VIRUS-INDUCED TUMOURS OF ANIMALS

The fundamental alteration of cell properties that accompanies virus-induced cell transformation is expressed in a variety of morphological, behavioural, and chemical ways. In particular, the transformed cell may possess surface proteins that are altered from the form found in normal cells; the cell may express embryonic proteins not normally present in differentiated cells; the cell may possess increased concentrations of normal cellular products; virus-cellular protein complexes may occur to form new antigenic determinants; and virus encoded proteins may be produced in or on the transformed cell [77,78]. Clearly, consideration of all these elements is not possible in the present discussion, and many further products of the transformed cell remain to be discovered. We propose to limit the discussion to some of the virus-induced products that induce an immune response in the host, for which identification indicates the virus as an aetiological factor in tumourigenesis.

Tumours induced by DNA viruses

Tumour (T) antigen

Studies with Polyomavirus, SV40, and adenovirus have shown that cells transformed in vitro and the cells of tumours induced by these viruses in experimental animals contain a virus-specific protein, termed the tumour or T-antigen, directly encoded from the transforming fraction of the virus nucleic acid [77]. Tumour-bearing animals develop a serum antibody to T-antigen and this antibody reacts with antigen extracted from tumour cells in complement fixation tests [79]: using such tests, the T-antigens induced by a single virus in cells of any species are identical but antigenically distinct from the comparable antigen induced by other transforming viruses. Thus, the T-antigens extracted from tumours induced by adenovirus type-12, SV40, and the avian adenovirus (CELO) react with sera from animals bearing homologous tumours, but not with sera from animals bearing heterologous tumours (table 11-4). The T-antigen can be extracted from tumour cells in a soluble form, and has been shown to have an MW of 70,000 to 100,000 daltons [80,81] and to bind to cell DNA [61]. Using an immunofluorescence test with sera from tumour-bearing animals, the T-antigen can be located within the nucleus of tumour cells [82]; however, the results of other studies have identified T-antigen in the cell cytoplasm or suggested that the antigen is synthesised in the cytoplasm and migrates to the nucleus or the plasma membrane [83,84]. The above studies have been carried out principally with SV40 virus, but it is probable that other oncogenic DNA viruses induce similar T-antigens with comparable properties.

Transplanation antigen (TSTA)

Immunization of experimental animals with SV40 or adenovirus type-12 has been shown to induce immunity to subsequent challenge with live, transplantable tumour cells induced by homologous virus; and similar protection could be shown following immunization with the killed homologous tumour cells [85–88]. These and other similar experiments clearly indicated the presence of a strong and specific virus-induced transplantation antigen (TSTA) on the cell surface. Since the size of the transforming fraction of the virus DNA is only

Table 11-4. Tumour (T) antigens in DNA virus-induced hamsters tumours

Sera from hamsters bearing tumours induced by:	CF-titre of antigen extracts of tumours induced by:		
	Adenovirus-12	SV40	CELO virus
Adenovirus-12	128	<4	<4
SV40	<4	32	<4
CELO virus	<4	<4	32
Normal serum	<4	<4	<4

compatible with the encoding of a protein MW of approximately 70 to 100,000 daltons, and this is the approximate size of the T-antigen, the TSTA must be encoded by the same DNA fraction as the T-antigen. The TSTA induced by SV40 virus has been solubilised from tumour cells and has a MW of 30,000 to 50,000 daltons [89,90].

The SV40-induced tumour model has been used to study the relationship between TSTA and T-antigens and, although distinguishable from each other on the basis of temperature sensitivity and serologically noncrossreactivity, both would appear to be coded for by the same early region of the SV40 genome [90,92]. Sera from SV40 tumour-bearing animals will precipitate out both T-antigens and t-antigens from SV40-infected or transformed cells [93–95], and this represents an essential step in studying further the immunological potential of these molecules. With the realisation that TSTA and T-antigens were coded for by the same segment of the SV40 genome, and therefore share a degree of homology, attempts were made to establish TSTA activity of purified T-antigen: the two activities were shown to copurify and the induction of transplant immunity has been achieved with low doses of the precipitate [96]. It is currently thought that tumour rejection sites are distributed over the entire T-antigen molecule but that only a portion of this molecule is required for TSTA activity. The above findings were substantiated using adenovirus 2-SV40 nondefective hybrid viruses, containing various lengths of the early SV40 DNA segment [91,97–99]; this has allowed a more precise determination of the relationship between TSTA activity and the T-antigen. Recently Tevethia et al. [100] have purified a T-related antigen, designated D2, from HeLa cells infected with adenovirus 2-SV40 hybrid virus (Ad2 + D2) and shown this product to be effective in mediating a tumour rejection response in mice. Whether the products of the various T-antigen sites so far identified differ in TSTA activity remains to be determined.

The demonstration that T-antigen can induce host immunocompetence is important, since this can now be proposed as the most likely mechanism whereby immunization with live virus promotes transplant immunity, although the nature of TSTA expression at the cell membrane remains unclear. Anti-T-antigen sera fails to react with the membranes of either SV40- or Polyomavirus-transformed cells, suggesting that either the TSTA represents an altered form of T-antigen or that the concentration of TSTA at the cell membrane is below the limits of detection by conventional assays for T-antigen [101].

Studies with hamster cells transformed by human Herpesviruses HSV-1 and HSV-2 have failed to detect proteins comparable to the T-antigen induced by Papovaviruses and adenoviruses: the transformed cells contain defective virus genomes, but the products of these genes are unknown [58]. Transplantation studies have shown that immunization of hamsters with irradiated HSV tumour cells induces immunity to subsequent challenge and this indicates the presence of a TSTA [90,102,103]: the transplantation antigen(s) is relatively weak, shows some degree of individual specificity, alters further for the cells of metastatic deposits, and has more in common with naturally arising or chemically induced tumours than those induced by other DNA viruses [45].

Tumours induced by RNA viruses

Tumours induced by C-type viruses have been shown to contain virus structural proteins on the plasma membranes, even in the absence of infective virus; and these proteins can induce an immune response [104]. Thus, the cells of tumours induced by various mouse leukaemia viruses contain virus-specific proteins that act as targets of immunological reactions and are specific for the inducing virus [105,106]. Similar studies with tumour cells induced by feline sarcoma virus or feline leukaemia virus have demonstrated the presence of virus proteins p30 or gp70 [107], and in some instances the protein is expressed on a high molecular weight polypeptide on the cell surface [108]. Both p30 and gp70 can induce immunity to virus infection [109,110]; however, immunization with antigens does not induce immunity to subsequent homologous tumour cell challenge [111]. This suggests that these virus antigens are not the targets of transplantation immunity reactions [101]. In attempts to identify transformation antigens (TSTA) on C-type virus-transformed cells, a mouse leukaemia cell line has been studied by one group of workers. Tumour cells were solubilised and the virus structural proteins p30 and gp70, the histocompatibility antigens, and the transplantation immunity antigen separated; subsequent study showed all these antigens to be distinct [101]. Transplantation immunity studies showed the TSTAs to be highly specific and that they did not induce immunity to tumour cells induced by agents other than viruses of the same group [101,111]. Determination of the molecular weight of the TSTA has not been possible due to incomplete solubilisation; it is possible that the virus-specific antigen is expressed on the tumour cell surface complexed to a host protein, as probably occurs for the TSTA induced by DNA viruses.

IMMUNE RESPONSES TO VIRUS-INDUCED TUMOURS

The host immune response to cancer cells is thought to be important in two respects: first, in preventing primary tumour development (immune surveillance), and second, in preventing metastases from the primary tumour. The recognition by the "immune" system of abnormal cell types is a prerequisite to the development of effective host response. Immunocompetence is mediated either by cells capable of specific antitumour activity, following encounter of newly expressed antigenic determinants on the cancer cells, or alternatively by effector cells recognising and causing lysis of abnormal cancer cells without requiring prior sensitisation to "tumour-associated antigens." The effector cells responsible for mediating this nonadaptive antitumour response are natural killer (NK) cells and cells of macrophage/monocyte lineage. A more concise account of the properties of these effector cells is given in chapter 2; our aim here is to give only those details relevant to virally induced neoplasia.

Adaptive immune responses

DNA virus-induced tumours

Tumours induced by DNA-containing viruses, and expressing virally determined cell products at their cell surface, are able to provoke a host immune response(s) that may be either humoral antibody-mediated or mediated by cells of the lymphoid system. The mechanism of induction of transplantation immunity has been widely studied, and many conclusions can be drawn regarding the specificity and nature of this response.

Using in vivo transplantation techniques, the specificity of immunity to DNA virus-induced tumour challenge has been determined. Unlike tumours induced by chemical carcinogens, the specificity of response is determined by the oncogenic agent. Thus, immunization induces specific resistance to those tumours expressing TSTA encoded for by the homologous virus; protection is restricted and is not afforded to cross-challenge with cells from tumours induced by other DNA viruses [86,112,113]. Adoptive transfer experiments, using lymphoid cells or serum from "immune" animals, have been used previously to study the nature of this transplantation immunity and the results have established a role for the cellular rather than humoral limb of the immune response in tumour rejection [114, 115]. It has been shown that spleen cells or peritoneal cells from immunised animals are capable of transferring immunocompetence to their normal, nonimmunised counterparts; the main effector cell is of T-cell lineage, probably a cytotoxic T-lymphocyte (Tc) [116–118]. Using an SV40-induced tumour model in hamsters, Blasecki [119] has more recently shown that sensitised T-lymphocytes can be induced in vivo by immunization with attenuated tumour cells, and in vitro by exposure of T-lymphocytes to TSTA present on tumour cells; similar findings have been reported for Polyomavirus-induced tumours [120]. T-lymphocytes sensitised in vivo are capable of mediating in vivo tumour rejection and responding in vitro to soluble TSTA [119]. This cytotoxic response is subject to genetic restriction [121,122]; thus, lymphocyte recognition of the TSTA molecule and homology between histocompatibility antigens expressed on the effector T-lymphocyte and the target cell is essential for cytolysis [123]. Cytotoxic T-lymphocytes reactive toward SV40 TSTA are capable of prolific growth in vitro in medium containing T-cell growth factor, termed interleukin 2 (IL-2) [124]. Individual lymphocytes expand under the influence of IL-2 and have been shown to be cytotoxic toward SV40 target cells homologous for H2 antigens. This approach has furthered our understanding of the antigenic determinants associated with the SV40 TSTA. T-lymphocytes cloned by this procedure were shown to possess cytotoxic activity for SV40 transformed cells, but only one of two clones reacted toward a human Papovavirus transformed cell line previously shown to express antigenic moieties cross-reactive with the SV40 T-antigen [124]. This would suggest that lymphocyte clones recognise different antigenic sites on the SV40 TSTA.

In tumour-bearer animals the induction of sensitised T-lymphocytes may be suppressed, either by inhibition of the afferent or efferent limbs of the immune system or by the development of suppressor mechanisms, mediated primarily through antigen-specific suppressor T-cells (Ts); indeed, several studies have shown the development of an anergic state in the tumour-bearer host [125–129]. That Ts-cells regulate the Tc antitumour response has been inferred from recent studies, and development of responsive Ts-cells in preference to Tc-cells may contribute to the development of anergy [119]. Evidence also shows that the effector function of lymphocytes from tumour-bearer animals is blocked [128], possibly by factors produced from tumour cells or host factors stimulated as a result of progressive tumour growth. This is an area where progress has been hampered by technical constraints, and the nature of "blocking" factors has not been clearly established.

The cellular reactivity to tumour antigens expressed on virus-induced tumours can be monitored in vitro using either cytotoxicity assays that demonstrate functional properties of lymphocytes or tests designed to measure sensitisation to antigen components. For example, macrophage migration inhibition has been used to demonstrate delayed hypersensitivity to antigens expressed on DNA virus-induced tumours [130,131] and to C-type retroviruses [132,133]. Koppi and his colleagues [134,135] have used the leukocyte adherence inhibition (LAI) test to monitor cell-mediated immune reactivity and to test for the presence of inhibitory serum components in Moloney murine sarcoma virus (M-MSV)-induced tumour models; it was shown that peritoneal cells harvested from virus-infected mice bearing progressor or regressor tumours were sensitised to tumour-associated antigens, and this was independent of H2 expression. Serum factors that block LAI were also reported, and at the height of tumour progression serum unblocking activity was evident. These authors suggest that serum-blocking factors resembled IJ region encoded products and that unblocking activity mimicked the effect of anti-idiotypic antibody [135], although no direct evidence concerning the identity of the factors has been given.

Many of the DNA-virus-induced tumour systems, although providing valuable insight into the mechanism of rejection, may represent poor models for the study of human neoplasia, since most of the viral agents associated with experimental tumours are not thought to be oncogenic for man. However, Herpesviruses may be important in the aetiology of some human cancers [49,136]. Elucidating the immune response to experimental tumours induced by these viruses may therefore be of value in furthering our understanding of human tumour immune responses. *Herpesvirus hominis*, type-1 and type-2, has been shown to transform mammalian cells in vitro, and inoculation of these cells into the appropriate host leads to the development of progressively growing neoplasms [45,48,102,137].

Unlike other DNA virus-induced tumours, HSV-transformed cells grow from low tumour inoculum and metastasise at low frequency from a primary tumour graft; the immunogenicity of these tumours has been studied, and inoculation of attenuated (15,000 rads X-irradiated) tumour cells shown to induce resistance to challenge with live homologous tumour cells and to provoke a degree of cross-immunity with other HSV-1 and HSV-2 transformed cells, but not tumours induced by other DNA viruses [103,138]. Further studies have been performed using the HSV-333-2-26 cell line, when comparison has been made of the immunogenic properties of the original parent tumour lines and sublines derived from lung metastases. A distinguishing feature of many of these in vivo cloned sublines is their increased metastatic potential compared with the parent tumour, following resection of subcutaneous tumour grafts [139]. Increased or altered metastatic ability of cells from nonviral tumour models has, at least in part, been inferred to be due to a decreased or altered TSTA expression on metastasising tumour cells [140]. Experiments have recently been performed to assess the immunogenic properties of the HSV-333-2-26 parent tumour compared with its metastatic sublines (Met A and Met B). In these studies Met A and Met B tumour cells were shown to possess a reduced immunogenicity, failing to induce host immunocompetence to homologous tumour cell challenge (figure 11–3). These tumours are not however devoid of TSTA, since parent-immune animals will reject a challenge inoculum of either Met A or Met B tumour cells (figure 11–4). These findings imply that the expression of TSTA on metastasising cells is insufficient to evoke a tumour rejection response but that its altered expression does allow recognition, and subsequent rejection, in immunocompetent animals. These results suggest a means of tumour cell escape from immune destruction in vivo and may represent an important property of cells destined to metastasise.

RNA virus-induced tumours

Cells transformed by the M-MSV complex are highly immunogenic, and host immunocompetence is induced during progressive in vivo tumour growth [141]. The Friend, Maloney

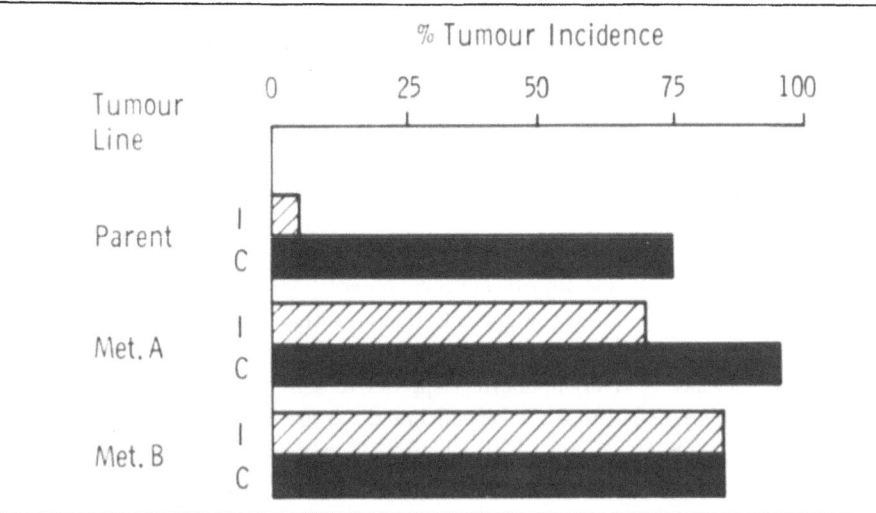

Figure 11-3. Tumour incidence in hamsters immunised against the HSV-333-2-26 parent tumour or two sublines (Met A and Met B) derived from spontaneous lung metastases of the parent tumour, and challenged with live homologous tumour cells. ⊿ Tumour takes in hamsters immunised with X-irradiated tumour cells X3; ■ Tumour takes in control (nonimmunised) hamsters; I immunized; C control.

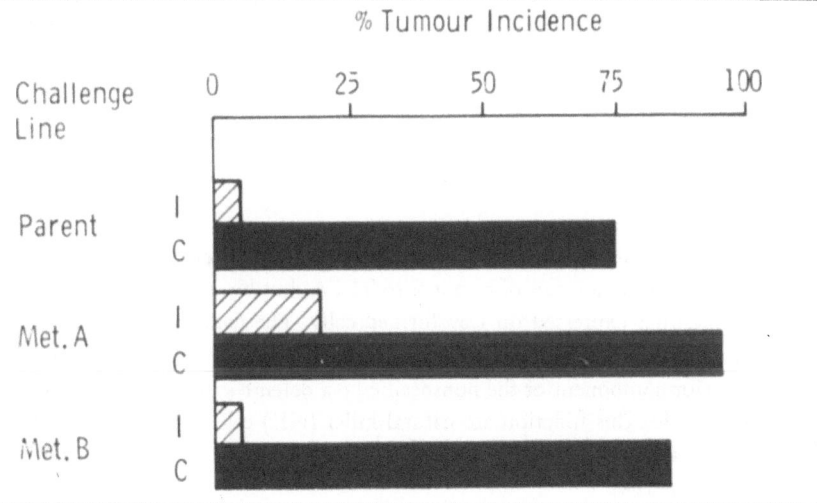

Figure 11-4. Cross-challenge experiment. Tumour incidence in hamsters immunised against the HSV-333-2-26 parent tumour and challenged with live tumour cells derived from the parent line, and Met A and Met B sublines. ⊿ Tumour takes in hamstes immunised with X-irradiated tumour cells X3; ■ Tumour takes in control (nonimmunised) hamsters I immunized; C control.

and Rauscher leukaemia viruses (FMR-LV) all readily induce Tc responses that show genetic restriction in mediating cytolytic activity [127,142,143]. As with DNA virus-induced tumours, Tc-mediating cytotoxicity to virus-induced murine leukaemia targets must recognise both the antigens encoded by the major histocompatibility complex and the antigen responsible for inducing sensitisation [121,122], although the nature of these target structures expressed on FMR-LV leukaemia cells is not clear. Enjuanes and Lee [144] have reported inhibition of Tc-lymphocyte reactivity using M-MLV gp 70, suggesting this glycoprotein to be the major component recognised by specifically cytotoxic lymphocytes; however, other studies [143] have failed to demonstrate inhibition of immune Tc-cell cytotoxicity using high titre anti-gp70 antisera, although antiserum with specificity for H2 antigens was shown to inhibit cytolysis [143,145]. In a more recent study, tunicamicin was used to inhibit gp70 antigen expression, but these investigations failed to demonstrate a linear relationship between gp expression and Tc killing [146]. The reduction in gp70 antigen expression proved to be incomplete and these observations could not account for the reduced level of lymphocyte activity, suggesting that an antigen other than M-MLV gp70 was acting as a recognition structure for Tc-lymphocyte killing.

The in vivo relevance of Tc-lymphocyte responses to cells transformed by FMR-LV viruses is clearly important but may not account for the entire immune response mounted by the host; serum antibody toward structural antigens, particularly to gp70, may have a decisive role in preventing proliferation of disease [147]. The therapeutic value of passive serum therapy, for example, has previously been reported—the beneficial activity stemming primarily from a reduction in virus burden, so reducing the immunosuppressive effect on viraemia and allowing the development of host antiviral responses and long-term resistance. In feline leukaemia (FeLV), antibody-dependent cellular cytotoxicity (ADCC) has been shown, and reactivity occurs toward the FOCMA-transplantation antigen expressed on FeLV transformed cells and not against structural components of the virus [148–150]. This may prove to be an important mechanism whereby antitumour antibody acts synergistically with mononuclear cells of the body to effect destruction of target cells, although the evidence suggesting a role for ADCC in tumour immunity is limited.

Nonadaptive immune responses

So far discussion has focused on specific host reactivity toward TSTA expressed at the cell surface of virally transformed cells. However, other lymphoid cells are capable of mediating tumour cell lysis, not as a result of response to TSTA, but by recognition of other receptor molecules sometimes expressed on transformed cells. The deliberate induction of specific immunocompetence is not required, and abnormal cell types are recognised by effector cells that form a major component of the nonspecific host defense system. The main effector cell types responsible for this function are natural killer (NK) cells and/or macrophages; their possible role as antitumour mechanisms in immune surveillance has been the subject of much debate [151–154].

NK-cell cytotoxicity can be observed against susceptible target cells upon co-culture with effector cells for four to six hours; in most studies radioisotope-labeled target cells are used and cell killing assessed by the release of radioisotope into the culture medium. Many virally induced leukaemias and lymphomas are lysed by NK-cells and have been extensively used for the detailed study of NK-cell function, their properties, and biological relevance. Several studies have shown that NK-cells, as well as cytotoxic T-lymphocytes, mediate killing of M-MSV-induced lymphomas [155–157], and as such they represent an important element of the host defense to tumours of viral as well as nonviral aetiology [158]. The role of NK-cells in preventing the occurrence of tumour metastases in tumour models of nonviral origin has been stressed [154]. In this respect evasion from NK-cells, possibly due to the failure of metastasising cells to express relevant receptor sites, may play a decisive role in allowing metastases to occur. Using the HSV-333-2-26 hamster tumour model, it has been shown that sublines established from lung foci possess an increased ability to metastasise to the lungs as well as other organs, and metastatic potential correlated with a greatly reduced susceptibility to lysis by hamster NK-cells [159]. Collectively, the results obtained with this tumour model suggest that alteration in the immunobiological properties of tumour cells that helps the cells evade immune recognition is of particular importance in allowing blood-borne metastatic spread of the tumour. The HSV-tumour system may prove an important model for studying human cancer, since the transforming virus has been implicated in the aetiology of human carcinomas.

VIRUSES AND HUMAN CANCER

Proof that viruses cause various forms of malignant diseases in a variety of animals has been obtained by direct experimentation; thus, purified viruses inoculated into susceptible animals can induce malignant cells, and the cells of the malignancy can be shown to contain virus or virus-induced products. This type of study has been used to identify numerous tumourigenic viruses in animal species. Similar investigations cannot be carried out in man; some authorities believe that the absence of proof that viruses are the cause of some natural cancers of man is due to the ethical constraints against the type of experiments that have provided conclusive evidence of association for many animal malignant diseases. The evidence implicating viruses in the aetiology of natural cancers of man rests almost entirely on circumstantial evidence of association. The viruses now thought to be possibly aetiologically associated with human cancers are shown in table 11-5. In all cases association is based on circumstantial evidence, but the weight of evidence in some cases is now heavy.

The Epstein-Barr virus (EBV) was first identified in cells established in vitro from a biopsy specimen of a Burkitt's lymphoma, a malignant B-cell lymphoma of children in central Africa and New Guinea [160]. Multiple copies of the virus DNA, existing as a circular episome [161], have been identified in the tumour cells from most biopsies, and similar

Table 11-5. Virus implicated in cancers of man

Agent	"Cancer"	Predisposing conditions
Epstein-Barr virus	Burkitt's lymphoma Nasopharyngeal carcinoma	? Malaria
Herpes hominis	Carcinoma cervix	Promiscuity/venereal infection
Papovaviruses (SV40, JC, BK)	Progressive multifocal encephalopathy	Immunosuppression
Unknown virus	Kaposi's sarcoma	Acquired immunedeficiency syndromes
Hepatitis B	Primary hepatocellular carcinoma	Chronic hepatitis B infection
Human Papillomaviruses	Genital tumours	Venereal infection
T-cell leukaemia virus	1. Sézary syndrome 2. Mycosis fungoids	—

results have been obtained for tumour cells from patients with nasopharyngeal carcinoma, but not for other malignant diseases [162]. In these geographic areas, EBV infection occurs early in life and persists as a chronic infection, occasionally flaring to infect contacts. Usually, and almost exclusively in other countries, infection is manifest as the common disease infectious mononucleosis, and it is now clear that the agent of Burkitt's lymphoma and glandular fever is one and the same [160,162]. The evidence supporting the aetiological role for EBV in Burkitt's lymphoma and nasopharyngeal carcinoma rests on the identification of virus DNA in tumour cells, on the presence of antibody to various EBV antigens in sera of patients, on the ability of EBV to transform B-lymphocytes in vitro, and on the observation that EBV can induce lymphomas in marmosets and primates [58]. However, the case is not completely satisfactory, since EBV DNA cannot be found in all tumours and not all patients with Burkitt's lymphoma possess serum antibodies to EBV. Since infectious mononucleosis has a world-wide distribution and Burkitt's lymphoma is associated with the same agent but is confined chiefly to Africa, a cofactor(s) is probably involved in the aetiology of Burkitt's lymphoma; the cofactor offering the best thesis for the aetiology of this lymphoma is endemic malaria. Thus, infection with EBV in most persons causes the self-limiting infection glandular fever; however, in areas where malaria is endemic, infection with EBV can occur in subjects who are immunosuppressed by concurrent malaria infection, and approximately one in 10,000 cases of dual infection may result in lymphoma [160]. This tentative and simplistic explanation of the role of EBV in Burkitt's lymphoma is thought by many to be the theory embracing most of the known information, but not all are in agreement. In addition, the theory offers no explanation for the role of EBV in nasopharyngeal carcinoma.

Epidemiological and virological investigations carried out during the last decade have produced a large body of circumstantial evidence suggesting that HSV is an aetiological factor in carcinoma of the cervix [163,164]. Thus, the incidence of antibody to HSV is higher in patients with carcinoma of the cervix than in matched controls [165,166], HSV polypeptides have been identified in cells from biopsy specimens grown in tissue culture [167], HSV viruses have been recovered from biopsy specimens [168], and HSV-specific DNA and RNA have been identified in tumour cells [169,170]. In addition, epidemiological studies have shown that the cervical cancer is more common in sexually active women with a history of venereal disease, in women whose sexual partners have malignant disease, and in the wives of men whose first wives died of carcinoma of the cervix; this evidence indicated a sexually transmitted agent in the aetiology of this cancer, and genital infection by HSV is relatively common [171]. In contrast, other studies have revealed anomalies in the above thesis. For example, not all studies have shown a higher incidence of HSV antibody in patients with cervical cancer [172,173]; antibodies to viruses other than HSV have been observed to occur with higher frequency in sera from women with carcinoma of the cervix, compared to controls [174]; and some authorities submit that identification of HSV-specific nucleic acids and polypeptides may indicate a venereal infection of cancer tissues, rather than being a causal factor in the malignancy [173].

The suggestion that human Papillomaviruses may be an aetiological factor in cancer of the cervix is relatively new, and evidence to support the hypothesis has been sought in studies similar to those described for HSV. Thus, a survey of the incidence of Papillomavirus infection in women with cervical cancer revealed that over 90% had associated Papillomavirus infection whilst the incidence was ony 12.5% in matched noncancer controls [175]; virus-specific Papillomavirus DNA has been identified in cells from urogenital tumours [176,177]; and occasionally genital warts have converted to malignant tumours [178]. This evidence, together with the results of other studies [179,180], has suggested that human Papillomaviruses, and particularly type 6 [177] associated with condylomata acuminata, may have an aetiological role in some genital tumours.

The recent explosive increase in the incidence of a severe variant form of Kaposi's sarcoma in homosexuals with acquired immunodeficiency syndrome in the United States and now elsewhere has clearly implicated a transmissible agent passed as a venereal infection in this group of subjects [181,182]. The malignancy has been associated with cytomegalovirus (CMV) infection, since this virus has been isolated from patients and high titres of serum antibody have been found more frequently in patients than in controls [183]; however, it is probable that CMV infection is a reactivation or a generalised primary infection of immune deficient subjects and hence a parallel event.

Epidemiological studies have shown that in areas of the world where the incidence of hepatitis B infection is high, there is an associated high incidence of hepatocellular carcinoma; that the incidence of hepatitis B soluble antigen in the serum of patients with hepatocellular carcinoma is aproximately 80%; and that hepatitis B infection precedes the development of the malignancy [184,185]. Using hybridization techniques, several groups have reported the presence of hepatitis B DNA sequences integrated into the human cell genome [186,187] and the cells contain virus-specific antigens [186]. The evidence supporting an aetiological role for hepatitis B virus in hepatocellular carcinoma is highly suggestive; however, an alternative hypothesis is that cirrhosis, which may be due to many causes and has been associated with an increased risk of this cancer, may also increase the susceptibility of the cancer cells to hepatitis B infection and virus persistence [188].

The fatal demyelinating disease progressive multifocal leucoencephalopathy (PML) is a rare condition only seen in immunosuppressed patients. From the brains of such patients, a Polyomavirus, termed JC virus, has been isolated [189]. In addition, a related virus, termed BK virus, has been isolated from patients undergoing immunosuppressive therapy or suffering from immunosuppressive diseases such as Hodgkin's disease or Wiskott-Aldrich syndrome, and the related virus SV40 has been isolated from the brains of patients with glioblastoma [190]. Serological studies indicate that antibody to JC virus is common in the human population—approximately 80% of adults have it [58], and virus DNA sequences have been identified in PML cells [189]. The evidence that these Polyomaviruses are aetiologically related to PML is similar to that for EBV and Burkitt's lymphoma; indeed, the mechanism could be as described above for the latter, with immunosuppression induced by preexisting disease or drugs and a common, subclinical Polyomavirus infection of man only inducing a rare malignancy in immunosuppressed patients.

Finally, Sézary syndrome is a rare form of leukemia of T-cells, and probably specifically of T-helper cells [191,192]; the disease being related to mycosis fungoides [193]. A unique leukemaeia virus has been isolated from the malignant cells; patients have antibody to this T-cell leukaemia virus; and antibody to virus is found in several populations from which the cases arise [194,195]. The evidence suggesting this virus as the cause of Sezary syndrome is accumulating rapidly, but the mechanism of tumourigenesis remains unknown.

The role(s) of virus infection in the aetiology of malignant diseases in man outlined above suggests some common factors. First, the agents involved tend to produce persistent infection, which may continue for months, years, and even for life. Second, the association of virus infection and malignant disease is seen predominantly in patients with an induced or natural immunosuppression, and this may be highly significant. Experimental tumours induced by viruses in animals are relatively strongly immunogenic; if this is true for virus-induced tumours of man, a state of relative immunosuppression would be required for tumour growth and progression, since the natural body immunity would normally cause rejection. Thus, the immunosuppression induced by chronic malaria, acquired immunodeficiency syndrome, and drug therapy may be essential to the development of Burkitt's lymphoma, Kaposi's sarcoma, and PML, respectively. Furthermore, it is possible that local immunodeficiency induced by chronic infections by such viruses as HSV and hepatitis B may allow cancers to arise at the relevant sites. Two possibilities are suggested: first, viruses may transform cells in patients or at sites in patients in which the immune response is unable to reject the growth and progression of the tumour cell; or second, virus infection may induce a state of general or local immune suppression that allows naturally occurring transformed cells to proliferate and progress without rejection. The finding of virus DNA sequences in tumour cells but not in surrounding normal tissue cells does not invalidate the latter possibility, since virus DNA may more easily integrate with the highly labile chromosome structure of tumour cells and not in more stable normal cells. Which of these two possibilities is relevant to the aetiology of human cancers is not known, and the answer may vary for different malignancies.

VIRUS-INDUCED ANTIGENS IN HUMAN CANCER CELLS

Some of the associations between viruses and human cancer are so recent that studies on virus-specific antigen induction in the malignant cells have not yet been initiated, let alone completed and confirmed. In addition, our present ignorance of this subject is compounded by the inability to perform the type of experiment that has proved so valuable in identifying virus-induced antigens present in experimental tumours of animals and in the recognition of transplantation antigens by transplantation immunity studies. It is not proven that naturally arising tumours of man are immunogenic or can stimulate an immune rejection response comparable to that seen in experimental virus-induced tumours of animals. However, virus-induced antigens have been reported in some human malignant cells, antibody reactions to these products have been demonstrated in some cases, and these immune reactions may act toward tumour cell rejection.

Of the viruses and the associated malignancies shown in table 11–5, little is known in many cases. Patients with Kaposi's sarcoma possess significantly higher titres of antibody to CMV than do control subjects [183]; however, this is probably an opportunist and synchronous infection. The virus and virus-induced antigens of this tumour in acquired immunodeficiency syndromes are as yet unknown. The T-cell leukaemia virus related to Sézary syndrome and mycosis fungoides has been isolated from the tumour cells, and virus particles have been observed in the cells of biopsy specimens. However, the virus and the antigens associated with this agent have not been characterized [194,195]. Patients with Sézary syndrome develop antibody to two virus structural proteins, termed p19 and p24, and it has been assumed that these two antigens are expressed in the tumour cells, are equivalent to the p30 and gp60 present in tumour cells induced by animal retroviruses, and induce antibody in the host [196]. Virus and virus-specific proteins of human Papillomavirus have been described in condylomatous lesions of the uterine cervix, but whether these antigens induce an immune response is not known [177,197]. Hepatitis B virus DNA has been identified in primary hepatocarcinoma cells, together with specific antigens of this virus; thus, both the soluble antigen HB_S and the core antigen HB_C have been identified in tumour cells, and the sera of patients may contain antibody to these antigens [198,199].

More complete studies have been carried out on HSV-induced antigens present in cells of carcinoma of the cervix. Thus, biopsy specimens grown in vitro have been shown to contain nonstructural virus-specific proteins [200,201], an early virus-specific antigen termed AG antigen [202], a virus-specific membrane antigen [203], a virus-specific antigen [204], and a tumour-associated antigen [205]. The relationship of these various findings is not clear, and theoretically the results may be for different virus-induced antigens or a single virus-specific protein detected with different reagents and techniques. The truth probably rests between these two extremes, and the HSV virus in cervical cancer cells encode for at least one virus-specific antigen, which is probably an early protein and may be a nonstructural protein.

The Papovaviruses SV40 and JC viruses have been recognised as infective agents within tumour cells, and virus-specific antigens have been identified in these cells [206,208]. Thus, a nonstructural T-antigen, equivalent to that described for SV40 and adenovirus-induced tumours of animals (see above), has been reported in meningiomas associated with SV40 [208] and in PML associated with JC virus [207]. In addition, virus structural antigens have been detected in the cells of both these tumours [206,208]. Again, the nature of the immune response to these antigens and the possible importance of these reactions to tumour cell rejection is unknown.

The antigens associated with EBV-infected cells of Burkitt's lymphoma and postnasopharyngeal carcinoma have been extensively analysed for virus antigens by many workers. The results indicate that all Burkitt's lymphoma cells possess EB nuclear antigen [209,210], and some if not all contain virus capsid protein [211], early antigen [212], and virus-specific membrane antigen [213]. Again, antibody to these antigens can be detected in the sera from patients, but the relevance of this response to tumour rejection remains to be determined. Other studies of EBV infected cells have demonstrated raised concentrations of polypeptide p53 in these cells, which is probably bound to EB nuclear antigen [214]; this finding is reminiscent of p53 protein bound to T-antigen in many experimental virus-induced tumours of animals and other models [215] and has drawn attention to the possible universal importance of this protein in the malignant process. Thus, binding of virus-induced proteins and naturally occurring p53 may result in excessive production of the latter substance in the cell, and it is the effects produced by increased p53 concentration that initiate the expression by the cells of cancerous properties. The p53 protein has been identified in a number of human tumours not associated with a virus aetiology, and antibody to this substance has been identified in sera from cancer patients [215].

IMMUNE RESPONSE TO HUMAN TUMOURS

Investigation into the immune response of TSTA of animal neoplasms has been made possible by the availability of syngeneic inbred strains of animals, which have allowed tumour transplantation experiments to be performed to establish the relevance of antitumour immune responses. Similar studies in humans are not possible, and our understanding of the immune responses to human cancer cells is therefore limited. The main questions to be answered relate to the presence of TSTA or virally determined antigens on human cancer cells and whether these evoke an immune response in the host. In this respect, it has proved difficult to relate particular immune responses—for example, cellular versus humoral antibody reactivity—with tumour rejection, or to recognise viral genome encoded products; much of the evidence suggesting host immunocompetence is based on in vitro findings, where it is difficult to draw conclusions as to the in vivo role of a given mechanism.

In spite of these drawbacks, the study of immune responses has allowed conclusions to be drawn regarding the aetiological significance of certain viruses, for example, the human T-cell leukaemia virus [195,216] where the detection of antibody has played a major role in suggesting viral aetiology. It must be stressed, however, that the functional integrity observed by in vitro testing helps little to determine the in vivo relevance of a given immune reaction. The following observations relate to those tumours where viral aetiology has been inferred, although in most cases not proven.

In human breast carcinoma patients, immune reactivity to antigens cross-reactive with murine mammary tumour virus (Mu-MTV) structural antigen gp52 has been observed [217,218]. Evidence has been presented showing that human breast carcinoma tissue, but not benign breast tissue, possesses antigenic determinants cross-reactive with Mu-MTV glycoproteins; Mu-MTV gp52 antigen has been localised in human breast carcinoma tissue using immunoperoxidase staining [219], and immune recognition of this antigen has been reported to be cellular as well as humoral. Black et al. [220], by leukocyte migration inhibition (LMI) testing, reported cell-mediated hypersensitivity reactions to a Mu-MTV glycoprotein in breast carcinoma patients with a good prognosis, although a subsequent study failed to confirm this finding [221].

Other tests demonstrating humoral antibody to Mu-MTV antigens have been used with some degree of success; these include indirect immunofluorescence, immune electronmicroscopy, and agglutination tests [217,222]. Antibody to Mu-MTV glycoproteins was demonstrated in the sera of a high proportion of patients with breast carcinoma; sera from patients with benign breast diseases and other malignancies, and from control subjects, showed considerably less reactivity to Mu-MTV antigens. On further analysis, no correlation could be inferred between antibody status and the stage of disease [217]. Furthermore, the reactive antibodies, which were shown to be IgG and IgM, could be removed from sera by absorption with gp52 or gp34 of Mu-MTV, or adsorption with Rauscher leukaemia virus, demonstrating the cross-reactive nature of the immune response. In a recent study reported by Holder and Wells [222], sera from 79% of patients with breast carcinoma showed antibody to Mu-MTV antigen as determined by immune electronmicroscopy, compared to 19% of normal subjects or patients with benign breast disease. Patients with breast carcinoma would appear to have antibody responses to antigens Mu-MTV, although the precise relevance of this immune response is not clear. Whether T-lymphocyte responses occur to these or similar antigenic determinants has not yet been studied.

Several lines of evidence suggest a relationship between Herpesviruses and human carcinoma—including HSV-2 with cervical carcinoma and EBV with nasopharyngeal carcinoma [223]. Much of the evidence for the involvement of HSV in cervical neoplasia stems from studies of the humoral antiviral antibody response in carcinoma patients [224–228]. Recent laboratory investigations have shown the presence of antibody to HSV-2 early antigen AG-4 to be of possible importance as a prognostic indicator, since sero-negative patients showed a relative increase in mortality compared with sero-positive patients, who showed an improved survival rate [227,228]. It is not clear whether the humoral response to AG-4 antigenic determinant operates as an effector mechanism in vivo or whether the presence of antibody reflects a level of general immunocompetence that may influence tumour progression.

Antibody to HSV has been documented by virus neutralisation testing and ADCC [225, 226,229,238], where higher antibody levels were shown for patients with cervical carcinoma than for control individuals or for patients with other malignancies [230,231]. A degree of correlation has been reported between anti-HSV antibody titres and the severity of disease, low levels of response being indicative of a bad prognosis. Antibody responses to CMV, as well as HSV, have been detected more frequently in the sera of women with cervical atypia than in the sera from healthy women with cervical disorders [225]. However, perhaps of more significance than the observed antiviral humoral response is the development of immunocompetence toward virally transformed cells. The antigenic specificities encoded for by the viral genome in transformed cells may be distinct from viral structural antigens, suggesting that the host response to viral components may be inadequate to deal effectively with neoplastic cells. Recent studies by Christenson [230] have shown that antibody present in the sera of women with cervical carcinoma can act synergistically with peripheral blood mononuclear cells to cause lysis of HSV-transformed cells through ADCC. The specificity of this reaction is determined by the antibody, but killing is effected through blood mononuclear cells. Further studies are required to determine the relative importance of this mechanism in vivo.

Considerable interest has been aroused about the significance of human BK and JC Papovaviruses as aetiological agents of cancer. The humoral antibody response to these viruses, which have previously been associated with progressive multifocal leukoencephalopathy and ureteric stenosis, is widespread in the community [231–234]. On serological evidence the BK virus would appear to cause peak infection at two years of age, and it is suggested that the immune system may be important in controlling virus reactivation/infection, since these agents are found in immunocompromised patients. Again it has proved difficult to determine the role of these viruses in human neoplastic disease, although the experimental oncogenicity of these viruses has been shown [189].

Studies on immunosuppressed groups of patients have provided a clue as to the importance of an intact immune defense system in preventing the development of neoplasia. In immunosuppressed patients (e.g., transplant recipients), reactivation of EBV, HSV, and Polyomaviruses occurs at a higher frequency than expected; in parallel, the prevalence of malignant lymphoma in these patients is 350 times more common than in the general population [235]. The suggestion can be made that immunocompetence, either specific or nonspecific, is necessary for effective human neoplasia to operate. The nature of the immunological surveillance, although not clear, may require functional NK-cells, macrophages, and possibly T-lymphocytes [152–154], and abrogation of these mechanisms, due to immunosuppression, would possibly allow oncogenic viruses or oncogenic virus-induced tumour cells to proliferate.

REFERENCES

1. Cairns J. The cancer problem. Sci Amer 233: 64–72, 1975.
2. Weisburgher JH, Williams GM. Metabolism of chemical carcinogens. In Becker FF (ed.), Cancer. Etiology; chemical and physical carcinogenesis. New York: Plenum Press, 1975.
3. Ellerman V, Bang O. Experimentelle leukaemie bei huhnern. Centr Bakteriol Abt 1: 559–601, 1908.
4. Rous P. A sarcoma of the fowl transmissible by an agent separable from the tumour cells. J Exp Med 13: 397–411, 1911.
5. Moses A. O virus do mixoma dos collhos. Mem Inst Oswald-Cruz. 3: 46–53, 1911.
6. Shope RE. Filterable virus causing tumour-like condition in rabbits and its relationship to virus myxomatosum. J Exp Med 56: 803–822, 1932.
7. Shope RE. Infectious papillomatosis of rabbits. J Exp Med 58: 607–625, 1933.
8. Furth J. Lymphomatosis, myelomatosis and endothelioma of chickens caused by a filterable agent. J Exp Med 58: 253–275, 1933.
9. Bittner JJ. Some possible effects of nursing on mammary gland tumour incidence in mice. Science 84: 162, 1936.
10. Lucké B, Carcinoma of the leopard frog: Its probable causation by a virus. J Exp Med 68: 457–468, 1938.
11. Sweet BH, Hilleman MR. The vacuolating virus SV40. Proc Soc Exp Biol Med 105: 420–427, 1960.
12. Rabson AS, O'Connor GT, Kirschstein RL, Branigan WJ. Papillary ependymomas produced in *Rattus (Mastomys) Natalensis* inoculated with vacuolating virus (SV40). J Natl Cancer Inst 29: 765–787, 1962.
13. Trenton JJ, Yabe Y, Taylor G. The quest for human cancer viruses. Science 137: 835–841, 1962.
14. Huebner RJ. Adenovirus-directed tumour and T-antigens. In Pollard M (ed.), Perspectives in virology. 5: 147–166, 1967.
15. Jordan WS, Badger GF, Dingle JH. A study of type-specific adenovirus antibodies in the first five years of life—Implications for the use of adenovirus vaccine. N Eng J Med 258: 1041–1044, 1958.
16. Tooze J. Structure and composition of polyoma, SV40 and the Papillomaviruses. In Watson J (ed.), Origins of human cancer. New York: Cold Spring Harbor, 1977.
17. Zur Hausen H. Human Papillomaviruses and their possible role in squamous cell carcinomas. Curr Top Microbiol Immunol 78: 1–30, 1977.
18. Stewart SE, Eddy BE, Borgese N. Neoplasms in mice inoculated with a tumour agent carried in tissue culture. J Nat Cancer Inst 20: 1223–1236, 1958.
19. Carr I, McGinty FM, Potter CW. Neoplastic metastasis of transplantable animal neoplasms. Experimenta 30: 185–186, 1974.
20. Huebner RJ. Tumours induced by adenoviruses. In Pollard M (ed.), Perspectives in virology. New York: Academic Press, 1967.
21. Sarma PS, Heubner RJ, Lane WT. Induction of tumours in hamsters with an avian adenovirus (CELO). Science 149: 1108, 1965.
22. Hull RN, Johnson IS, Cuthbertson CG, Reimer CB, Wright HF. Oncogenicity of the simian adenoviruses. Science 150: 1044–1046, 1965.
23. Gilden RJ, Kern J, Beddow TG, Heubner RJ. Bovine adenovirus type 3: Detection of specific tumour and T-antigens. Virology 31: 727–729, 1967.
24. Brandt CD, Kim HW, Varsosky AJ, Jeffries BC, Arrobio JO, Rindge B, Parrott RH, Chanock RM. Infections in 18,000 infants and children in a controlled study of respiratory tract disease. I Adenoviruses. Amer J Epidemiol 90: 484–500, 1969.
25. Potter CW, Sheddon WIH. The distribution of adenovirus antibodies in normal children. J Hyg (Camb.) 61: 155–160, 1963.
26. Potter CW, Schild GC. Antibodies in human sera to adenoviruses (types 7, 12, and 18). Arch Ges Virusforsch 18: 80–87, 1966.
27. Green M, Mackey JK. Are oncogenic human adenoviruses associated with human cancer? Cold Spring Harbor Conf. Cell Proliferation 4: 1027–1031, 1977.
28. Rafferty KA. The cultivation of inclusion-associated viruses from Lucké tumours frogs. Ann NY Acad Sci 126: 3–21, 1965.
29. Naegele RF, Granoff A, Darlington RW. The presence of the Lucké Herpesvirus genome in induced tadpole tumours and its oncogenicity. Proc Natl Acad Sci (USA) 71: 830–834, 1974.
30. Purchase HG. Marek's disease virus and the Herpesvirus of turkeys. Prog Med Virol 18: 178–197, 1974.
31. Payne LN, Biggs PM. Studies on Marek's disease. II. Pathogenesis. J Natl Cancer Inst 39: 281–291, 1967.
32. Hunt RD, Melendez LV, Garcia G, Trum BF. Pathologic features of *Herpesvirus ateles* lymphoma in cotton-topped marmosets (Saguinas oedipus). J Natl Cancer Inst 49: 1631–1638, 1972.

33. Niven JSF, Armstrong JA, Andrewes CH, Pereira HG, Valentine RC. Subcutaneous growths in monkeys produced by a poxvirus. J Path Bact 81: 1–14, 1961.
34. Blair FB. The mammary tumour virus (MTV). In Current topics in microbiology. New York: Springer Verlag 45: 1–69, 1968.
35. Hageman PC, Calafat J, Daams JH. The mouse mammary tumour viruses. In Emmelot P, Bentvelsen P (eds.), RNA viruses and the host genome in oncogenesis. Amsterdam: North Holland, 1972.
36. Panem S, Reynolds JT. Retrovirus expression in normal and pathogenic processes of man. Fed Proc 38: 2674–2678, 1979.
37. Essex M, Cotter SM, Hardy WD, Hess P, Jarrett W, Jarrett O, Mackey L, Laid H, Perryman L, Olsen RG, Young DS. Antibody titres in cats with naturally occurring leukaemia, lymphoma and other diseases. J Nat Cancer Inst 55: 463–467, 1975.
38. Theilen GH, Wolfe LG, Rabin H, Deinhardt F, Dungworth DL, Fowler ME, Gould D, Cooper R. Biological studies of four species of nonhuman primates with simian sarcoma virus. Bibl Haematol 39: 251–257, 1973.
39. McAllister RM, Nicolson MO, Reed G, Kern J, Gilden RV, Huebner RJ. Transformation of rodent cells by adenovirus 19 and other group D adenoviruses. J Natl Cancer Inst 43: 917–922, 1969.
40. Ankerst J, Jonsson N, Kjellen L, Norrby E, Sjogren HO. Induction of mammary fibroadenomas in rats by adenovirus type 9. Int J Cancer 13: 286–290, 1974.
41. Monoz N. Effect of Herpesvirus type 2 and hormonal imbalance in uterine cervix of the mouse. Cancer Res 33: 1504–1508, 1973.
42. Wentz WB, Facog JW, Reagan JW, Heggie AD. Cervical carcinigenesis with herpes simplex virus type 2. Amer J Obs Gyn 46: 117–121, 1975.
43. Potter CW. Some aspects of the role of viruses in cancer. Postgrad Med J 55: 150–158, 1979.
44. Boyd AL. Characterization of single-cell clonal lines derived from HSV-2 transformed mouse cells. Intervirol 6: 156–167, 1975.
45. Potter CW, Shortland JR, Mousway KM, Rees, RC. Comparative studies of transformed hamster cells by Herpesvirus hominis types 1 and 2. Brit J Exp Path 63: 285–298, 1982.
46. Todaro, GJ, Green H, Swift MR. Susceptibility of human diploid fibroblast strains to transformation by SV40. Science 153: 1252–1254, 1966.
47. Butel JS, Brugge JS, Noonan CA. Transformation of primate and rodent cells by temperature-sensitive mutants of SV40. In Tumour Viruses (Cold Spring Harbour Symp.) 34: 25–36, 1974.
48. Duff R, Rapp F. Oncogenic transformation of hamster cells after exposure to herpes simplex virus type 2. Nature 233: 48–50, 1971.
49. Rapp F, Westmoreland D, Cell transformation by DNA-containing viruses. Biochimica Biophysica Acta 458: 167–211, 1976.
50. Aaronson SA. Susceptibility of human cell strains to transformation by simian virus SV40 and simian virus deoxyribonucleic acid. J Virol 6: 470–475, 1970.
51. Casto BC, Adenovirus transformation of hamster embryo cells. J Virol 2: 376–383, 1968.
52. Sambrook J. Transformation by Polyomavirus and simian virus 40. Adv Cancer Res 16: 141–180, 1972.
53. Rabson AS, Kirchstein RL. Induction of malignancy in vivo in newborn hamster kidney tissue infected with simian vacuolating virus (SV40). Proc Soc Exp Biol Med 111: 323–328, 1962.
54. Jensen F, Koprowski H, Ponton JA. Rapid transformation of human fibroblast cultures by simian virus 40. Proc Nat Acad Sci 50: 343–348, 1963.
55. Todaro GJ, Aaronson SA. Human cell strains susceptible to focus formation by human adenovirus type 12. Proc Nat Acad Sci 61: 1272–1278, 1968.
56. Green M. DNA and RNA tumour viruses—molecular events of virus replication and cell transformation and role in human cancer. Adv Pathbiol 2: 10–23, 1976.
57. Galloway DA, McDougall JK. Transformation of rodent cells by a cloned DNA fragment of herpes simplex virus type 2. J Virol 38: 749–760, 1981.
58. Wyke JA. Oncogenic viruses. J Pathol 135: 39–85, 1981.
59. Sambrook J, Westphal H, Srinvasan PR, Dulbecco R. The integrated state of viral DNA in SV40-transformed cells. Proc Nat Acad Sci 60: 1288–1295, 1968.
60. Butel JS, Brugge TC, Noonan CA. Transformation of primate and rodent cells by temperature sensitive mutants of SV40: Cold Spring Harbour Symp. Quant Biol 39: 25–31, 1974.
61. Carroll RB, Smith AG. Monomer molecular weight of T antigen from simian virus 40-infected and transformed cells. Proc Soc Exp Biol, Med 73: 2254–2258, 1976.
62. Rubin H, Figge J, Bladon MT, Chen LB, Ellman M, Bikel I, Farrel M, Livingston DM. Role of small t antigen in the acute transforming activity of SV40. Cell 30: 469–480, 1982.
63. Levine AJ. Transformation-associated tumour antigens. Adv. Cancer Res 37: 75–109, 1982.

64. Hanafusa H. Cell transformation by RNA tumour viruses. In Fraenkel-Conrat H, Wagner R (eds.), Comprehensive virology. New York: Plenum Press, vol 10, 1977.
65. Vogt PK. The genetics of RNA tumour viruses. In Fraenkel-Conrat H, Wagner R (eds.), Comprehensive virology. New York: Plenum Press, vol 10, 1977.
66. Hunter T, Sefton BM. Transforming gene product of Rous sarcoma virus phosphorylates tyrosine. Proc Natl Acad Sci 77: 1311–1315, 1980.
67. Hayman MJ. Transforming proteins of avian retroviruses. J Gen Virol 52: 1–14, 1981.
68. Brugg JS, Erikson RL. Identification of a transformation specific antigen induced by avian sarcoma virus. Nature 269: 346–348, 1977.
69. Duesbery PH. Transforming genes of retroviruses. Cold Spring Harbour Symp. Quant Biol 44: 13–21, 1980.
70. Shih TY, Weeks MO, Young HA, Scolnick EM. Identification of a sarcoma virus coded phosphoprotein in the non-producer cells transformed by Kirsten or Harvey murine sarcoma viruses. Virology 96: 64–79, 1979.
71. Graf T, Beug H. Avian leukaemia viruses. Interaction with their target cells, in vivo and in vitro. Biochim Biophys Acta 516: 269–299, 1978.
72. De Larco JE, Tadaro GJ. Growth factors from murine sarcoma virus-transformed cells. Proc Nat Acad Sci 75: 4001–4005, 1978.
73. Langan T. Malignant transformation and protein phosphorylation. Nature 286: 329–330, 1980.
74. Weil R. Viral "tumour antigen": A novel type of mammalian regulator protein. Biochim Biophys Acta 516: 310–388, 1978.
75. Hayward WS, Weel BG, Astrin SM. Avian lymphoid leukosis is correlated with the appearance of discrete new RNAs containing viral and cellular genetic information: In Neth R, Gallo R (eds.), Modern trends in human leukaemia. Munich: Bergerman Verlag, 1981.
76. Stephenson JR. Type C virus structural and transformation-specific proteins. In Stephenson JR (ed.), Molecular biology of RNA tumour viruses. New York: Academic Press, 1980.
77. Old LJ, Stockert E. Immunogenetics of cell surface antigens of mouse leukaemia. Anns Rev Genet 11: 127–160, 1977.
78. Coggin JH, Ambrose KR. Embryonic and foetal determinants on virally and chemically induced tumours. Methods Cancer Res 18: 371–389, 1979.
79. Black PH, Rowe WP, Turner HC, Huebner RJ. A specific complement-fixing antigen present in SV40 tumour and transformed cells. Proc Nat Acad Sci 50: 1148–1156, 1963.
80. Potter CW, McLaughlin BC, Oxford JS. Simian virus 40-induced T and tumour antigen. J Virol 4: 574–579, 1969.
81. Ahmed-Zadeh C, Allet B, Greenblatt J, Weil R. Two forms of the simian virus-40-specific T-antigen in abortive and lytic infection. Proc Nat Acad Sci 73: 1097–1101, 1976.
82. Pope JH, Rowe WP. Detection of specific antigen in SV40-transformed cells by immunofluorescence. J Exp Med 120: 121–128, 1964.
83. Schild GC, Oxford JS, Potter CW. Changes accompanying long-term tissue culture of an adenovirus type 12 tumour cell line. Brit J Cancer 22: 798–807, 1968.
84. Anderson JL, Martin RG, Chang C, Mora PT, Livingstone D. Nuclear preparations of SV40-transformed cells contain tumour specific transplantation antigen activity. Virology 76: 420–425, 1977.
85. Girardi AJ. Prevention of SV40 virus oncogenesis in hamsters. I. Tumour resistance induced by human cells transformed by SV40. Proc Nat Acad Sci 54: 445–451, 1965.
86. Potter CW, Hoskins JM, Oxford JS. Immunological relationship of some oncogenic DNA viruses. I. Transplantation immunity studies. Arch Ges Virusforsch 27: 73–86, 1969.
87. Zarling JM, Tevethia SS. Transplantation immunity to simian virus-40 transformed cells in tumour bearing mice. I. Development of cellular immunity to simian virus 40 tumour specific transplantation antigens during tumourigenesis by transformed cells. J Natl Cancer Inst 50: 137–147, 1980.
88. Tevethia SS, Greenfield RS, Flyer DC, Tevethia MJ. SV40 transplantation antigen: Relationship to SV40-specific proteins. Cold Spring Harbour Symp. Quant Biol 44 (Pt. 1): 235–242, 1980.
89. Smith RW, Morganroth J, Mora PT. SV40 virus-induced tumour specific transplantation antigen in cultured mouse cells. Nature 227: 141–145, 1971.
90. Rogers MJ, Low LW. Immunogenic properties of a soluble tumour rejection antigen (TSTA) from a simian virus 40-induced sarcoma. Int J Cancer 23: 89–96, 1979.
91. Lewis AM Jr, Rowe WP. Studies of nondefective adenovirus 2-simian virus 40 hybrid viruses. VIII. Association of simian virus 40 transplantation antigen with a specific region of the early viral genome. J Virol 12, 836–840, 1973.
92. Girardi AJ, Defendi V. Induction of SV40 transplantation antigen (TrAg) during the lytic cycle J Virol 42, 688–698, 1970.

93. Tegtmeyer P, Schwatz M., Collins JK, Rundell K. Regulation of tumour antigen synthesis by simian virus 40 gene. J Virol 16: 168–178, 1975.

94. Crawford LV, Pim DC, Lane DP. An immunochemical investigation of SV40 T antigens. II. Quantitation of antigen and antibody activities. Virology 100: 314–325, 1980.

95. Greenfield RS, Flyer DC, Tevethia SS. Demonstration of unique and common antigenic sites located on the SV40 large T and small t antigens. Virology 104, 312–322, 1980.

96. Chang C, Martin RG, Livingston DM, Luborsky SW, Hu C, Mora PT. Relationship between T-antigen and tumour specific transplantation antigen in simian virus 40 transformed cells. J Virol 29: 69–75, 1979.

97. Morrow JF, Berg P, Kelly TJ Jr., Lewis AM Jr. Mapping of simian virus 40 early functions on the viral chromosome. J Virol 12, 653–658, 1973.

98. Jay G, Jay FT, Chang C, Friedman RM, Levrin AS. Tumour specific transplantation antigen: Use of the $Ad2^+$ ND_1 hybrid virus to identify the proteins responsible for simian virus 40 tumour rejection and its genetic origin. Proc Natl Acad Sci 75, 3055–3059, 1978.

99. Jay G, Jay FT, Chang C, Levine AS, Friedman RM. Induction of simian virus 40-specific tumour rejection by the $Ad2^+$ ND_2 hybrid virus. J Gen Virol 44: 287–296, 1979.

100. Tevethia SS, Flyer DC, Trian R. Biology of simian virus 40 (SV40) transplantation antigen (TrAG). Virology 107: 13–23, 1980.

101. Law LW, Rogers MJ, Apella E. Tumour antigens in neoplasms induced by chemical carcinogens and by DNA and RNA-containing viruses: Properties of the solubilised antigens. Adv Cancer Res 32: 201–215, 1980.

102. Duff R, Doller E, Rapp F. Immunologic manipulation of metastases due to Herpesvirus transformed cells. Science 180: 79–81, 1973.

103. Mousawy KM, Rees RC, Potter CW. Immunogenic properties of hamster tumours of Herpesvirus hominis aetiology. Cancer Immunol Immunother 8: 119–126, 1980.

104. Baver H. Virion and tumour antigens of C-type RNA tumour viruses. Adv Cancer Res 20: 275–341, 1975.

105. Old LJ, Boyse EA, Stockert E. The G(Gross) leukaemia antigen. Cancer Res 25: 813–819, 1965.

106. Geering G, Old LJ, Boyse EA. Antigens of leukaemia induced by naturally occurring murine leukaemia virus: Their relation to the antigen of Gross virus and other murine leukaemia viruses. J Exp Med 124: 753–772, 1966.

107. Grant CK, De Noronha F, Tusch C, Michalek MT, McLane MF. Protection of cats against progressive fibrosarcomas and persistent leukaemia virus infection by vaccination with feline leukaemia cells. J Natl Cancer Inst 65: 1285–1291, 1980.

108. Ledbetter J, Nowinski RC, Emery S. Viral proteins on the surface of murine leukaemia cells. J Virol 22: 65–73, 1977.

109. Hunsmann G, Moennig V, Schafer W. Properties of mouse leukaemia viruses. IX. Active and passive immunization of mice against friend leukaemia and isolated viral GP_{71} glycoprotein and to corresponding antiserum. Virology 66: 327–329, 1975.

110. De Noronha F, Baggs, R, Schafer W, Bolognesi DP. Prevention of oncornavirus-induced sarcomas in cats by treatment with antiviral antibodies. Nature 267: 54–56, 1977.

111. Rogers MJ, Law LW, Appella E. Solubilized TSTA and the major viral structural proteins gp70 and p30 in the immune response to murine leukaemia induced by Friend and Rauscher virus. Int J Cancer 20: 303–308, 1977.

112. Rees RC, Potter CW, Shelton J. The specificity of cellular immune reactions to three DNA virus-induced tumours as measured by the macrophage migration inhibition test. Europ J Cancer 11: 79–86, 1975.

113. Sjogren HO, Minowada J, Ankerst J. Specific transplantation antigens of mouse sarcomas induced by adenovirus type 12. J Exp Med 125: 689–701, 1967.

114. Rees RC, Potter CW. In vivo studies of cell-mediated and humoral immune responses to adenovirus 12-induced tumour cells. Ach Ges Virusforsch 41: 116–126, 1973.

115. Blasecki JW, Tevethia SS. Restoration of specific immunity against SV40 tumour-specific transplantation antigens to lymphoid cells from tumour-bearing mice. Int J Cancer 16: 275–283, 1975.

116. Gooding LR. Specificities of killing by cytotoxic lymphocytes generated in vivo and in vitro to syngeneic SV40 transformed cells. J Immunol 118: 920–927, 1977.

117. Gooding LR. Specificities of killing by T-lymphocytes generated against syngeneic SV40 transformants: Studies employing recombinants with the H2 complex. J Immunol 122: 1002–1008, 1979.

118. Gooding LR. T-lymphocyte effectors generated against SV40 transformed cells. J Immunol 121: 2328–2336, 1979.

119. Blasecki JW. Functional analysis of lymphoid cell subpopulations involved in rejection of tumours induced by simian virus 40. In Streilen JW, Hart DA, Stein-Streilen J, Duncan WR, Billingham RE (eds.), Hamster immune responses in infections and oncologic diseases. New York: Plenum Press, 1981, pp. 123–134.

120. Allison AC. Immune responses to polyoma virus-induced tumours. In Klein G. (ed.), Viral oncology. New York: Raven Press, 1980, pp. 481–488.
121. Schroder JW, Henning R, Molner RJ, Edelman GM. The recognition of H2 and viral antigens by cytotoxic T-cells. Cold Spring Harbour, Quant Biol 41: 547–558, 1976.
122. Doherty PC, Gotle D, Trinchieri G, Zinkernagel RM. Models for recognition of virally modified cells by immune thymus-derived lymphocytes. Immunogenetics 3: 517–524, 1976.
123. Gooding LR, Edwards CB. H-2 antigen requirements in the in vitro induction of SV40-specific cytotoxic T-lymphocytes. J Immunol 124: 1258–1262, 1980.
124. Campbell AE, Foley FM, Tevethia SS. Demonstration of multiple antigenic sites of the SV40 transplantation rejection antigen by using cytotoxic T-lymphocyte clones. J Immunol 130: 490–492, 1983.
125. Mitulska ZB, Smith C, Alexander P. Evidence for an immunological reaction of the host directed against its own actively growing primary tumour. J Natl Cancer Inst 36: 29–35, 1966.
126. Barski G. Youn JK. Evolution of cell-mediated immunity in mice bearing an antigenic tumour. Influence of tumour growth and surgical removal. J Natl Cancer Inst 43: 111–112, 1969.
127. Herberman RB, Aoki T, Nunn ME, Lavrin DH, Soares N, Gazdar A, Holden H, Chang KSS. Specificity of ^{51}Cr-release cytotoxicity of lymphocytes immune to murine sarcoma virus. J Natl Cancer Inst 53: 1103–1111, 1974.
128. Blesecki JW, Tevethia SS. In vitro studies on the cellular immune response of tumour-bearing mice to SV40-transformed cells. J Immunol 114, 244–249, 1975.
129. Zarling JM, Tevethia SS. Transplantation immunity to Simian virus-40-transformed cells in tumour-bearing mice. I. Development of cellular immunity to Simian virus 40 tumour-specific transplantation antigen during tumourigenesis by transplanted cells. J Natl Cancer Inst 50: 137–147, 1973.
130. Rees RC, Potter CW. Immune response to adenovirus 12-induced tumour antigens, as measured in vitro by the macrophage migration inhibition test. Europ J Cancer 9: 497–502, 1973.
131. Blesecki JW, Tevethia SS. In vitro assay of cellular immunity to tumour-specific antigen(s) of virus-induced tumours by macrophage migration inhibition. J Immunol 110: 590–594, 1973.
132. Mortensen RF, Ceglowski WS, Friedman H. In vitro assessment of cellular immunity to Rauscher leukaemia virus. J Immunol 111: 657–660, 1973.
133. Datta SK, McCormick KJ, Trentin JJ. Induction of tumour-specific cell-mediated immunity by a non-infectious type-C virus. Infect Immun 33: 126–129, 1981.
134. Koppi TA, Halliday WJ. Regulation of cell-mediated immunologic reactivity to Moloney murine sarcoma virus-induced tumours. I. Cell and serum activity detected by leukocyte adherence inhibiton. J Natl Cancer Inst 66: 1089–1096, 1981.
135. Koppi TA, Halliday WJ, McKenzie IF. Regulation of cell-mediated immunologic reactivity to Moloney murine sarcoma virus-induced tumours. II. Nature of blocking and unblocking factors in serum. J Natl Cancer Inst 66: 1097–1102, 1981.
136. Nahmias AJ, Sawanabori S. The genital herpes-cervical cancer hypothesis—10 years later. Prog Exp Tumour Res 21: 117–125, 1978.
137. Shortland J, Mousway KM, Rees RC, Potter CW. Tumourigenicity of Herpesvirus hominis type 2 transformed cells (line 333-8-9) in adult hamsters. J Path 129: 169–178, 1979.
138. Mousway KM, Rees RC, Potter CW, Shortland JR. Immune response of hamsters to transplanted herpesvirus induced tumours. In Letnansky (ed.), Biology of the cancer cell. Kugler Medical Publ, 1980, pp. 127–132.
139. Walker JR, Rees RC, Teale DM, Potter CW. Properties of a Herpesvirus-transformed hamster cell line. I. Growth and culture characteristics of sublines of high and low metastatic potential. Europ J Cancer Clin Oncol 18: 1017–1026, 1982.
140. Gorlik E, Fogel M, Baetselier P, Katzav S, Feldman M, Segal S. Immunobiological diversity of metastatic cells. In Liotta LA, Hart IT (eds.), Immune invasion and metastases. The Hague: Martinus Nijhoff, 1982, pp. 133–146.
141. Levy JP, Leclerc JC. The murine sarcoma virus induced tumour: Exception or general model in tumour immunology. Adv Cancer Res 24: 1–66, 1977.
142. Gomard E, Duprez V, Reme T, Colombani MJ, Levy JP. Exclusive involvement of H-2d^b or H-2K^d products in the interaction between T-killer lymphocyte and syngeneic H-2^b and H-2^d viral lymphomas. J Exp Med 146: 909–922, 1977.
143. Gomard E, Levy JP, Plata F, Henin Y, Duprez V, Bismuth A, Reme T. Studies on the nature of the cell surface antigen reacting with cytolytic T-lymphocytes in murine oncornavirus-induced tumours. Europ J Immunol 8: 228–236, 1978.
144. Enjuanes L, Lee I. Antigenic specificities of the cellular immune response of C57Bl/6 mice to the Moloney leukaemia/sarcoma virus complex. J Immunol 122: 665–674, 1979.

145. Zarling DA, Keshet I, Watson A, Bach FH. Association of mouse major histocompatibility and Rauscher murine leukaemia virus envelope glycoprotein antigens on leukaemia cells and their recognition by syngeneic virus-immune-cytotoxic T-lymphocytes. Scand J Immunol 8: 497–508, 1978.

146. Watson A, Bach FH. The role of gp70 in the target antigen recognised by murine leukaemia virus immune cytotoxic T-lymphocytes. Int J Cancer 26: 483–494, 1980.

147. Collins JJ, Sanfilippo F, Tsong-Chou L, Ishizaki R, Metzgar RS. Immunotherapy of murine leukaemia. I. Protection against Friend leukaemia virus-induced disease by passive serum therapy. Int J Cancer 21: 51–61, 1978.

148. Charman HP, Kim N, Gilden RV, Hardy WD Jr, Essex M. Humoral immune response of cats to feline leukaemia virus: Comparison of responses to the major structural protein p30 and to a virus-specific cell membrane antigen (FOCMA). J Natl Cancer Inst 57: 1095–1099, 1976.

149. Grant CK, Pickard DK, Ramaika C, Madewell BR, Essex M. Complement and tumour antibody levels in cats, and changes associated with natural feline leukaemia virus infection and malignant disease. Cancer Res 39: 75–81, 1979.

150. Grant CK, Essex M, Gardner MB, Hardy WD Jr. Natural feline leukaemia virus infection and the immune response of cats of different ages. Cancer Res 40: 823–829, 1980.

151. Herberman RB, Holden HT. Natural cell-mediated immunity. Adv Cancer Res 27: 305–377, 1978.

152. Rees RC, Underwood JCE. Tumour immunology. In Hancock BW (ed.), Assessment of tumour response. The Hague/Boston/London: Martinus Nijhoff, 1982, pp. 181–210.

153. Herberman RB. Natural killer cells and other natural effector cells. New York: Academic Press, 1982.

154. Hanna N. The role of natural killer (NK) cells in the control of tumour metastasis. In Liotta LA, Hart IR (eds.), Tumour Invasion and Metastases. The Hague: Martinus Nijhoff, 1982, pp. 29–41.

155. Fernandez-Cruz E, Halliburton B, Feldman JD. In vivo elimination by specific effector cells of an established syngeneic rat Moloney virus-induced sarcoma. J Immunol 123: 1772–1777, 1979.

156. Platta F, MacDonald, HR, Sordat B. Studies on the distribution and origin of cytolytic T-lymphocytes present in mice bearing Moloney murine sarcoma virus (MSV)-induced tumours. Bibl Haematol 43: 274–277, 1976.

157. Becker S, Klein E. Defective cytotoxic T-cell generation in Moloney murine sarcoma virus-infected A/Sn mice. J Natl Cancer Inst 65: 811–816, 1980.

158. Stutman O. Natural and induced immunity to mouse mammary tumours and the mammary tumour virus (MuMTV). Springer Semin Immunopathol 4: 333–372, 1982.

159. Teale DM, Rees RC, Clark A, Walker JR, Potter CW. Reduced susceptibility of NK cell lysis of hamster tumours exhibiting high levels of spontaneous metastasis. Cancer Letters (in press).

160. Epstein MA, Achong BG. The Epstein-Barr virus. Berlin: Springer Verlag, 1979.

161. Lindahl T, Adams A, Bjursell G, Bornkamn GW, Kaschka-Dierick C, Jehn V. Covalently closed circular duplex DNA of Epstein-Barr virus in a human lymphoid cell line. J Mol Biol 102: 511–530, 1976.

162. Lindahl T, Klein G, Reedman BM, Johannson B, Singh S. Relationship between Epstein-Barr (EBV) DNA and the EBV-determined nuclear antigen (EBNA) in Burkitt lymphoma and other lymphoproliferative malignancies. Int J Cancer 13: 764–772, 1974.

163. Josey WE, Nahmias AJ, Naib ZM. Viruses and cancer of the lower genital tract. Cancer 38: 526–533, 1976.

164. Melnick JL, Adam E. Epidemiological approaches to determining whether Herpesvirus is the etiological agent of cervical cancer. Prog Exp Tumour Res 21: 49–69, 1978.

165. Nahmias AJ, Naib ZM, Josey W. Epidemiological studies relating genital herpes to cervical cancer. Cancer Res 3: 1111–1117, 1974.

166. Rawls WE, Adam E. Herpes simplex viruses and human malignancies. In Hiatt, HH, Watson JD, Winston JA (eds.), Origins of Human Cancer. Cold Spring Harbour 4: 1133–1155, 1977.

167. Melnick JL, Adam E, Lewis R, Kaufman RH. Cervical cancer cell lines containing Herpesvirus markers. Intervirology 12: 111–114, 1979.

168. Aurelian L. Virions and antigens of Herpesvirus type 2 in cervical carcinoma. Cancer Res 33: 1539–1547, 1973.

169. Frankel N. Roizman B, Cassai E, Nahmias A. A DNA fragment of herpes simplex 2 and its transcription in human cervical cancer tissue. Proc Natl Acad Sci 69: 3784–3789, 1972.

170. Jones JW, Fenoglio CM, Shevchok-Chaban M, Maitland NJ, McDougall JK. Detection of herpes simplex virus type 2 ^{m}RNA in human cervical biopsies by in situ cytological hybridization. IARC Sci Publ 24: 917–925, 1979.

171. Kessler I. Human cervical cancer as a venereal disease. Cancer Res 36: 783–791, 1976.

172. Ishiguro T, Ozarki Y. Antibodies to herpes simplex virus in cervical cancer. Adv Obstet Gynecol (Jpn) 30: 9–13, 1978.

173. Ory H. Conger B, Richart R, Barron B. Relation of type 2 Herpesvirus antibodies to cervical neoplasia: Barbados, West Indies, 1971. Obstet Gynecol 43: 901–904, 1974.

174. Vestergaard BF, Hornsleth A, Pedersen SN. Occurrence of herpes- and adenovirus antibodies in patients with carcinoma of the cervix uteri. Cancer 30: 68–74, 1972.

175. Reid R, Stanhope CR, Herschman BR, Booth E, Phibbs GD, Smith JP. Genital warts and cervical cancer. Cancer 50: 377–387, 1982.

176. Green M, Brackman KH, Sanders PR, Loewenstein PM, Freel JH, Eisinger M, Switlyx SA. Isolation of a human Papillomavirus from a patient with epidermodysplasia verruciformis. Proc Natl Acad Sci 79: 4437–4441, 1982.

177. Gissmann L, de Villiers EM, Zur Hausen H. Analysis of human genital warts (condylomata acuminata) and other genital tumours for human Papillomavirus type 6 DNA. Int J Cancer 29: 143–146, 1982.

178. Zur Hausen H. Human Papillomaviruses and their possible role in squamous cell carcinomas. Curr Top Microbiol Immunol 78: 1–30, 1977.

179. Orth G, Faure M, Jablonska S, Brylak K, Croissant O. Viral sequences related to a human skin Papillomavirus in genital warts. Nature 275: 334–336, 1978.

180. Zur Hausen H. Condylomata acuminata and human genital cancer. Cancer Res 36: 794, 1976.

181. Friedman-Kien AE. Disseminated Kaposi's sarcoma syndrome in young homosexual men. J Amer Acad Dermatol 5: 468–471, 1981.

182. Hymes KB, Greene JB, Marcos A, William DC, Cheung T, Prose NS, Ballard H, Laubenstein LJ. Kaposi's sarcoma in homosexual men. Lancet 2: 598–600, 1981.

183. Giraldo G, Beth E, Henle W, Henle G, Mike V, Safai B, Huraux JM, McHardy J, de The G. Antibody patterns to Herpesviruses in Kaposi's sarcoma. Int J Cancer 22: 126–131, 1978.

184. Tong MG, Sun SC, Schaeffer BT. Hepatitis-associated antigen and hepatocellular carcinoma in Taiwan. Ann Intern Med 75: 687–691, 1971.

185. Beasley RP, Hwana LY, Lin CC, Chien CS. Hepatocellular carcinoma and hepatitis B virus. A prospective study of 22,707 men in Taiwan. Lancet 2: 1129–1133, 1981.

186. Edman JC, Gray P, Valenzuela P, Rall LB, Rutter WJ. Integration of hepatitis B virus sequences and their expression in a human hepatoma cell. Nature 286: 535–538, 1980.

187. Brechot C, Pourcel C, Louise A, Rain B, Tiollais P. Presence of integrated hepatitis B virus DNA sequences in cellular DNA of human hepatocellular carcinoma. Nature 286: 533–535, 1980.

188. Johnson PJ, Williams R. Of woodchucks and man: The continuing story of hepatitis B and hepatocellular carcinomas. Brit Med J 284: 1586–1588, 1982.

189. Howley PM. DNA sequences of human Papovavirus BK. Nature 284: 124–125, 1980.

190. Schernecks S, Rudolph M, Geissler E. Isolation of an SV40-like Papovavirus from a human glioblastoma. Int J Cancer 24: 523–531, 1979.

191. Brovet JC, Flandrin G, Seligmann M. Indication of the thymus derived nature of the proliferating cells in six patients with Sézary's syndrome. N Eng J Med 289: 341–344, 1973.

192. Thivolet J, Fulton R, Souteyrand P, Gaucherand M, Claudy A. Sézary syndrome: Relative increase in .T helper lymphocytes demonstrated by monoclonal antibodies. Acta Derm Venereal 62: 337–340, 1982.

193. Edelson RL. Cutaneous T cell lymphoma: Mycosis fungoides, Sézary syndrome and other variants. J Amer Acad Dermatol 2: 89–106, 1980.

194. Neth R, Gallo RC, Graff K, Mannweiler K. Regulation of human T-cell proliferation: T-cell growth factor and isolation of a new class of type-C retroviruses. In Winkler K (ed.), Modern trends in human leukaemia 4: 502–514, 1981.

195. Blattner WA, Kalyanaraman VS, Robert-Guroff M, Lister A, Galton DAG, Sarin PS, Crawford MH, Catousky D, Greaves M, Gallo RC. The human type-C retrovirus HTLV in blacks from the Caribbean region and relationship to adult T-cell leukaemia/lymphoma. Int J Cancer 30: 257–264, 1982.

196. Bishop JM. Retrovirus and cancer genes. Adv Cancer Res 37: 1–32, 1982.

197. Syrjanen KJ. Demonstration of human Papillomavirus antigen in the condylomatous lesions of the uterine cervix. Lancet 2: 125–127, 1982.

198. Maupas PH, Goudeau A, Coursaget P, Chiron JP, Drucker J, Barin F, Perrin J, Denis F, Diopmar I. Hepatitis B virus infection and primary hepatocarcinoma. In Essex M, Tadoro G, Zur Hausen H (eds.), Viruses and naturally occurring cancer. Cold Spring Harbour Conference on Cell Proliferation 7: 481–506, 1980.

199. Normura A, Grant N, Stemmerman N, Wasnick RD. Presence of hepatitis B surface antigen before primary hepatocellular carcinoma. JAMA 247: 2247–2249, 1982.

200. Melnick JL, Adam E, Lewis R, Kaufman RH. Cervical cancer cell lines containing Herpesvirus markers. Intervirol 12: 111–114, 1979.

201. Dreesman GR, Burch J, Ada E, Kaufman RH, Melnick JL, Powell KL, Purifoy DJ. Expression of Herpesvirus-induced antigens in human cervical cancer. Nature 283: 591–593, 1980.

202. Smith CC, Aurelian L, Gupta PK, Frost JK, Rosenhein NB, Klacsmann K, Geddes S. An evaluation of herpes simplex virus antigenic markers in the study of established and developing cervical neoplasia. Anal-Quant Cytol 2: 131–143, 1980.

203. Hollinshead AC, Tarro C. Soluble membrane antigens of LIP and cervical carcinomas. Science 179: 698–700, 1973.

204. Gall SA, Haines HG. Cervical carcinoma antigen and the relationship to HSV-2. Gynecol Oncol 2: 451–459, 1974.

205. Notter MF, Docherty JJ, Mortel R, Hollinshead AC. Detection of herpes simplex virus tumour-associated antigen in uterine cervical cancer tissue. Gynecol Oncol 6: 574–581, 1978.

206. Weiner LP, Herndon RM, Johnson RT. Viral infections and demyelinating diseases. N Eng J Med 288: 1103–1110, 1973.

207. Weiner LP, Narayan O. Virological studies in progressive multifocal leukoencephalopathy. Prog Med Virol 18: 229–240, 1974.

208. Weiss AF, Portmann R, Fischer H, Simon J, Zang KD. Simian virus 40-related antigens in three human meningiomas with defined chromosome breaks. Proc Natl Acad Sci 72: 609–613, 1975.

209. Pope JH, Horne MK, Wetters EJ. Significance of a complement-fixing antigen associated with herpes-like virus and detected in the Raji cell line. Nature 222: 186–187, 1969.

210. Reedman BM, Klein G. Cellular localisation of an Epstein-Barr virus (EBV)-associated complement-fixing antigen in producer cells and non-producer lymphoblastoid cell lines. Int J Cancer 11: 499–520, 1973.

211. Zur Hausen H. Biochemical approaches to detection of Epstein-Barr virus in human tumours. Cancer Res 36: 678–681, 1976.

212. Henle W, Henle G, Zagac B, Pearson G, Waubke R, Scriba M. Differential reactivity of human serums with early antigens induced by Epstein-Barr virus. Science 169: 188–189, 1970.

213. Svedmyr E, Jondal M. Cytotoxic effector cells specific for B cell lines transformed by Epstein-Barr virus are present in patients with infectious mononucleosis. Proc Natl Acad Sci 72: 1622–1628, 1975.

214. Levine AJ. Transformation-associated tumour antigens. Adv Cancer Res 37: 75–109, 1982.

215. Crawford LV, Pim DC, Gurney EG. Goodfellow P, Taylor-Papadimitrou A. Detection of a common feature in several human tumour lines—A 53,000-dalton protein. Proc Natl Acad Sci 787: 41–45, 1981.

216. Catovsky D, Greaves MF, Rose M, Galton DAG, Goolden AWG, McCluskey DR, White JM, Lampert I, Bourikas G, Ireland R, Bridges JM, Blather WAC, Gallo RC. Adult T-cell lymphoma leukaemia in blacks from the West Indies. Lancet 1: 639–643, 1982.

217. Tomana M, Kajdos AH, Niedeimeier W, Durkin WJ, Mestecky J. Antibodies to mouse mammary tumour virus-related antigen in sera of patients with breast carcinoma. Cancer 47: 2696–2703, 1981.

218. Zachrau RE, Black MM, Dion AS, Shore B, Isac M, Andrade AM, Williams CJ. Prognostically significant protein components in human breast cancer tissue. Cancer Res 36: 3143–3146, 1976.

219. Mesa-Tejada R, Oster MW, Fenoglio CM, Majidson J, Spiegelman S. Diagnosis of primary breast carcinoma through immunochemical detection of antigen related to mouse mammary tumour virus metastatic lesions: A report of two cases. Cancer 15: 261–268, 1982.

220. Black MM, Zachrau RE, Dion AS, Shire B, Fine DL, Leis HP Jr, Williams CJ. Cellular hypersensitivity to gp55 of R111-murine tumour virus and gp55-like protein of human breast cancers. Cancer Res 36: 4137–4142, 1976.

221. Cannon GB, Barsky SH, Alford TC, Jerome LF, Tinley V, McCoy JL, Dean JH. Cell-mediated immunity to mouse mammary tumour virus antigens by patients with hyperplastic benign breast disease. J Natl Cancer Inst 68: 935–943, 1982.

222. Holder WD Jr, Wells SA Jr. Antibody reacting with the murine mammary tumour virus in the serum of patients with breast carcinoma: A possible serological detection method for breast carcinoma. Cancer Res 43: 239–244, 1983.

223. Hewetson JF, Levine PH, Neubàuer RH. Rubin H. Discordant Epstein-Barr virus molecular antigen (EBNA) antibody patterns in nasopharyngeal carcinoma. Int J Cancer: 581–585, 1982.

224. Falaky IHE, Vestergaard BF. IgG-, IgA- and IgM-antibodies to herpes simplex virus type 2 in sera from patients with cancer of the uterine cervix. Europ J Cancer 13: 247–251, 1977.

225. Pasca AS, Kummerlauder L, Pejtsik B, Pali K. Herpesvirus antibodies and antigens in patients with cervical anaplasia and in controls. J Natl Cancer Inst 55: 775–781, 1975.

226. Cristenson B. Antibody-dependent cell-mediated cytotoxicity to HSV transformed cells in the course of cervical carcinoma. Am J Epidemiol 115: 556–568, 1982.

227. Arsenakis M, May JT, Cauchi MN. Antibody to AG-4 and survival of carcinoma of the cervix patients. Lancet 2: 437, 1981.

228. Heise ER, Kucera LS, Raben M, Homesley H. Serological response patterns to herpes virus type 2 early and late antigens in cervical carcinoma patients. Cancer Res 39: 4022–4026, 1979.

229. Christenson B, Espmark A. Long-term follow-up studies on herpes simplex antibodies in the course of cervical cancer. II. Antibodies to surface antigen of herpes simplex virus infected cells. Int J Cancer 17: 318–325, 1976.

230. Christenson B. Antibody-dependent cell-mediated cytotoxicity to herpes simplex virus type 2 infected target cells, in the course of cervical carcinoma. Amer J Epidem 108: 126–135, 1978.

231. Notter MFD, Docherty JJ. Reaction of antigens isolated from herpes simplex virus-transformed cells of squamous cell carcinoma patients. Cancer Res 36: 4394–4401, 1976.

232. Brown P, Tsai T, Gajdusek DC. Seroepidemiology of human Papovaviruses. Discovery of virgin populations and some unusual patterns of antibody prevalence among remote peoples of the world. Amer J Epidem 102: 331–340, 1975.

233. Gardner SD. Prevalence in England of antibody to human Polyomavirus (BK). Brit Med J 1: 77–78, 1973.

234. Padgett BL, Walker DL. New human Papovaviruses. Progr Med Virol 22: 1–35, 1976.

235. Penn I. Tumours arising in organ transplant recipients. Adv Cancer Res 28: 31–61, 1978.

12. Immunotherapy

B.W. HANCOCK
T.J. PRIESTMAN

INTRODUCTION

Traditionally, and based mainly on the acceptance of the theory of tumour immunosurveillance, it has been envisaged that the application of immunological concepts to the control of malignancy is both pertinent and feasible. The basic optimistic aims of therapy have been (1) to restore immunocompetence in immunodeficient patients together with prevention of immunosuppression by conventional anticancer therapies and (2) to modulate or potentiate specific or nonspecific antitumour immune responses. Various categories of immunotherapy have been defined and are summarized simplistically:

1. *Nonspecific:*
   a. local: BCG, DNCB.
   b. systemic: BCG, C.parvum, levamisole, thymic hormones, poly A/poly U, streptococcal extract, synthetic activators, differentiation agents.
2. *Specific:* tumour cell "vaccines."
3. *Adoptive:* interferons, transfer factor, immune RNA, lymphokines.
4. *Passive:* antitumour antibodies.

Obviously, the categories overlap, since with our increasing knowledge of tumour immunology it has become evident that most forms of therapy are in fact multifactoral in their effect. It is now also recognised that the term *immunotherapy* encompasses treatment methods that modify not only immune but other biological responses to cancer.

B.W. Hancock and A.M. Ward (eds.), Immunological Aspects of Cancer. Copyright © 1985, Martinus Nijhoff Publishing, Boston/Dordrecht/Lancaster.

Hersh [1] has suggested a modified classification of immunotherapy in the light of recent developments: (1) tumour specific immunotherapy (active, involving immunisation with tumour antigen vaccines; and passive, serotherapy with antitumour antibodies); (2) effector cell activation using microbiological or synthetic agents that can activate nonspecific host defenses such as NK-cells, macrophages, reticuloendothelial clearance; (3) cytokine therapy using the natural products of the host immune system (interferon, transfer factor, lymphokines) as cytotoxic or immunoregulatory agents; (4) immunomodulation using natural (e.g., thymic hormones) and synthetic (e.g., levamisole, isoprinosine) immunorestorative agents, or depletive techniques (plasmapheresis, plasma immunoabsorption) to remove blocking factors; (5) tumour cell differentiation agents (e.g., retinoids).

Against the scientific background of tumour immunology we must keep in mind the fact that the history of cancer immunotherapy in the clinical setting has been inglorious to say the least. It is by no means a new subject; indeed in 1806 [2] the Medical Committee of the Society for Investigating the Nature and Cure of Cancer seriously considered and rejected the possibility of altering the body's natural response to cancer. Clinical trials have been undertaken, therefore, since the last century, and most of the results have been inconclusive. Nevertheless, over the past three decades more and more space has been taken in cancer journals and books by articles and chapters on immunity in cancer, and despite this extensive coverage of the subject clinical achievements have been few.

NONSPECIFIC IMMUNOTHERAPY

The interest in nonspecific immunotherapy follows studies in the 1920s by Coley, who noted that tumours sometimes regressed when they became infected or if infection was present in the vicinity. Subsequently, it was shown that postoperative empyema improved survival in lung cancer [3]. Such beneficial effects seem to be mediated by nonspecific mechanisms such as via macrophage and natural killer (NK) cell activation.

Nonspecific local immunotherapy

Local nonspecific immunotherapy has been used mainly with cutaneous or other superficial lesions. Agents such as BCG (*Bacillus Calmette-Guérin*), DNCB (dinitrochlorobenzene), viruses, and bacterial antigens have been injected into small primary or secondary tumour lesions (melanoma, squamous cell carcinoma, lymphoma), and there are many reports of regression of such lesions following treatment [e.g., 4,5]. These agents work by inducing an acute local inflammatory response and particularly by activating macrophages; they are therefore acting as bystanders rather than having any significant effect on the tumour-host immunity relationship. This procedure therefore is unlikely to have any effect on the course of the cancer or survival of the patient.

Nonspecific systemic immunotherapy

Systemic nonspecific immunotherapy using active immunomodulators has been the most popular form of immunotherapy used in clinical practice; such treatment represents over two-thirds of the studies on immunotherapy reported in the 1960s and 1970s. In general terms, the idea is to increase general immunocompetence and to increase reticuloendothelial activity.

BCG

The vast majority of studies in nonspecific systemic immunotherapy have been with BCG. Early studies showed that administration of BCG to mice increased their resistance to transplantable tumours; this effect seems to be mediated through a wide range of immunomodulating effects including enhancement of cell-mediated and humoral immunity and activation of macrophages and NK-cells. Mathé et al. in 1969 [6] described good results with BCG therapy in acute lymphoblastic leukaemia. However, these early encouraging results have not been matched by the results from other trials [7,8], and the undoubted therapeutic benefits of multiple chemotherapy in leukaemia have now overridden the questionable additional advantages of adjuvant immunotherapy.

In melanoma, BCG has been used as therapy in recurrent disease and as an adjuvant for "high-risk" primary lesions [9,10,11]. Some of the earlier studies suggested an undoubted benefit from immunotherapy [9,10]; unfortunately, in these studies the results were compared with those seen in historical controls, making the reliability of such comparative findings doubtful. Of the randomised studies only one [11] showed benefits from BCG. In acute myeloid leukaemia, BCG has been used in combination with chemotherapy and irradiated leukaemic blast cells [12]; the advantages for those patients having immunotherapy were marginal.

BCG immunotherapy has also been applied in lung cancer. In the much publicized study of McKneally et al. [13,14], intrapleural BCG resulted in a 93%-disease-free rate at two years compared with a 67%-disease-free rate in randomised cases treated by surgery alone. Unfortunately, other studies have failed to show any effect on survival following intrapleural BCG [e.g., 15]. One of the big problems with many of these studies is that quite often the dosages and strains of BCG were different, and this of course could have a vital influence on outcome.

BCG therapy is not without side effects [16]. Systemic infection or anaphylaxis may occur, and mild fever and malaise with ulceration of the injection site are to be expected. Of more sinister importance, however, is the possibility that certain dosages (usually low) of BCG may actually potentiate tumour growth.

The initial interest in a methanol extract residue of BCG (MER-BCG), which was thought to be more immunostimulatory than ordinary BCG [17], has not been maintained in view of studies that have shown little clinical benefit and enhanced local toxicity.

Cornebacterium parvum (C.parvum)

C.parvum has also been shown experimentally to enhance transplantable tumour rejection in rodents and has been thought to have immunomodulatory effects comparable to or better than BCG. A large study of 414 patients with various metastatic cancers suggested that patients who received immunotherapy and chemotherapy survivied longer than those receiving chemotherapy alone [18]. Unfortunately, since that time many studies have failed to confirm any benefit, with the possible exception of the use of intrapleural or intraperitoneal C.parvum in malignant ascitic and pleural effusions; the recurrence of effusions was reduced though there was no effect on survival [19].

Levamisole

Levamisole, an effective synthetic antihelminthic agent with supposedly few toxic effects, has been shown to stimulate immune responses by unknown mechanisms. Experimental studies in animals suggest that tumour growth is inhibited and that there is an increase in survival in treated animals. Favourable results have been reported using levamisole in patients with carcinoma of the breast [20] and bronchus [21]. Most studies have shown no advantage, however [22]; for example, a recently reported randomised trial of levamisole versus placebo as adjuvant therapy in 203 patients with malignant melanoma showed no benefit for levamisole [23]. Some investigators have also demonstrated a higher recurrence rate in levamisole-treated patients [24] and an unacceptable incidence of toxicity (white blood cell depression and cardiorespiratory problems) [25,26]. (Isoprinosine, another synthetic immunomodulator, also awaits definitive evidence that it can benefit patients with cancer.)

Thymic hormones

Thymosin, an active polypeptide hormone, has been shown to convert featureless null cells into T-cells and therefore was greeted excitedly in the field of immunotherapy. Preliminary studies in disseminated malignancy [27], small cell lung carcinoma [28], and head and neck cancer [29] have shown favourable results but, in the light of experience with other forms of immunotherapy where initial optimism has been overshadowed by subsequent negative findings, we must await data from further randomised and controlled clinical trials. It is now recognised that thymostimulin and thymosin fraction 5, the agents used in many studies, are mixtures of polypeptides, some potentially antagonistic; studies are now underway with pure, more potent fractions [30]. Also, in some studies thymic hormones have been combined with steroids or cytotoxic agents, which, if incorrectly timed, may kill the lymphocytes as they respond to the hormones [31].

Poly A/poly U

Another nonspecific immune response modifier that has been used in the clinical situation is polyadenylic/polyuridylic acid (poly A/poly U); this agent was tested in a randomised trial of 300 patients and reported to be a simple nontoxic and efficient adjuvant treatment in operable breast cancer [32]. Further studies using this agent are awaited.

Streptococcal extract

Recently, Japanese workers [33] have demonstrated improved palliation and survival in patients with malignant ascites (usually secondary to gastric carcinoma) treated with intraperitoneal streptococcal extract (OK-432). In this controlled study of nearly 200 patients, immunological indices improved at follow-up only in those patients responding to treatment.

Synthetic cell activators

Many investigators are now assessing synthetic polymers with macrophage or NK-cell activating potential [1]; macrophage activators have also been encapsulated into liposomes with good effect in experimental tumour systems. As yet there is no evidence of clinical efficacy.

Differentiation agents

A number of agents (e.g., retinoids) have been shown to induce tumour cell differentiation; their role in the prevention and treatment of cancer is being assessed.

SPECIFIC ACTIVE SYSTEMIC IMMUNOTHERAPY

Studies earlier this century [34,35] reported that attempts at immunising against tumours using autologous or allogeneic tumour tissue were impracticable and unsuccessful. Likewise, in 1962, a large study of 232 cases of gynaecological cancer treated with autologous tumour vaccine (intact tumour cells + Freund's adjuvant) concluded that the vaccines failed to alter the course of the disease [36].

A prerequisite for successful specific immunotherapy is the expression on tumour cells of a tumour-associated antigen against which a rejection response can be initiated. With immunogenic animal tumours, adjuvant therapy using BCG mixed with tumour cells enhances specific transplant resistance. However, it is not yet firmly established that human cancer cells possess transplantation rejection antigens, and this helps to explain the very limited success of specific therapy in human cancer.

In leukaemia, as well as showing improved survival with BCG alone, Mathé et al. [6] combined BCG with irradiated tumour cells in patients in complete remission after cytotoxic chemotherapy, with favourable results. Other studies, however, have not confirmed a major advantage to this form of treatment [7,8].

In acute myeloid leukaemia, Powles et al. [12] used BCG and irradiated leukaemic blast cells and concluded that there was no improvement over chemotherapy alone in first remission duration, though there might be an improvement in survival duration after relapse.

Virus-infected tumour cells (viral oncolysates) have been used for immunisation of patients after conventional anticancer treatment. Early clinical results suggest that this is a useful approach to immunotherapy [1]. It is thought that virus infection of the cancer cells makes them more immunogenic and hence more susceptible to the host immune defenses.

ADOPTIVE IMMUNOTHERAPY

Adoptive immunotherapy, the transfer of immunity by lymphocytes or their products, has been extensively used in animal studies but has proved of little help clinically because of the lack of compatible donors (to avoid host versus graft and graft versus host reactions). More promising is the use of lymphokines and other white cell products.

Interferons

Experiments reported during the 1960s and 1970s demonstrated that interferons had antitumour activity in a wide range of laboratory models. The mechanism of this activity remains unclear, for although interferons have a stimulatory effect on a number of components of the immune system, including macrophage phagocytosis and natural killer cells, they also have a growth inhibitory effect when added to tumour cells growing in vitro, indicating a direct cytotoxic effect. In addition, the observation that interferons alter certain cell membrane characteristics of tumour cells—for example, enhancing expression of H2 antigens—has led to the suggestion that interferon administration may render malignant cells more antigenic and thus more susceptible to the body's natural defense mechanisms.

Human interferons have classified as α, β, and γ. α-interferons are produced by white blood cells in response to a challenge by virus; this process is regulated by 16 different genes, resulting in production of a range of α-interferon polypeptides with molecular weights between 18,000 and 25,000. Three types of α-interferon have so far been used in clinical trials: leucocyte (αLe), lymphoblastoid (αLy), and recombinant. αLe and αLy are both mixtures of α-polypeptides, whereas the recombinant material has been produced by cloning a single gene in *E.coli* bacteria to produce the α-2 subtype. It is still too early to say whether there is any clear therapeutic difference between these various preparations. β-interferons, produced by fibroblasts when cultured with virus, have been used in a number of clinical studies but appear to be highly unstable and thus have minimal activity. γ-interferons are produced by lymphocytes, following stimulation by certain mitogens such as concanavalin A, phytohaemagglutinin, and *C.parvum*. The first γ-interferons are just entering clinical evaluation; thus no results are available as yet.

The antitumour activity of α-interferons has now been explored in a wide range of human cancers. Unequivocally negative results have been reported in advanced lung cancer (both small cell [37] and nonsmall cell [38] varieties), colorectal cancer [39], gastric cancer [40], and acute myeloid leukaemia [41]. Very limited activity, with response rates of 2 to 5%, has been demonstrated in malignant melanoma [42,43], and rather higher rates of 10 to 15% regression have been seen in hypernephroma [44,45,46]. Response rates of 20 to 25% have been reported in breast cancer [47] and multiple myeloma [48,49,50], although in the former benefit has been confined to patients with cutaneous or lymph node involvement and in the latter a prospectively randomised series has shown the results of interferon administration to be significantly worse than conventional chemotherapy with melphalan and prednisone [50]. These have all been studies in advanced tumours, and only one study—a Scandinavian study in osteogenic sarcoma [51]—has reported, inconclusively, on the use of interferon as an adjuvant in early stage disease.

α-interferons do have a number of side effects, including fever, malaise, anorexia, nausea, mental confusion (accompanied by bizarre EEG changes), myelosuppression, hepatotoxicity, hypocalcaemia, and hyperkalaemia as well as possible clotting disturbance and cardiotoxicity. Although these are largely dose-related, they are similar with all three α-preparations and even at very low doses might well still prove sufficiently troublesome to limit their use in long-term adjuvant or maintenance situations.

Rather more encouraging results have been obtained in two virally related tumours: juvenile laryngeal papilloma and multiple Kaposi's sarcoma associated with acquired immunodeficiency syndrome (AIDS). In both conditions a viral aetiology is strongly suspected, although the causative agent remains to be identified. In juvenile laryngeal papilloma, interferon administration results in control of the disease in the great majority of cases, although long-term maintenance is necessary to prevent relapse [52]. Initial results in Kaposi's sarcoma in AIDS have indicated complete responses in 20% of patients and partial remission in a further 15% [53]; these findings have stimulated an intensive evaluation of interferon in this otherwise untreatable condition, which is, particularly in the United States, a growing health concern.

In addition to these results there have been anecdotal reports of responses in ovarian carcinoma and lymphoma and formal evaluations in these conditions are currently in progress. At present, however, the results in common tumours have been disappointing and, with the possible exception of renal cell cancer, there is no evidence of interferon improving on the results of established treatment. The possibility remains that combining interferons with conventional therapy might enhance response rates, but care will have to be exercised to avoid undue toxicity [54].

Transfer factor

Transfer factor is a low-molecular-weight substance consisting of a short polypeptide chain joined to three or four RNA bases. It allows the specific transfer of cellular immunity by means of a cell-free nonantigenic extract. Its exact action is unknown, but it undoubtedly improves T-cell immunity and is concerned with the collaboration between T-cells and other cells in the immune system. The main application has been in the treatment of congenital immunodeficiency syndromes [55]. Preliminary laboratory tests suggested that transfer factor could be prepared for the treatment of cancer [56,57]; with such preparations donor lymphocytes showed vigorous inhibition of tumour cell growth in vitro. A number of studies have suggested that transfer factor can stimulate specific-cell-mediated immunity in patients with cancer and produce a clinical effect on the tumour under certain circumstances [see 58 for review]. The success of this form of therapy seems to depend on the patients' acquiring and maintaining cellular immunity [59].

Unfortunately, most studies have been rather small or nonrandomised; two randomised studies with melanoma [60] and osteogenic sarcoma [61] showed no benefit for transfer factor therapy. The most relevant clinical use of transfer factor in cancer, however, seems to be in the prevention of infections such as varicella/zoster in leukaemia [62] and possibly other malignancies.

Immune RNA

It has been known for some time that it is possible to transfer subcellular RNA fractions of specifically immune lymphoid cells from one species to another, thus conferring cell-mediated immunity. In the clinical context, one study [63] has been reported using immune RNA in disseminated renal cell carcinoma, the RNA having been obtained from lymphocytes taken from sheep immunised with renal carcinoma cells; the results were favourable when compared with historical controls.

Other lymphokines

Other lymphokines and cytokines (products of cells in general) are being assessed as biological response modifiers; early studies suggest that certain of these substances (e.g., interleukins, colony-stimulating factors) may be beneficial to the host-tumour interaction by immune enhancement [30], but the results of clinical trials using better defined materials are awaited.

PASSIVE IMMUNOTHERAPY

The failure of direct administration of immunotherapeutic agents may be due in part to intrinsic defects in the ability of the patient's immune system to respond. Hence, passive immunotherapy is an area that has undergone much experimental and clinical research with some success over the past 80 years [64]. In particular, the idea of using specific antitumour antibodies to target other toxic reagents such as drugs to the tumour, i.e., the magic bullet, has attracted much interest. Experimentally, beneficial effects have been shown using this technique [65], but its application in the therapy of human cancer has been more difficult since in the past a reliable method of producing sufficient quantities of antibody with the desired specificity has not been available. However, production of monoclonal antibodies has recently revolutionized this area of immunotherapy. Full details of monoclonal antibodies are given in chapter 8, but briefly the technique, based on Kohler and Milsteins' method [66], involves the fusion of suitably immunised rodent spleen cells to myeloma cell line grown in vitro. The resulting hybridomas are tested for antibody production, cloned, and then grown in quantity for bulk antibody production. The place for such monoclonal antibodies in the diagnosis and therapy of cancer is now the subject of intensive research, which though still in its infancy, is already showing considerable promise. To give one example, a monoclonal antiidiotype antibody has been recently used in treating a patient with B-cell lymphoma in which only the malignant clone of lymphocytes carried the idiotype [67]; this is an almost unique example of tumour-specific immunotherapy. The use of specific monoclonal antibodies could also avoid the theoretical risk involved in the passive administration of antisera; that is, the antibodies, rather than destroying the tumour cells, may block the effective action of the normal immune system.

ADJUVANT IMMUNOTHERAPY: A CRITICAL OVERVIEW

Based on the belief that the lower the tumour burden the greater the chance of successful immunotherapy, studies have been carried out exploring the role of various immunomodulators in preventing relapse in high-risk patients who have rendered clinically disease-free by prior surgery, radiation, or chemotherapy. Many of these series have been anecdotal or uncontrolled, but in three conditions—carcinoma of the bronchus, acute leukaemia, and malignant melanoma—sufficient data have now accumulated from prospectively randomised studies to allow a preliminary evaluation of adjuvant immunotherapy.

McKneally's trial of intrapleural BCG following resection of bronchogenic carcinoma gave great encouragement: in patients with stage 1 disease, with a median follow-up of 12 months, no recurrences or deaths were reported among 17 recipients of BCG, whereas 9 of 22 controls had relapsed and 5 of these had died [13]. Even at four years' follow-up the results were still encouraging, with the recurrence rate in treated patients being only 33% compared to 62% in the controls [14]. Unfortunately, studies subsequently undertaken in both the United Kingdom [15] and the United States [68] have been unable to reproduce these results and, despite differences in detail of study design and materials, must cast serious doubts on the validity of McKneally's original observations. Another study reporting positive results in early lung cancer gave levamisole after resection and claimed a survival advantage in those patients weighing less than 70 kg [21]. Once again, confirmatory trials, this time in the United Kingdom [26] and Belgium [69], have failed to reproduce the original findings; the U.K. series actually demonstrated a significantly reduced survival in the levamisole-treated patients. Randomised trials have been carried out with C.parvum in resectable lung cancer using both the intrapleural route [70] and specific active immunotherapy, inoculating the vaccine intradermally with autologous irradiated tumour cells [71]; both studies showed no benefits from the immunotherapy.

In acute lymphoblastic leukaemia (ALL) a report by Mathé et al., in 1969, claimed improved survival when BCG was given as maintenance therapy following chemotherapy-induced remission [6]. Multicentre studies in the United Kingdom [7] and the United States [8] failed to confirm these observations and, although it has been argued that differences in BCG strain and administration techniques might have influenced the outcome, there has been little recent interest in adjuvant immunotherapy for ALL. Studies of acute myeloblastic leukaemia (AML) have used both specific immunotherapy (using irradiated leukaemic cells or neuraminidase-treated cells) and nonspecific immunomodulators (BCG, MER-BCG, C.parvum, and levamisole) either combined with chemotherapy or given alone in order to maintain remission after initial induction therapy. Overall, with the possible exception of the neuraminidase series, there has been no impact on duration of remission or relapse-free survival [72] although some series have shown that total survival-time is marginally prolonged due to an increase in postrelapse survival, possibly due to an apparently higher response rate to second-line chemotherapy. Increase in postrelapse survival, however, offers no prospect of cure, and the realisation that prolonged intensive cytotoxic therapy or bone marrow transplantation might result in long-term survival in AML has, in the last two to three years, focused attention on these two approaches to the virtual exclusion of adjuvant immunotherapy [73,74].

Trials assessing BCG as an adjuvant to surgery in operable malignant melanoma were reviewed in 1980 [75]. At that time six studies were considered of which two showed a benefit from BCG and four were negative. Unfortunately, the two trials claiming improved results were based on historical controls, whereas the negative series were prospectively randomised and thus infinitely more reliable. Since that time there have been negative reports from randomised studies with BCG and cytotoxics in combination [76], C.parvum [77], transfer factor [60], and levamisole [23]. One additional series using BCG alone has indicated a significant reduction in loco-regional recurrence although the influence of this on survival is not yet clear [77].

In some of the series considered here meticulous analysis of subgroups has revealed an advantage for certain patients following adjuvant immunotherapy. In others promising trends, which were not statistically significant, have been reported, and in yet others postrelapse survival has been increased. These observations, however, fail to remove on overwhelming pessimism about adjuvant immunotherapy in its present forms. When one adds in the negative data from randomised studies in breast [24] and large bowel carcinomas [79], then the conclusion must be that such treatment has little to offer and some major new initiative is needed to rekindle interest in this therapeutic approach.

CONCLUSIONS

The motivation for research into tumour immunology has always been the development of immunological methods for the treatment of cancer. As we have seen to date, however, immunotherapy in human cancer has not proved to be universally or consistently successful. Experimental protocols devised in animal models, in which immunisation protects against tumours, have been highly successful; regression of established tumours has been far less easy to achieve, however, and, as with so much in tumour immunology, extrapolation from animal models to human cancer has not proved simple. Such therapy is ineffective against large tumour burdens such as those that are inevitably present when the patient first presents with clinical evidence of cancer. It is most likely to be successful when there is a minimal tumour load, that is, when the primary tumour has been removed by surgery, radiotherapy, or chemotherapy and only small areas of disease persist; the critical range for tumour cell acceptance or rejection seems to be 10^5 to 10^7, depending on the immunologic state of the host. The timing of therapy is probably also vital; in theory it would be inappropriate to give active immunotherapy during a course of chemotherapy or radiotherapy, which in itself is likely to be severely immunodepressive. However, unlike conventional therapies the potential efficacy is largely independent of cell cycle kinetics, hence the possible, though so far disappointing, role as an adjuvant to other therapies (as previously discussed).

Immunotherapy has always drawn criticism on the basis that much of the work has been on laboratory models completely irrelevant to the human situation, that clinical trials have been poorly designed or anecdotal, and that exaggerated claims have been made for its success and have been largely unsupported by the few controlled randomised studies conducted [80,81,82]. Against this background of what has been termed "old" immunotherapy [30], current research into monoclonal antibodies and biological response modifier therapies, so-called "new" immunotherapy, is being conducted.

Major advances in technology have already improved our understanding of immunological mechanisms in cancer—cellular interactions, mediators, helper and suppressor cell systems, and specific antigens—and should help us put new theories into practice [83]. Laboratory investigations in future studies must be appropriate to the clinical situation, and immunotherapy trials must be large, well controlled, and randomised. Only then will we be able to decide whether immunotherapy in cancer is truly an impossible dream for oncologists [84].

REFERENCES

1. Hersh EM. Current status of immune therapy and biological therapy of human cancer. A brief review and an evaluation of future prospects. In Spitzy KH, Karrer K (eds.), *Proceedings of the 13th International Congress of Chemotherapy*, 1983, pp. 1/64–1/75.
2. Report of the Medical Committee of the Society for Investigating the Nature and Cure of Cancer. Edinburgh Med Surg J 2: 382–389, 1806.
3. Ruckdeschel JC, Codish SD, Stranahan A, McKneally MF. Postoperative empyema improves survival in lung cancer: Documentation and analysis of a natural experiment. N Engl J Med 287: 1013–1017, 1972.
4. Morton DL. Immunological studies with human neoplasms. J Reticuloendothel Soc 10: 137–160, 1971.
5. Mastrangelo MJ, Clark WH Jr, Bellet RE, Berd D. Cutaneous malignant melanoma diagnosis, prognosis, and conventional medical therapy. In Terry WD, Windhorst D (eds.), Immunotherapy of cancer; present status of trials in man. New York: Raven Press, 1978, pp. 1–17.
6. Mathé G, Amiel JL, Schwarzenberg L, Schneider M, Cattan A, Schlumberger JR, Hayat M, Vassal F. Active immunotherapy for acute lymphoblastic leukaemia. Lancet 1: 697–699, 1969.
7. Medical Research Council. Preliminary report by the Leukaemia Committee and Working Party on Leukaemia in Childhood. Treatment of acute lymphoblastic leukaemia—comparison of immunotherapy (BCG), intermittent therapy and no therapy after a five months intensive cytotoxic regimen (Concord Trial). Br Med J 4: 189–194, 1971.
8. Heyn RM, Joo P, Karon M, Nesbit M, Shore N, Breslow N, Weiner J, Reed A, Hammond D. BCG in the treatment of acute lymphocytic leukaemia. Blood 46: 431–442, 1975.
9. Gutterman JU, Mavligit G, McBride C, Frei E III, Freireich EJ, Hersh EM. Active immunotherapy with BCG for recurrent malignant melanoma. Lancet 1: 1208–1212, 1973.
10. Eilber FR, Morton DL, Holmes EC, Sparks FC, Ramming KP. Adjuvant immunotherapy with BCG in the treatment of regional-lymph-node metastases from malignant melanoma. N Engl J Med 294: 237–240, 1976.

11. Wood WC, Cosimi AB, Carey RW, Kalufman SD. Randomised trial of adjuvant therapy for "high risk" primary malignant melanoma. Surgery 83: 677-681, 1978.

12. Powles RL, Crowther D, Bateman CJT, et al. Immunotherapy for acute myelogenous leukaemia. Br J Cancer 28: 365-376, 1973.

13. McKneally MF, Maver C, Kausel HW. Regional immunotherapy of lung cancer with intrapleural BCG. Lancet 1: 377-379, 1976.

14. McKneally MF, Maver C, Lininger L, Kausel HW, Mellduff JB, Older TM, Foster ED, Alley RD. Four-year follow-up on the Albany experience with intrapleural BCG in lung cancer. Thorac Cardiovasc Surg 81: 485-492, 1981.

15. Lowe J, Iles PB, Shore DF, Langman MJ, Baldwin RW. Intrapleural BCG in operable lung cancer. Lancet 1: 11-14, 1980.

16. Sparks FC, Silverstein MJ, Hunt JS, Haskell CM, Pilch YH, Morton DI. Complications of BCG in immunotherapy in patients with cancer. N Engl J Med 289: 827-830, 1973.

17. Mikulski SM, Muggia FM. The biologic activity of MER-BCG in experimental systems and preliminary clinical studies. Cancer Treat Rev 4: 103-117, 1977.

18. Israel L. Report of 414 cases of human tumours treated with corynebacteria. In Halpern B (ed.), *Corynebacterium parvum*: Applications in experimental and clinical oncology. New York: Plenum Press, 1975, pp. 389-401.

19. Webb HE, Oaten SW, Pike CP. Treatment of malignant ascitic and pleural effusions with *Corynebacterium parvum*. Br Med J 1: 338-340, 1978.

20. Rojas AF, Mickiewicz E, Feierstein JN, Glait H, Olivari AJ: Levamisole in advanced human breast cancer. Lancet 1: 211-213, 1976.

21. Amery WK. Final results of a multi-centre placebo-controlled levamisole study of resectable lung cancer. Cancer Treat Rep 62: 1677-1683, 1978.

22. Spitler LE, BCG, levamisole and transfer factor in the treatment of cancer. Prog Exp Tumour Res 25: 178-192, 1980.

23. Spitler LE, Sagebiel R. A randomized trial of levamisole versus placebo as adjuvant therapy in malignant melanoma. N Engl J Med 303: 1143-1147, 1980.

24. Executive Committee of the Danish Breast Cancer Co-operative Group. Increased breast cancer recurrence rate after adjuvant therapy with levamisole. Lancet 2: 824-827, 1980.

25. Retsas S, Phillips RH, Hanham IW, Newton KA. Agranulocytosis in breast cancer patients treated with levamisole. Lancet 2: 452-453, 1978.

26. Anthony HM, Mearns AJ, Mason MK, Scott DG, Moghissi K, Deverall PB, Rozyki ZJ, Watson DA. Levamisole and surgery in bronchial carcinoma patients: Increase in deaths from cardio-respiratory failure. Thorax 34: 4-12, 1979.

27. Costanzi JJ, Cagliano RG, Delaney F, Harris N. Thurman GB, Sakai H, Goldstein A, Loukas D, Gohen GB, Thomson PD. The effect of thymosin on patients with disseminated malignancies. Cancer 40: 14-19, 1977.

28. Lipson SD, Chretien PB, Makuch R, Kenady DE, Cohen MH. Thymosin immunotherapy in patients with small cell carcinoma of the lung. Cancer 43: 863-870, 1979.

29. Wara WM, Wara WD, Neely MH, Amman AJ. Head and neck cancer treatment with thymosin. Proc Am Assoc Cancer Res 22: 375, 1981.

30. Oldham RK, Smalley RV. Immunothreapy: The old and the new. J Biol Resp Modif 2: 1-37, 1983.

31. Editorial. Which thymic hormone? Lancet 1: 1309-1311, 1983.

32. Lacour J, Lacour F, Spira A, Michelson M, Petit JY, Delage G, Sarrazin D, Contesso G, Viguier J. Adjuvant treatment with polyadenylic-polyuridylic acid (polyA/polyU) in operable breast cancer. Lancet 2: 161-164, 1980.

33. Torisu M, Katano M, Kimura Y, Itoh H, Takasue M. New approach to management of malignant ascites with a streptococcal preparation, OK-432. I. Improvement of host immunity and prolongation of survival. Surgery 93: 357-364, 1983.

34. Coca AF, Dorrance GM, Lebredo MG. Vaccination in cancer. Z Immun Exp Ther 13: 343-385, 1912.

35. Leitch A. Discussion of the present position of cancer research. Br Med J 2: 656-658, 1920.

36. Graham JB, Graham RM. Autogenous vaccine in cancer patients. Surg Gynecol Obstet 114: 1-4, 1962.

37. Jones DH, Bleehen NM, Slater AJ, George PJ, Walker JR, Dixon AK. Human lymphoblastoid interferon in the treatment of small cell lung cancer. Br J Cancer 47: 361-366, 1983.

38. Krown SE, Stoopler S, Cunningham-Rundles S. Oettgen F. Phase II trial of human leukocyte interferon in non-small cell lung cancer. Proc Am Assoc Cancer Res 21: 179, 1980.

39. Chaplinski T, Laszlo J, Moore J, Schneider W. Phase II trial of interferon in metastatic colon carcinoma. Proc Am Soc Clin Oncol 2: 130, 1983.

40. Priestman TJ. Unpublished observations.
41. Rohatiner AZ, Balkwill J, Lister TA. Interferon in acute myelogenous leukaemia. Mod Trends Hum Leuk 5: 56–58, 1983.
42. Krown SE, Burk M, Kirkwood JM, Kerr D, Nordlund JJ, Morton DL, Oettgen F. Human leukocyte interferon in malignant melanoma. Proc Am Assoc Cancer Res 22: 158, 1981.
43. Retsas S, Priestman TJ, Newton KA, Westbury G. Evaluation of human lymphoblastoid interferon in advanced malignant melanoma. Cancer 51: 273–276, 1983.
44. Krown SE, Einzig AI, Abramson JD, Oettgen HF. Treatment of advanced renal cell cancer with recombinant leukocyte A interferon. Proc Am Soc Clin Oncol 2: 58, 1983.
45. Quesada JR, Gutterman JV, Swanson D, Trindale A. Antitumour effects of partially pure human leukocyte interferon in renal cell carcinoma. Proc Am Assoc Cancer Res 23: 143, 1982.
46. Retsas S, Priestman TJ, Newton KA. Treatment of metastatic renal cell carcinoma with human lymphoblastoid interferon: A phase II study. Proc Am Soc Clin Oncol 2: 132, 1983.
47. Borden EC, Holland JF, Gutterman JV, Wiener L, Chang Y-C, Patel J. Leukocyte derived interferon (alpha) in human breast cancer: The American Cancer Society Phase II Trial. Ann Int Med 97: 1–7, 1982.
48. Gutterman J, Blumenschein G, Alexanian R, Yap H, Buzdar A, Cabanillas F, Hortabagyi G, Hersh E, Rasmussen S, Harman M, Kramer M, Pestka S. Leukocyte interferon-induced tumour regression in human metastatic breast cancer, multiple myeloma and malignant lymphoma. Ann Int Med 93: 399–406, 1980.
49. Alexanian R, Gutterman J, Levy H. Interferon treatment for multiple myeloma. Clin Haematol II: 211–220, 1982.
50. Mellstedt H, Ahre A, Bjorkholm M, Johansson B, Strander H. Brenning G, Engstedt L, Gahrton G, Holm G, Lehrner R, Longvist B, Nordenskjold B, Killander A, Stalfeldt A-M, Simonsson B, Ternstedt B, Wadmana B. Interferon therapy of patients with myeloma. In Terry W, Rosenberg S (eds.), Immunotherapy of human cancer. New York: Elsevier North Holland, 1982: pp. 387–391.
51. Strander H, Einhorn S. Interferon therapy in neoplastic diseases. Philos Trans R Soc Lond B299: 113–117, 1982.
52. Haglund S, Lundquist PG, Cantell K, Strander H. Interferon therapy in juvenile laryngeal papillomatosis. Arch Otolaryngol 107: 327–332, 1981.
53. Krown SE, Real FX, Cunningham-Rundles S, Myskowski A, Koziner B, Fein S, Mittelman A, Oettgen HF, Safai B. Preliminary observations on the effect of recombinant leukocyte A-interferon in homosexual men with Kaposi's sarcoma. New England J Med 308: 1071–1076, 1983.
54. Priestman TJ. The present status of clinical studies with interferons in cancer in Britain. Philos Trans R Soc Lond B299: 119–214, 1982.
55. Lawrence HS. Transfer factor. Adv Immunol 2: 195–266, 1969.
56. Levin AJ, Spitler LE, Wybran J, Fudenberg HH, Hellstrom I, Hellstrom KE. Treatment of osteogenic sarcoma with tumour specific transfer factor. Clin Res 20: 568, 1972.
57. Spitler LE, Levin AS, Blois S, et al. Lymphocyte responses to tumour-specific antigens in patients with malignant melanoma and results of transfer factor therapy. J Clin Invest 51: 92a, 1972.
58. Al-Sarraf M, Baker LH. Transfer factor. Cancer Treat Rev 6: 209–215, 1979.
59. Kirkpatrick CH. Therapeutic potential of transfer factor. N Eng J Med 303: 390–391, 1980.
60. Bukowski RM, Deodhar S, Hewlett JS, Greenstreet R. Randomized controlled trial of transfer factor in stage II malignant melanoma. Cancer 51: 269–272, 1983.
61. Gilchrist GS, Ivins JC, Ritts RE, Pritchard DJ, Taylor WF, Edmonson JM. Adjuvant therapy for non-metastatic osteogenic sarcoma: An evaluation of transfer factor versus combination chemotherapy. Cancer Treat Rep 62: 289–294, 1978.
62. Steele RW, Myers MG, Vincent MM. Transfer factor for the prevention of varicella/zoster infection in childhood leukaemia. N Engl J Med 303: 355–359, 1980.
63. Ramming KP, Dekernion JB. Immune RNA therapy for renal cell carcinoma. Ann Surg 186: 459–467, 1977.
64. Rosenberg SA, Terry WD. Passive immunotherapy of cancer in animals and man. Adv Cancer Res 25: 323–388, 1977.
65. Ghose T, Norvell ST, Guclu A, Cameron D, Bodurtha A, MacDonald AS. Immunochemotherapy of cancer with chlorambucil-carrying antibody. Br Med J 3: 495–499, 1972.
66. Kohler G, Milstein C. Continuous cultures of fused cells secreting antibody of predefined specificity. Nature 256: 495–497, 1975.
67. Miller RA, Maloney DG, Warnke R, Levy R. Treatment of B cell lymphoma with monoclonal anti-idiotype antibody. N Eng J Med 306: 517–522, 1982.
68. Mountain CF, Gail MH. Surgical adjuvant intrapleural BCG treatment for stage 1 non-small cell lung cancer: Preliminary report of the National Cancer Institute Lung Cancer Study Group. J Thorac Cardiovasc Surg 82: 649–653, 1981.

69. Van Houtte P, Bondue H, Rocmans P, Michel J, Wybran J, Dalesio O, Balikdjian D, Vanderhoeft P, Kenis Y. Adjuvant immunotherapy by levamisole in resectable lung cancer. Europ J Cancer 16: 1597–1601, 1980.

70. Stjernsward J. Adjuvant immunotherapy in operable lung cancer. In Proceedings of the Second International Conference on the Immunotherapy of Cancer, NCI, Bethesda, 1980, p. 36.

71. Souter RG, Gill PG, Gunning AJ, Morris PJ. Failure of specific active immunotherapy in lung cancer. Br J Cancer 44: 496–503, 1981.

72. Foon KA, Gale RP. Controversies in the therapy of acute myelogenous leukemia. Am J Med 72: 963–979, 1982.

73. Preisler HD. Therapy for patients with acute myelocytic leukemia who enter remission: Bone marrow transplantation or chemotherapy? Cancer Treat Rep 66: 1467–1473, 1982.

74. Goldman JM. Adult acute leukaemia: Prospects for cure. Br Med J 283: 1205–1206, 1981.

75. Terry WD. Immunotherapy of malignant melanoma. N Engl J Med 303: 1174–1175, 1980.

76. Karakousis CP, Holtermann OA, Berger J. Adjuvant treatment of malignant melanoma with DTIC + BCG or estracyt. Proc Am Soc Clin Oncol 2: 227, 1983.

77. Balch CM, Smalley RV, Bartolucci AA, Burns D, Presant C, Durant JR. A randomised prospective clinical trial of adjuvant C.parvum immunotherapy in 260 patients with clinically localized melanoma (stage I). Cancer 49: 1070–1084, 1982.

78. Paterson AH, Willans D, Jerry LM, Hanson J, McPherson TA. BCG immunotherapy of malignant melanoma. Proc Am Soc Clin Oncol 2: 240, 1983.

79. Gilbert JM. Adjuvant chemotherapy of large bowel cancer. Cancer Treat Rev 9: 195–228, 1982.

80. Woglom WH. Immunity to transplantable tumours. Cancer Rev 4: 129, 1929.

81. Alexander P. Back to the drawing board—The need for more realistic animal model systems for immunotherapy. Cancer 40: 467–470, 1977.

82. Hewitt HB. A critical examination of the foundations of immunotherapy for cancer. Clin Radiol 30: 361–369, 1979.

83. Berken A. Case for adoptive immuotherapy in cancer. Lancet 2: 1190–1192, 1982.

84. Priestman TJ. Immunotherapy for cancer: The impossible dream? Surg Rev 3: 1–24, 1982.

13. CANCER IMMUNOLOGY AND THE PRACTISING CLINICIAN

I.H. MANIFOLD

INTRODUCTION

A vast and rapidly enlarging literature is accumulating on the many experimental aspects of the host's attempted defense against malignancy. The final outcome of this battle will probably determine the ultimate fate of an individual cancer patient. This chapter, however, will be concerned largely with aspects of tumour immunology, which, although they might be described as mere skirmishes in the above battle, are of considerable relevance to the clinician's everyday practice. Immunosuppression, immunosurveillance, immunodiagnosis, and immunotherapy, though discussed more fully in other chapters of the book, will be overviewed as they affect the clinician, and some aspects of tumour natural history will be considered in the light of a supposed, host-immune response.

IMMUNOSUPPRESSION

The immune defense mechanisms of patients may be impaired by multiple factors, both disease and treatment related, at different stages of their disease. This suppression may be manifested by an increased incidence of infection and can be routinely assessed by a variety of relatively noninvasive, laboratory techniques.

Lymphocyte responses are now known to be regulated in vitro by a bewildering network of helper and suppressor cells, from both macrophage and lymphocyte lines, which themselves rely on further cellular interactions for their induction and activities. The complexity of intercellular cooperation in vivo is likely to be much greater than has been demonstrated in vitro. For instance, some regulatory systems are crucially dependent on local cell density for their activity [1]. Many of these regulatory functions are mediated by secreted soluble

B.W. Hancock and A.M. Ward (eds.), Immunological Aspects of Cancer. Copyright © 1985, Martinus Nijhoff Publishing, Boston/Dordrecht/Lancaster.

factors [2] as well as cell contact. The availability of monoclonal antibody labels for helper and suppressor lymphocyte subsets, as well as for activated and nonactivated cells [3], may be expected to elucidate further the mechanisms of immunosuppression in the near future.

As the complexity of the immune system is increasingly discovered, more and more possible immunosuppressive factors are revealed. Taking as an example the decreased cell-mediated immunity of Hodgkin's disease, lymphocyte depletion [4], inherent lymphocyte defects [5], circulating suppressor cells [6], and plasma inhibitors [7] have all been incriminated.

Effects of immunosuppression

The effects of immunosuppression are what most concern the clinician. Defects of cell-mediated immunity (CMI) are found particularly in Hodgkin's disease; in some non-Hodgkin's lymphomas; and, often combined with depressed humoral immunity, after treatment and in many patients with advanced disease.

Opportunistic infections occur sometimes by normal commensals. The following are among the more important:

1. Reactivations may occur of herpes zoster/varicella—both in the form of localised "shingles" and as more generalised, occasionally life-threatening, infections of skin, lungs, and other organs—and of herpes simplex which as herpes labialis is relatively common and which may rarely become generalised; herpes encephalitis is usually fatal. The recent therapeutic innovation, acyclovir, should always be considered for use against these viruses in immunosuppressed patients.
2. Candidiasis, usually presenting orally, occasionally genitally, may spread to the oesophagus and other parts of the gastrointestinal tract and may eventually become generalised.
3. *Pneumocystis carinii,* a protozoan, produces pulmonary infection with severe dyspnoea and rigors. There may be a characteristic chest x-ray appearance (diffuse perihilar opacities), and firm diagnosis relies on lung biopsy. In the situation that often prevails, however, where the patient is extremely ill, it is wiser to treat with high-dose co-trimoxazole without attempting invasive investigations.
4. Tuberculosis may occur in the generalised "miliary" form or as bone involvement in the immunosuppressed host.
5. Other infections include cytomegalovirus, other atypical pneumonias, and other types of fungal infection such as Aspergillus and Cryptococcus. The latter may cause a fatal meningitis.

The relationship of impaired CMI to disease extent and prognosis is not simple. Again, taking Hodgkin's disease as an intensively investigated example, immunosuppression is broadly correlated with disease stage [8]. However, it is a well-known observation that there are patients with early disease and marked immunosuppression and vice versa. Pretreatment peripheral anergy, in early studies, was not found to correlate with subsequent prognosis after treatment [9]. More recently, in studies of over 500 patients, Kaplan suggested that pretreatment results of skin tests might have limited prognostic importance

[10]. In contrast, improvement in skin testing during treatment may be associated with a better prognosis [11,12]. De Sousa et al. [13] reached similar conclusions with lymphocyte transformation, but this association of improvement of immune function and prognosis has been disputed by other studies [14,15].

Impaired humoral immunity is seen classically in chronic lymphocytic leukaemia, in multiple myeloma, after treatment, and in advanced disease. Bacterial ("coccal") infections and Pneumocystis may result.

Immunosuppression results after all major treatment modalities

Lymphocytes are exquisitely sensitive to radiation, tending to suffer an intermitotic death within one or two days after relatively low doses of x-rays. This is in contrast to epithelial cells, which tend to die during or after subsequent mitoses, after times depending on the tissue turnover rate and after rather higher radiation doses. Peripheral lymphocyte counts may start to fall one to two days after the start of wholebody or total-nodal irradiation, and any large-field course of conventional radiotherapy may profoundly depress circulating lymphocyte numbers. B-cells tend to recover (with possible overshoot) more quickly than T-cells, which may remain reduced for up to several years posttreatment [14]. Circulating antibody levels and immunoglobulin synthesis by plasma cells tend to be relatively more radioresistant [16]. Radiotherapy alone in patients with Hodgkin's disease does not depress antibody levels, chemotherapy alone only marginally so, but the combination markedly decreases levels [17].

CMI as manifested by lymphocyte transformation may be depressed after radiation for prolonged periods of one or even several years [14,18]. The latter study showed normal skin testing, however, emphasizing the complexity of the situation.

Combination chemotherapy depresses primarily CMI—especially regimens involving prolonged and high-dose prednisolone. The effect on humoral immunity is less marked unless in conjunction with radiotherapy (see earlier discussion). Further, the effect is more marked on humoral immunity when chemotherapy is combined with splenectomy [19]. The duration of depressed CMI may be prolonged for up to five years after chemotherapy for Hodgkin's disease [20].

Acute myelosuppression, the most immediately dangerous aspect of which is granulocytopenia, is possible after most of the commonly used chemotherapy agents—with the exception of vincristine, prednisolone, and, relatively so, of bleomycin. It also occurs following irradiation. Bacterial septicaemias may then result from initial infections of urinary or respiratory tract, or skin, and may be lacking in classical features such as pyrexia or pus-formation. Infusions of human white cells have successfully been used in the acutely septicaemic, leukaemic patient as a short-term measure [21], but their prophylactic use is probably of no value [22,23]. The general principles of treatment remain early detection of infection and administration of complementory combinations of broad sepctrum antibiotics for a sufficient length of time.

Major surgery may have an immunosuppressive effect, by a variety of possible mechanisms. Two aspects are of particular interest. First, splenectomy is associated with an increased risk of septicaemia during subsequent treatment of malignancy. There has long been interest in the phagocytosis-stimulating peptide, tuftsin, produced by the spleen [24].

Second, fibronectin (cold-insoluble globulin, LETS protein, α_2SB glycoprotein) is a plasma and cell-surface protein that also acts as a nonimmune-specific opsonin and regulator for clearance of particulate debris by the mononuclear phagocyte system. Fibronectin levels are depressed in cases of widespread malignancy [25], and further decrease is possible after traumatic events such as surgery [26].

In summary, any patient with advanced malignant disease is likely to have suppression of all aspects of the immune system from a variety of causes:

1. Presenting disease.
2. Modes of therapy (chemotherapy, radiotherapy, and surgery).
3. Nutritional impairment (anorexia, dysphagia, and malabsorption).
4. Consequences of organ failure, secondary to disease or treatment (hepatic failure, renal failure, marrow failure).
5. Breakdown of local and nonspecific host defense mechanisms: impaired cough reflex (laryngeal nerve palsy, sedatives, postoperative pain); effects of immobility on respiratory and urinary tract; penetration of mucosal and epidermal barriers due to poor oral hygiene or pressure sores.

Attempts to reverse the immunosuppression have been varied and largely unsuccessful. Two recent methods may yet see further development.

1. The use of indomethacin to block the prostaglandin-mediated suppressor cell system [27].
2. The use of the immunostimulating tumour lymphocyte product, transfer factor [28].

The complications of immunosuppression in the patient who is still being actively treated may present an exciting, therapeutic challenge. However, it is important to recognise that in the advanced and incurable case, there comes the point where severe infection is best regarded as a part of the dying process. The aim of treatment is then to palliate. This should mean achieving the maximum relief of symptoms with the least upset and inconvenience. Even then, the use of antibiotics and antiviral agents may be necessary to achieve this palliation.

IMMUNOSURVEILLANCE

The early theories were based on lymphocyte-mediated mechanisms eliminating newly arising malignant cells; an impairment of immunity would then lead to increased malignancy. This is the classical immune surveillance mechanism, as proposed by Burnett [29]. This concept has been cited in the past as an explanation for the increased incidence of malignancy seen in states such as renal dialysis and transplantation [30] and treated malignancy [31,32]. However, the spectrum of increased incidence of tumours is narrow [33], such as leukaemias in the case of anticancer [31,32] and non-Hodgkin's lymphomas and carcinomas of skin in the case of renal patients [34]. Other possible mechanisms of carcinogenesis are present in these situations, for example, cytotoxic mutagenic drugs, the original disease processes, and excessive immune stimulation from organ grafts. Thus, the simple concept of immunosurveillance has fallen out of favour. Other surveillance mechanisms have been proposed based, for instance, on nonspecific macrophage cytotoxicity [35]. This represents a phyllogenetically more primitive system than immune-specific lymphocyte mechanisms and would not be open to the same criticisms as would the original immunosurveillance theory. There is some evidence, based on the histology of premalignant conditions of the liver and gastrointestinal tract, for a role of macrophages in tumour surveillance that is not immune-specific [36].

IMMUNODIAGNOSIS

Two aspects will be considered. First, much effort has been expended in attempting to develop an immune-based test that will detect the presence of malignancy in a patient. This is founded on the hope that the presence of a tumour will have produced some generalized sensitization or alteration in the immune system. Extracts from common tumours have been prepared, and stored, to be used as test reagents, usually with patients' peripheral leucocytes. Macrophage electrophoretic mobility and leucocyte migration inhibition are examples of this approach. It is a reasonable comment that none of these procedures has yet given results that are sufficiently discriminating or reproducible between different laboratories to be of consistent clinical value. Experimental techniques are complex and variable. Like good wine, these methodologies do not travel well!

Second, it seems more likely at present that clinical benefit will be gained from recent imaging developments, whereby antibodies (particularly monoclonal) to tumour determinants have been developed and isotopically labeled. The gamma-camera enables detection and localisation of specific malignant deposits in the patient. This has been achieved for carcinoma of the colon [37] and for choriocarcinoma using βHCG [38].

IMMUNOTHERAPY

The promise shown by this modality in in vitro systems has not yet resulted in widely accepted, consistently useful additions to the treatment options for patients. Properly randomised, controlled trials of the well-known nonspecific immune stimulants, BCG and levamisole, have on the whole failed to yield unequivocally positive results. Interferon, while apparently responsible for some isolated responses [39], has yet to become of proven value.

This situation may have arisen because the experimental animal systems in which the early, more spectacular results were obtained cannot be extrapolated to man. Tumours were studied that were induced by oncogenic viruses and had exceptional antigenicity, and others may have developed antigenicity during repeated in vivo/in vitro passage. These systems have only limited similarities to "wild" spontaneously arising malignancy in man.

A more recent hope for the future of useful immunotherapy comes with the development of monoclonal antibodies that, it is hoped, are tumour-specific [40]. Potent cellular toxins, attached to the antibodies, could thus be specifically targeted. This has been attempted but the method, in general, will need to circumvent at least three problems:

1. The relatively poor antigenicity of human tumours.
2. The possibility that tumour determinants, assumed to be tumour-specific antigens, are, in fact, normal molecules that are merely inappropriately expressed, with reference

to the tumour's tissue of origin. This could be compared to the ectopic hormone secretion exhibited by some tumours and would result in possible side effects from cross-reaction with the relevant normal tissues.

3.   The necessity of finding antigens specific to a given tumour type, rather than to normal tissue, but present in many patients with the tumour. The alternative would be to find methods of rapidly developing antibodies unique to each patient.

Unless such problems are overcome, some authorities may retain their disillusionment with immunotherapy [41] and others will continue to view it as a future dream [42]. In the meantime, clinicians will reluctantly continue to adopt the role of a "wet blanket" in the eyes of some of their patients. Their occasional overenthusiasm over "new discoveries" popularised by the media needs to be tactfully and sympathetically tempered by common-sense and realism.

IMMUNOLOGICAL PHENOMENA

Some malignancies are prone to eccentric natural histories:

1.   *Dormancy:* Distant metastases become evident after many disease-free years. This is seen with carcinoma of breast and malignant melanoma.
2.   *Latency:* Prostatic carcinoma may exist in a histologically malignant but clinically benign form for many years.
3.   *Spontaneous regression* [43]: This occurs rarely and mostly in a limited group of malignancies, including malignant melanoma, renal cell carcinoma, choriocarcinoma, and neuroblastoma.

These phenomena have often been explained on the basis of an immunological battle between the host and occult malignancy, which in the case of dormancy is eventually lost, in latency is in a state of equilibrium, and in spontaneous regression is eventually won. However, in some cases, at least, alternative mechanisms are likely, such as altered host-endocrine status or based merely on altered tumour growth kinetics [44].

Whatever this mechanism, such erratic tumour behaviour creates difficulties in counseling the patient. A happy medium must be achieved between, on the one hand, giving an unfounded pronouncement that the patient with a tumour with a long natural history is definitely cured after a relatively short period of disease-free follow-up, and, on the other, producing a pessimistic outlook preoccupied with the perpetual spectre of recurrence.

REFERENCES

1.   Laughter AH, Twomey JJ. Suppression of lymphoproliferation by high concentrations of normal human mononuclear leukocytes. J Immunol 119: 173–179, 1977.
2.   Aarden LA, Brunner TK, Cerottini JC, et al. Letter to the editor. Revised nomenclature of antigen-nonspecific T-cell proliferation and helper factors. J Immunol 123: 2928–2929, 1979.
3.   Reinherz EL, Scholssman SF. The characterization of function of human immunoregulatory T lymphocyte subsets. Immunol Today 2: 69–75, 1981.
4.   Young RC, Corder MP, Berard CW, DeVita VT. Immune alterations in Hodgkin's disease. Effect of delayed hypersensitivity and lymphocyte transformation on course and survival. Arch Int Med 131: 446–454, 1973.
5.   Aisenberg AC, Weitzman S, Wilkes B. Lymphocyte receptors for concanavalin A in Hodgkin's disease. Blood 51: 439–443, 1978.

6. Goodwin JS, Messner RP, Bankhurst AD, Peake GT, Saiki JH, Williams RC. Prostaglandin-producing suppressor cells in Hodgkin's disease. N Engl J Med 297: 963–968, 1977.
7. Sugden PJ, Lilleyman JS. Impairment of lymphocyte transformation by plasma from patients with advanced Hodgkin's disease. Cancer 45: 899–905, 1980.
8. Hancock BW, Bruce L, Sugden P, Ward AM, Richmond J. Immune status in untrated patients with lymphoreticular malignancy—A multifactoral study. Clin Oncol 3: 57–63, 1977.
9. Corder MP, Young RC, Brown RS, DeVita VT. Phytohaemagglutinin-induced lymphocyte transformation: The relationship to prognosis of Hodgkin's disease. Blood 39: 595–601, 1972.
10. Kaplan HS. The nature of the immunologic defect. In Hodgkin's disease, 2nd ed. Cambridge MA: Harvard University Press, 1980, pp. 236–279.
11. Ciampelli E, Pelu G. Comportamenta della intradermoreazione alla tuberculina nei pazienti affetti da morbo di Hodgkin trattata radiologicamente. Radiol Med 49: 683–690, 1963.
12. Jackson SM, Garrett JD, Craig AW. Lymphocyte transformation changes during the clinical course of Hodgkin's disease. Cancer 25: 843–850, 1970.
13. De Sousa M, Tan C, Tan R, Dupont B, Good RA. Immunological parameters of prognosis in childhood Hodgkin's disease. Proc Am Soc Clin Oncol 19: 333, 1973.
14. Fuks Z, Strober S, Bobrove AM, Sasazuki T, McMichael A, Kaplan HS. Long-term effects of radiation on T and B lymphocytes in peripheral blood of patients with Hodgkin's disease. J Clin Invest 58: 803–814, 1976.
15. Holm G, Perlmann P, Johansson D. Impaired phytohaemagglutinin-induced cytotoxicity in vitro of lymphocytes from patients with Hodgkin's disease or chronic lymphocytic leukaemia. Clin Exp Immunol 2: 351–360, 1967.
16. Duncan W, Nias AHW. Early response of normal tissues. In Clinical Radiobiology. Edinburgh: Churchill Livingstone, 1977, pp. 94–95.
17. Weitzman SA, Aisenberg AC, Siber GR, Smith DH. Impaired humoral immunity in treated Hodgkin's disease. N Eng J Med 297: 245–248, 1977.
18. Hancock BW, Heath J, Sugden P, Milford Ward A. The effects of radiotherapy on immunity in patients with localized carcinoma of the cervix uteri. Cancer 43: 118–123, 1979.
19. Hancock BW, Bruce L, Dunsmore IR, Ward AM, Richmond J. Follow-up studies on the immune status of patients with Hodgkin's disease after splenectomy and treatment, in relapse and remission. Br J Cancer 36: 347–354, 1977.
20. Hancock BW, Bruce L, Dunsmore IR, Ward AM, Richmond J. Immunity in Hodgkin's disease after 5 years remission. Br J Cancer 46: 593–600, 1982.
21. Higby DJ, Burnett D. Granulocyte transfusion: Current status. Blood 55: 2–8, 1980.
22. Schiffer CA, Aisner J, Poly PA, Schimpff SC, Wiernik PH. Alloimmunization following prophylactic granulocyte transfusion. Blood 54: 766–744, 1979.
23. Strauss RG, Connett JE, Gale RP, Bloomfield CD, Herzig GP, McCullough J, Maguire LC, Winston DJ, Ho W, Stump DC, Miller WV, Koepke JA. A controlled trial of prophylactic granulocyte transfusions during initial induction chemotherapy for acute myelogenous leukaemia. N Engl J Med 305: 597–603, 1981.
24. Constantopoulos A, Najjar VA, Wish JB, Necheles TH, Stolbach LL. Defective phagocytosis due to tuftsin deficiency in splenectomized subjects. Am J Dis Child 125: 663–665, 1973.
25. Stathakis NE, Fountas A, Tsianos E. Plasma fibronectin in normal subjects and in various disease states. J Clin Pathol 34: 504–508, 1981.
26. Saba TM. Prevention of liver reticuloendothelial systemic host defence failure after surgery by intravenous opsonic glycoprotein therapy. Ann Surg 188: 142–152, 1977.
27. De Shazo RD. Indomethacin-responsive mononuclear cell dysfunction in Hodgkin's disease. Clin Immunol Immunopathol 17: 66–75, 1980.
28. Khan A, Hill JM, MacLellan A, Loeb E, Hill NO, Thaxton S. Improvement in delayed hypersensitivity in Hodgkin's disease with transfer factor: Lymphopheresis and cellular immune reactions of normal donors. Cancer 36: 86–89, 1975.
29. Burnett FM. Immunological surveillance in neoplasia. Transplant Rev 7: 3–20, 1971.
30. Matas AJ, Simmons RL, Kjellstrand CM, Buselmeier TJ, Najarian JS. Increased incidence of malignancy during chronic renal failure. Lancet 1: 883–886, 1975.
31. Valagussa P, Santoro A, Kenda R, Fossati Bellani F, Franchi F, Banfi A, Rilke F, Bonadonna G. Second malignancies in Hodgkin's disease: A complication of certain forms of treatment. Br Med J 216–219, 1980.
32. Berk PD, Goldberg JD, Silverstein MN, Weinfeld A, Donovan PB, Ellis JT, Landaw SA, Laszlo J, Najean Y, Pisciotta AV, Wasserman LR. Increased incidence of acute leukemia in polycythemia vera associated with chlorambucil therapy. N Engl J Med 304: 441–447, 1981.
33. Leading article. Immunological deficiency and the risk of cancer. Br Med J 2: 654, 1977.

34. Kinlen LJ, Sheil AGR, Peto J, Doll R. Collaborative United Kingdom-Australasian study of cancer in patients treated with immunosuppressive drugs. Br Med J 2: 1461–1466, 1979.
35. Evans R, Alexander P. Mechanisms of extracellular killing of nucleated mammalian cells by macrophages. In Nelson DS (ed.), Immunobiology of the macrophage. London: Academic Press, 1976, pp. 535–576.
36. Manifold IH, Triger Dr, Underwood JCE. Kupffer-cell depletion in chronic liver disease: Implications for hepatic carcinogenesis. Lancet 2: 431–433, 1983.
37. Farrands PA, Perkins AC, Pimm MV, Hardy JD, Embleton MJ, Baldwin RW, Hardcastle JD. Radioimmunodetection of human colorectal cancers by an anti-tumour monoclonal antibody. Lancet 2: 397–400, 1982.
38. Begent RHJ, Searle F, Stanway G, Jewkes RF, Jones BE, Vernon P, Bagshawe KD. Radioimmuno-localization of tumours by external scintigraphy after administration of ^{131}I antibody to human chorionic gonadotrophin: Preliminary communication. J Royal Soc Med 73: 624–630, 1980.
39. Sikora K, Smedley H. Interferon and cancer. Br Med J 286: 739–740, 1983.
40. Miller RA, Maloney DG, Warnke R, Levy R. Treatment of B cell lymphoma with monoclonal anti-idiotype antibody. N Engl J Med 306: 517–522, 1982.
41. Hewitt HB. A critical examination of the foundations of immunotherapy for cancer. Clin Radiol 30: 361–369, 1979.
42. Priestman TJ. Immunotherapy for cancer: The impossible dream? In Lumley & Craven (eds.), Surgical review III. London: Pitman Medical, 1982, pp. 1–24.
43. Everson TC, Cole WH. Spontaneous regression of cancer. Philadelphia: W.B. Saunders, 1966.
44. Tubiana M, Malaise EP. Growth rate and cell kinetics in human tumours: Some prognostic and therapeutic implications. In Symington T, Carter RL (eds.), Scientific foundations of oncology. London: Heinemann, 1976, pp. 126–136.

INDEX